Cicely Saunders –
founder of the hospice movement

GW00776120

Cicely Saunders –
founder of the hospice movement
Selected letters 1959–1999

David Clark
Professor of Medical Sociology and Director, Institute for Health
Research and International Observatory on End of Life Care,
Lancaster University, UK

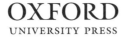

OXFORD

UNIVERSITY PRESS

Great Clarendon Street, Oxford OX2 6DP

Oxford University Press is a department of the University of Oxford.
It furthers the University's objective of excellence in research, scholarship,
and education by publishing worldwide in

Oxford New York

Auckland Bangkok Buenos Aires Cape Town Chennai
Dar es Salaam Delhi Hong Kong Istanbul Karachi Kolkata
Kuala Lumpur Madrid Melbourne Mexico City Mumbai Nairobi
Sao Paulo Shanghai Taipei Tokyo Toronto

and an associated company in Berlin

Oxford is a registered trade mark of Oxford University Press
in the UK and in certain other countries

Published in the United States
by Oxford University Press Inc., New York

A catalogue record for this title is available from the British Library

Library of Congress Cataloging in Publication Data
(Data available)

ISBN 0 19 856969 6
EAN 978 0 19 856969 5

Typeset by EXPO Holdings, Malaysia
Printed in Great Britain
on acid-free paper by Biddles Ltd, King's Lynn

Foreword

Balfour Mount, Montreal, Canada

The life work of Dame Cicely Saunders led to the creation of St. Christopher's Hospice in London, the development of the international Hospice/Palliative Care movement, the birth of Palliative Medicine as a new medical specialty and a decrease in suffering around the world. Sir Isaac Newton wrote, 'If I have seen further it is by standing on the shoulders of giants.' While giants are a rare breed, the twentieth century saw several physicians who qualify based on their contributions to the relief of human suffering. The list includes Alexander Fleming, Frederick Banting, Jonas Salk and Cicely Saunders. Fleming, Banting and Salk are remembered because of their discoveries – penicillin, insulin and the killed-virus vaccine against poliomyelitis, respectively. Dame Cicely's contribution differs in kind. She has been the catalyst for a paradigm shift in global health care.

In 'The Structure of Scientific Revolutions,' Thomas Kuhn argues that scientific research and thought are shaped by 'paradigms', or conceptual world views born out of formal theories, classic experiments and trusted methods. He questions the traditional view that scientific progress represents a gradual, value neutral, cumulative acquisition of knowledge as the result of objective, rationally chosen, experimental strategies. Instead, he argues, the accepted paradigm determines what is seen as being important and relevant, the kind of questions scientists ask, and the experiments they perform. A shift in the paradigm, Kuhn asserts, alters fundamental assumptions concerning the issues under consideration and gives rise to new research directions and strategies, new standards of evidence and a general reframing of priorities so that the new paradigm is incompatible with the old.

During the first decades of the latter half of the twentieth century, deficiencies in the care of the dying were documented to be endemic in Western health care and beyond. On assessing this conundrum John Hinton observed, 'We emerge deserving of little credit: we who are capable of ignoring the conditions which make muted people suffer. The dissatisfied dead cannot noise abroad the negligence they have experienced.' Strained communications between patient, family and professional care givers were shown to lead to isolation and distrust. Symptom control was found to be inadequate and psychosocial and spiritual needs were too often ignored.

There was a clear need to extend the horizons of healthcare beyond the reductionist biomedical model to the more inclusive perspective of whole person care, to move beyond an exclusive focus on disease, pathophysiology, curing and quantity of life to include consideration of experienced illness, suffering, the art of caring and quality of life.

Cicely Saunders was born on June 22, 1918. Though shy and unsure of herself in adolescence, her leadership potential was evident at an early age, leading her headmistress to write prophetically, 'I should be greatly surprised if anything deterred her once she had decided to embark on a piece of work.' Cicely was accepted in the St. Thomas's Nightingale

School of nursing in 1940 at the age of twenty-two. However, chronic disability due to back pain cut short her nursing career, leading to training as a medical social worker or 'lady almoner' as they were then known. In 1947 she was appointed assistant almoner at St. Thomas's. Within a year Cicely had started working evenings as a hospice volunteer at St. Luke's Hospital, originally 'Home for the Dying Poor.' A clear sense of vocation nurtured by that bedside experience, her deepening Christian faith and the advice of a mentor, then precipitated yet another career change. She read Medicine at Thomas's in order to start a 'home' for the dying and frail elderly. Her impressive determination in these studies led one of her tutors to comment 'her industry is overpowering.' She qualified in 1957 at the age of thirty-nine. In 1958, her paper 'Dying of Cancer' was published in the St. Thomas's Hospital Gazette and in 1959, 'Care of the Dying' in Nursing Times.

What personal qualities enabled the staggering productivity that was to ensue? In 'Cicely Saunders, Selected Letters, 1959–1999' we are privileged to enter the private world of a dynamic, highly effective leader. A candid picture of her motivations, priorities and actions emerges. Her legendary determination and vision, her warmth and enthusiasm, confident humility, sense of humour, curiosity and attention to detail shout from every page. She repeatedly stresses that her role has been to reshape, not innovate. Always ready to acknowledge her patients as the 'founders of hospice' and the importance of her mentors and team, she observes, 'What have I that I have not received?', and again, 'There are not many original ideas in the world. One only brings together things culled from here and there, shakes the kaleidoscope and finds a new pattern.' To paraphrase Churchill, 'Some kaleidoscope! Some pattern!' St. Christopher's Hospice was her kaleidoscope, Hospice/Palliative Care the pattern she so carefully created.

The letters in this book will be important to a variety of audiences. With their wide ranging topics, clarifying detail and robust candidness, this lively corpus offers rich rewards for both the general reader and those with specialized interests. For those working in Palliative /Hospice Care, Dame Cicely's letters are a touchstone against which one can reflect on subsequent developments from a personal, programmatic, or broader perspective. For scholars concerned with the changing aspects of death in society, those responsible for political and policy decisions and medical historians, these letters are a precious resource, for they provide a window on a healthcare revolution that has touched countless lives. Indeed, these pages provide an intimate picture of an ambassador for change and insight regarding the dynamics of leadership. They also will be of interest to students of the Cartesian dualism / whole-person-care dialectic, team functioning, organizational theory and expressions of religious conviction in the context of a pluralistic society.

The global paradigm shift to the healthcare pattern developed in Dame Cicely's kaleidoscope did not happen as the result of random good fortune. Each reader will glean his or her own list of personal attributes that contributed to Dame Cicely's success. I have been struck by her dogged determination to bring to her mission a sense of balance in body, mind and spirit. That balance has been hard-won. Along the way she has remained open to lead and be led. This is wonderfully captured in her letter of 31 July 1964 to The Most Reverend the Lord Archbishop Anthony Bloom, written a full three years prior to the opening of St. Christopher's. 'We have been looking and praying for the right person to take over as Chairman for a very long time.' 'Looking'; 'praying'; 'for a very long time'! Active searching is coupled with openness to the Way, in an attitude of patience. Attention to process, presence and patience, with tenacity and clarity of purpose as resources for the journey.

During the four decades in which these letters were written, St. Christopher's continued to expand and modify its programs. Currently, it addresses the needs of 1,600 patients and their families each year. The 48 beds complement a home care program following 500 patients on any one day and a day centre for 20 patients, five days a week. In addition, the St. Christopher's team continues an active research program into all aspects of Hospice Care and annually accommodates 2,000 visitors and hosts 80 conferences and workshops. During the same decades the St. Christopher's model of comprehensive patient and family care has spread around the world. Well in excess of 8,000 hospice/palliative care programs in 100 countries have now been established.

As impressive as the statistics are, numbers do not convey the significance of Dame Cicely's work. Compassion cannot be tabulated in columns, nor are we yet able to assign a p value to the significance of diminished suffering. These letters have helped to shape medical history. We are indebted to Dame Cicely and David Clark for this precious gift.

Spring 2002

Acknowledgements

A great many people, in ways seen and unseen, have assisted in this endeavour. My interest in the life and work of Cicely Saunders forms part of a larger project on the history of hospices, palliative care, and related fields and this has enjoyed considerable support from the Wellcome Trust to which I remain constantly grateful; I particularly want to thank John Malin, who, during his time at the Trust, provided both a steady eye and measured guidance, which were so helpful to me over a number of years.

I am fortunate indeed to be based in the Sheffield Palliative Care Studies Group where colleagues from the clinical disciplines, from the social sciences, and from the humanities make up my day-to-day working world. I am grateful to them all for their constant encouragement and intellectual stimulation. Several within our group over the years have made particular contributions which have made this book possible: Clare Humphreys, Rachael Marples, and Michelle Winslow have each given direct assistance in various ways and I thank them for their help.

At the University of Sheffield I was also fortunate in being able to take advantage during the year 2000 of a period of study leave in order to undertake the core work for this project; I am grateful to two successive Deans in the School of Medicine for supporting me in this way. Above all, however, it has been Margaret Jane at Sheffield who has unflaggingly and with enormous dedication produced and refined the entire manuscript from so many rough drafts and photocopies. Without her involvement, quite simply the project could not have come to fruition. I extend to her my warmest thanks and appreciation, as always.

At Oxford University Press, Catherine Barnes and her colleagues have shown tremendous enthusiasm for this project, and their interest has done much to help me finish off a work which has been several years in the making. I am particularly grateful to Kate Smith for her assiduous help on the proofs.

Much more than others in which I have been involved, this book is also caught up with my family life. Certainly it cluttered up the dining-room table for many months. Also it was being prepared at a time when our home was affected by illness, by death, and by bereavement. So it will always have some very special associations. My daughter Rachel Clark helped me with it throughout this time and did huge amounts of careful photocopying, in the process becoming expert herself in the book's subject matter. I thank her for her kindness and for keeping the whole thing moving, even when the spirit flagged.

At St Christopher's Hospice, Christine Kearney has been a constant source of help, and I am indebted to her for sharing so much of her knowledge as well as for giving practical assistance.

Finally, there is one person without whom truly this book could never have existed. Dr Cicely Saunders wrote all the letters. She worked tirelessly to realize the vision that is contained within them and she inspired so many others to go into the work of hospice and palliative care. From the outset she has been doubtful that her correspondence will be of interest to others. Naturally, I hope that the reaction to this book will prove her wrong. It has been my privilege to work with her on this project, though she has shown no inclination to influence my choice of correspondence or my interpretations. Her letters, so engagingly written, so full of energy and commitment, so practical and yet so reflective, deserve a wide reading. I hope, therefore, that she will feel satisfied with the products of my labours here and I take this opportunity to thank her for everything she has taught me along the way.

David Clark
Dalswinton, Dumfriesshire
February 2002

Contents

Plates

1   David Tasma (d. 1948): the inspiration for Cicely Saunders' subsequent work with the dying.

2   Antoni Michniewicz (d. 1960): cared for by Cicely Saunders in St Joseph's Hospice, and with whom she developed a deep and intense relationship in the final months of his life.

3   With Rosetta Burch (left) at a wedding in the early 1950s.

4   Sister Mary Antonia gives a cup of tea to a dying patient at St Joseph's Hospice, Hackney, c.1963.

5   With two patients at St Joseph's on their golden wedding anniversary; he is in the bed where Antoni Michniewicz was cared for.

6   Receiving the OBE on 9 March 1965, with her mother (left) and niece, Penelope (right). Permission sought.

7   Awarding nursing prizes at London's Royal Marsden Hospital, probably 1965.

8   Lord Thurlow and Cicely Saunders dig the first spit to mark the start of building at St Christopher's Hospice, Sydenham, on 22 March 1965. Reproduced with permission granted from Nursing Times.

9   Florence Wald (left) and Elisabeth Kübler-Ross (right), pictured at the Yale University meeting of April 1966, at which they met with Cicely Saunders and Colin Murray Parkes.

10 With Lord Thurlow (centre) and Almon Pepper (left) at the dedication and laying of the hospice foundation stone, 22 July 1966. Reproduced with permission granted from Nursing Times.

11 Olive Wyon, theologian and adviser to Cicely Saunders, on 22 July 1966 at the dedication of the hospice.

12 St Christopher's under construction, spring 1967. Reproduced with permission granted from Nursing Times.

13 St Christopher's soon after opening.

14 Sister Zita Marie Cotter, who came from the USA to work at St Christopher's soon after its opening.

15 Receiving her first honorary degree, at Yale University, on 9 June 1969.

16 Dame Albertine Winner at the official opening of St Christopher's Study Centre in 1973. Reproduced with permission granted from Nursing Times.

17 With Miss Betty Lestor and Carlton Sweetser in front of St Christopher's Chapel, Hyden, Kentucky, USA, 1978. Reproduced with permission granted from Gabrielle Beasley.

18 Drinks in the office, mid-1970s.

19 Dr Sam Klagsbrun visited the hospice annually to give organizational advice and was appointed Visitor in 1975.

20 Dr Gillian Ford, long-term friend of Cicely Saunders and supporter of St Christopher's, in 1979.

21 With her husband Marian Bohusz-Szyszko, outside their home in Sydenham. Reproduced with permission granted from David L. Goldin.

22 Over the years, fundraising was always a feature of life at St Christopher's. With (left to right) Tom West, Tom Breen, George Moore (of Help the Aged), and Eleri Price. Reproduced with permission granted from Help the Aged.

23 With (left to right) Robert Dunlop, Jacqui Field, Jo Hockley, and Judith Reddie at their book launch, 1990.

24 Speaking at the Second Congress of the European Association of Palliative Care, Brussels, 1992. Reproduced with permission, copyright DANN.

25 Grace Goldin – a friend for over thirty years, photographer, poet, and historian. Pictured outside her home in Swarthmore, Pennsylvania, USA.

26 David Tasma's window.

27 Despite periods of major illness in later life, Marian Bohusz-Szyszko was able to continue painting with vigour and enthusiasm.

28 Balfour Mount and daughter Bethany, mid-1990s. It was he who in 1975 began to popularize the term 'palliative care'.

29 Making a clear point.

30 Surrounded by friends and colleagues at a conference to mark her eightieth birthday, Royal College of Physicians, June 1998.

Introduction

The main duty of one who edits another's letters is to intrude as little as possible upon what they have to tell us. I therefore do not propose to offer too many distractions from the fascinations which this correspondence of Cicely Saunders contains. As a researcher, however, I do feel obliged to give some account of my methods and this should in turn help the reader to make sense of what is presented. I harboured the ambition of producing an edited volume of the letters of Cicely Saunders from the point, in the mid-1990s, when I first realized the extent of what she had written, coupled with the discovery that much of it was still extant. Since that time, as part of a wider project on the history of hospices, palliative care, and related fields, based at the University of Sheffield, UK, I have tried in various ways to understand and analyse the particular contribution of Cicely Saunders.

It has become a commonplace to regard her as the founder of the modern hospice movement: a woman of resilience and vision who, having trained as a nurse, social worker, and then physician, dedicated the remainder of her life to the care of the dying; a woman whose reputation has gone well beyond the healthcare field in which she has worked so tirelessly; a woman who has had very special relationships with three Polish men; a woman of deep Christian faith; a woman who has persistently opposed euthanasia. Several have written about her. She herself has spoken and published a great deal. Yet my own view is that much remains to be understood. This volume of letters is one step in that direction.

I have chosen here to allow her letters to tell their own story, but I also recognize the pervasiveness of the editorial hand. So let me explain how I have undertaken this work.

In 1998 I supervised the cataloguing of Cicely Saunders' personal papers. Since that date further materials have been added to the collection, which currently stands at about eighty archive boxes. Her correspondence goes back in the main to the late 1950s and is still growing. This book concentrates on the forty years 1959–99. Covering that period I estimate there are some 7000 of her letters among her papers. This is by no means a complete picture. In some places (though not many) small gaps occur for no apparent reason. Elsewhere, it is clear that material has been at some point discarded. Moreover, to colleagues who became personal friends, many letters have been written by hand, with no copy preserved. The papers from which I have drawn therefore tend to reflect a professional life in which letters are typed by secretaries and copies are filed and retained. That is not to say that they do not contain remarkable personal insights, or that her correspondents do not write to her by hand and in a personal way; several do so. My choice here, however, has been made from Cicely Saunders' own typed (occasionally handwritten) and preserved letters. I have made no attempt to seek out from their recipients other letters which she has written, but copies of which she has not kept. Moreover, I have selected only from letters written by Cicely Saunders herself. No letters are included here written *to* her, so this is a narrative in her voice only. In this way I have made a selection covering about one-tenth of the total.

From within such a corpus, how did selection proceed? I have to say that for this I used no protocol or formula. Rather, I have built on my growing knowledge of Cicely Saunders and the hospice movement to create a particular kind of narrative. This book should therefore be regarded as one sort of perspective on the life of Cicely Saunders, as seen through a selection of her correspondence. It may serve as a source book for further analysis, but the careful scholar will prefer the original documents for this.

I have chosen to depict a narrative which does several things. It begins by revealing something of the motivation of Cicely Saunders to study the problem of caring for dying people and then to act upon her knowledge. Alongside this it opens up the sense of calling that motivated this purpose. It also shows how a strategy was developed which allowed a rather idiosyncratic and personal vision to be put into operation with help from others. We see the achievements which took place long before St Christopher's Hospice received its first patients, and it becomes clear that the opening in 1967 should be regarded not as the start of the modern hospice movement, but rather as the conclusion to the first stage of its development.

Within this a picture emerges in which St Christopher's is seen as part of a wider network, not just within the United Kingdom, but also around the world. We understand the connectedness and the personal, professional, and institutional links that were developed, and we see the consequences that resulted. We gain insight into the expanding knowledge base of the hospice and the transition to a wider perspective in the form of palliative care. There are letters which deal with the growing professionalization of the work, and with the establishment of national and international palliative care organizations. We learn of working parties and research collaborations, of lecture tours and conference engagements. There are insights into the friendships made along the way.

Over time we read about the changing role which Cicely Saunders had in the hospice she founded, as well as in the wider movement. The letters pay testimony to the numerous honours and prizes that have been bestowed upon her in so many places. We also gain a powerful insight into her inner convictions: the evangelical Christianity which is touched by Catholicism, the gradual broadening of her spiritual path, the importance of prayer and religious reading in daily life. Likewise we learn of the things against which she sets her face: euthanasia, inadequate care, a lack of respect for personhood. There are insights too into three men, all Polish, who in different ways had such a formative influence on her adult life, and one of whom she eventually married. With this marriage came a new domesticity and a pleasure in companionship. In time it also brought direct experience of the informal carer's role. Then, after the death of her husband, she re-emerges from the home once again to travel the world, to write, to lecture, and to enjoy continued plaudits and acclaim.

All of these elements I have tried to capture in my choice of letters. Reading them is, I believe, a privilege, for in some ways they serve as a journal or diary. Set out in chronological order, rather than by recipient, they tell a compelling story. They can be read from beginning to end, or a particular time period can be explored in detail. The indices give the names of every person to whom a letter is included and can be searched by those interested in particular individuals and topics. Many well-known names in the history of hospice and palliative care are in evidence. Beyond these are letters to numerous men and women in different parts of the world who have only walk-on parts in hospice history, but with whom Cicely Saunders corresponded and had interesting ideas to exchange. In several cases I do not know who they are.

Apart from leaving out formal salutations and valedictions, I have made a principled decision not to abridge or edit the letters, so occasional irrelevancies and infelicities will result. Here and there, to preserve privacy, the names of patients, their family members, and some others have been anonymized. The footnotes which I have added are intended to guide the reader through the terrain and, perhaps, to stimulate further reading. Occasionally, in square brackets, I have added to a letter in order to increase intelligibility. The early letters are in the main addressed from St Joseph's Hospice, Hackney; from St Mary's Hospital; or from Cicely Saunders' own home in Connaught Square, London. After 1967 they are mostly from St Christopher's Hospice. A few were typed by Cicely Saunders herself, but mostly she was helped by secretaries, and it is appropriate to acknowledge: Jenny Powley, Harnia Tokarska, and Kitty Cole, all of whom, using a manual typewriter, typed letters from recorded tapes, often on the kitchen table at Connaught Square; subsequently she was assisted at St Christopher's by Freda Saunders, Jenny Jameson (later Chambers), and Monica Steadman, and in particular by Christine Kearney, who became her secretary and personal assistant from 1980.

Finally, I have grouped my choice of letters into three time periods: the years leading up to the opening of St Christopher's Hospice; those in which Cicely Saunders was its Medical Director; and her years as its Chairman, up to 1999. I have prefaced each of these with a short essay intended to give some insight into the main features and preoccupations of the period. I hope that these will serve to orientate the reader, but they are by no means essential to an appreciation of the letters, which need no one but their author to tell their tale.

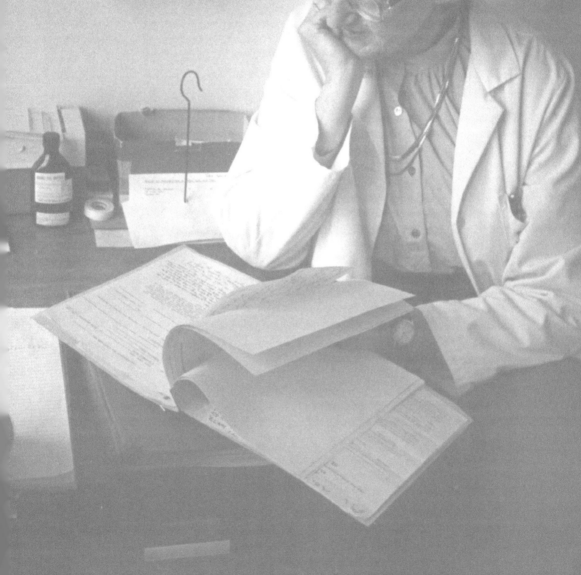

Part 1

Realizing a vision (1959–1967)

In the summer of 1957, just before she qualified in medicine at the age of thirty-nine, Cicely Saunders was also working on her first publication. Its contents set out the entire basis for a new approach to the care of dying people. By the time of its appearance the following year in the *St Thomas's Hospital Gazette*, the foundations for her life's work were fully in place. She had studied philosophy and economics at Oxford; trained as a nurse, though had to give up because of a back injury; she had been employed as an almoner; and was about to take up the work of a physician. In fact she would be the first modern doctor to dedicate her entire career to caring for those at the end of life. So this important first paper gave clear notice of her intentions:

> It appears to me that many patients feel deserted by their doctors at the end. Ideally the doctor should remain the centre of a team who work together to relieve where they cannot heal, to keep the patient's own struggle within his compass and to bring hope and consolation to the end (Saunders 1958: 46).

Here, then, was an ambition of singular proportions which would require a monumental transformation in professional knowledge, attitudes, and behaviour for its realization. In Cicely Saunders it was to draw on a powerful combination of personal motivations, professional aspirations, and a sheer determination to see her ideas through, no matter what efforts might be required.

By the late 1950s the British National Health Service had been in existence for more than a decade; it formed part of a welfare state pledged to provide care 'from the cradle to the grave'. Yet the new health service had done nothing to promote the care of its dying patients. Instead, the thrust of policy was moving towards acute medicine and rehabilitation. Yes, there was increasing awareness of the demographic changes which would lead to far more elderly people in the population, but the consequences for their care, and in particular for those affected by malignant disease, received scant attention. Cicely Saunders was one of a handful of clinicians on both sides of the Atlantic who began to take a special interest in the care of the dying. In letters written in the late 1950s, we see her eagerly seeking out published work on the subject, following up the authors, and endeavouring to build up a picture of what was known and, more importantly, what remained to be understood.

Around the world at this time no more than a dozen homes for the dying were in existence. Mostly founded in the late nineteenth century, they combined concerns which were religious, philanthropic, and moral, and gave special attention to the needs of the poor and disadvantaged. Their efforts were mostly directed towards nursing care, with little medical involvement. It was in two such homes in London that Cicely Saunders had gained her early insights. In 1948, working as a medical almoner in a large hospital, she had cared for one David Tasma, a dying Jewish émigré from Poland. It was a brief but extremely intense relationship in which they even discussed together the idea that she might one day found a home where others like him could find peace in their final days. Famously, he left her £500 and the injunction: 'I'll be a window in your home.' Soon afterwards she began voluntary nursing at St Luke's Hospital in Bayswater. On qualifying in medicine, she took up a research position at St Mary's Hospital, London, and began work at St Joseph's Hospice in the East End, where, under the direction of the Irish Sisters of Charity, the hospice served one of the poorest communities in the city of London. St Joseph's, Hackney, provided

Cicely Saunders first with a source of inspiration about how dying people might be cared for elsewhere, and also a testing ground for the development of her own clinical ideas. It was here, building on older traditions of religious care and solicitude, and introducing methods of recording clinical information in charts and notes, that she began to develop a modern strategy for hospice care which would be transforming in its scope. In so doing she felt moved by a clearly articulated sense of personal calling, which from an early stage led to the belief that her ideas could be generalized and taken up in many other settings. Initially, however, her energies focused on a single goal: the creation of the world's first modern hospice, one which would not only provide excellent clinical care, but would combine this with teaching and research. Accordingly, the late 1950s saw her embark upon a nearly decade-long programme that culminated in the opening of St Christopher's Hospice, and thereby set in train a social movement which would transform thinking about the care of the dying, worldwide.

Professional innovation

How best to summarize some of the ideas developed by Cicely Saunders in this decade after 1958? An immediate guide can be found in the fifty-six published articles, pamphlets, and reviews she published during the period (Clark 1998a). Her experience as nurse, almoner, and doctor brings a remarkable breadth to these writings, even from the earliest years, and it is these professions that constitute her principal audience at first. In some of the writings her work is then further extended to the wider public, and in particular to a Christian readership. From the very beginning patient narratives were a feature of her writing and the careful depiction of individual cases provides us with insights into a developing and multi-faceted approach to the care of dying people. These articles, reviews, published letters, and pamphlets were often hard won. They are written with a felicity and sure-footedness that belies the drafting and re-drafting and last-minute revisions to which she was particularly prone. These were years of rapid escalation in her knowledge base. In 1959 it had been an enormous struggle to cite forty references in her chapter for Ronald Raven's six-volume set on *Cancer* (Saunders 1960a); but in 1967 her pamphlet on *The management of terminal illness*, combined from three articles in the *British Journal of Hospital Medicine*, could contain reference to 184 published works (Saunders 1967a). By such means a new field of healthcare practice began to be defined.

In parallel with the publications, and as we see so clearly in the letters reproduced here, there was also a growing schedule of talks, lectures, and teaching sessions. A letter of thanks from the organizer of a district nurse refresher course held in Northern Ireland in 1962 typifies the reaction of colleagues:

> It was wonderful to learn that those suffering great pain can be free from that pain, and yet remain alert, that the personality and dignity of the dying can be preserved, and that you have a real answer to the problem of euthanasia. What hope you have given us!

Similarly her series of six articles which first appeared in *Nursing Times* in 1959 (Saunders 1960b) and an article in the *American Journal of Nursing* (Saunders 1965) stimulated postbags which astounded their editors. Lecture tours to the United States took place in 1963, 1965, and 1966, each one leading to wider recognition, whilst at St Joseph's itself regular ward rounds for medical students were having an imperceptible influence on formative attitudes, which would sometimes be manifested only years later.

A passage from a talk given by Cicely Saunders at St Mary's Hospital, London, in 1961 gives some clues to her underlying approach; describing her work at St Joseph's she states: 'I am fortunate too … above all, in being a doctor who isn't in a hurry, so that I have time to know and enjoy my patients.' Indeed, most unusually for a doctor of the period, she was in the habit of tape-recording conversations with patients – about their illnesses, their families, the things which concerned them. It is these patients and their experiences which are so central to the ideas developed by Cicely Saunders during this period and which were presented so vividly in her teaching and publications. From these narratives a new philosophy and practice of terminal care was forged. Here was swept aside the resigned admission to the patient that 'there is nothing more we can do', replaced instead by the positive assertion that 'we must think of new possibilities of doing everything'. Nowhere is this optimism better demonstrated than in Cicely Saunders' concept of 'total pain' which was developed over these years (Clark 1999).

The interest in pain can be traced through the publications of the decade. At first, two clear principles emerge: an orientation to the prevention rather than the alleviation of pain, coupled with a thorough understanding of available pain-relieving drugs. Thus:

> We should anticipate distress and pain by our treatment so that the patient does not continually do so himself … If pain is constantly allowed to occur, each time the patient has to ask for something to relieve it. Not only does he then make it worse by his fear and tension but he is reminded of his dependence upon the drugs and the person who gives them to him (Saunders 1966: 139).

At the same time the drugs given must be appropriate. So she distinguishes between mild, moderate, and severe pain and discusses the use of aspirin and codeine in tablet form, as well as the Brompton Mixture and the relative merits of morphine and diamorphine by injection. The result was a hard-headed approach to pain management ('constant pain needs constant control') in a method of regular giving where strong opiates were used with confidence and fears of addiction or 'unwanted elation' politely dismissed.

The ideas about pain relief did not stop there. Beyond regular giving and the frank use of narcotics was a recognition of the link between physical pain and mental distress. So by 1963 she could suggest that 'Mental distress may be perhaps the most intractable pain of all' for which 'Listening has to develop into real hearing' (1963a: 197). Indeed, physical and mental suffering are seen almost dialectically: each capable of influencing and shaping the other. So in a letter to the *British Medical Journal* in the same year she argues that: 'If physical symptoms are alleviated then mental pain is lifted also' (1963b: 746). Such an approach required attention to the meaning of pain, leading to a medicine capable of an orientation to suffering which allows the finest human sentiments to shine through. In this way pain is seen as something indivisible from the body and the personality, but also as something caught up in wider social circumstances. When a patient told Cicely Saunders 'all of me is wrong' or another said that 'it was *all* pain' it became increasingly apparent that the required response included a breadth of vision for its understanding and huge versatility in its alleviation.

As early as 1964 the concept of 'total pain' had been described in its full form and was taken to include physical symptoms, mental distress, social problems, and emotional difficulties. The emerging field of terminal care had now been furnished with one of its most important and enduring concepts and at the same time a profound challenge had been issued to the Cartesian body–mind dualism of modern medical practice.

Practical accomplishments

Such clinical innovations, combined with the associated teaching and writing may already seem like a heavy programme for one newly qualified in medicine. Yet it was during these same years that Cicely Saunders was pursuing a major practical project in order to create the physical environment in which her ideas about the care of the dying could be developed more fully.

As we can see from some of the letters presented here, the first clear evidence of her strategic intentions came in the second half of 1959, when over the space of a few months she circulated to several friends and associates a ten-page document, seeking their reaction. It was entitled *The scheme* and it set out *de novo* the structure and organization of a modern terminal care home containing sixty beds, together with staffing levels, capital and revenue costs, and contractual arrangements. By the end of the year the 'home' in question had a name: St Christopher's Hospice. The patron saint of travellers would thus accompany those making their final earthly journey. Soon a small but enthusiastic group of supporters had been formed, including: Dr H. L. Glyn Hughes (author of a recent report on the state of terminal care in Britain); Betty Read (head almoner at St Thomas's Hospital); and Jack Wallace (an evangelical friend and lawyer). The group was then joined by Evered Lunt (Anglican Bishop of Stepney); Sir Kenneth Grubb (of the Church Missionary Society); and, very significantly, Dame Albertine Winner (Deputy Chief Medical Officer). By early 1961 there were architectural drawings of the hospice and its estimated cost was £376,000, though in the inflationary environment of the times the architect warned 'prices are rising daily!'

From the earliest days small donations and gifts played their part in the fundraising effort, and each of these would be acknowledged with scrupulous attention and courtesy. There was also a systematic campaign targeted on the major charitable trusts, London's merchant companies, and the upper echelons of the British establishment. 'I am lobbying the peers at the moment', she wrote enthusiastically to Jack Wallace in February 1961. During the next three years over £330,000 was raised in this way. By 1966, however, with building at the chosen location in Sydenham well underway and the estimated project budget now in excess of £400,000, there was still a considerable shortfall and the national financial climate was not favourable. In a letter to Sir Kenneth Grubb of June 1966 she noted that: 'St Christopher's is getting very large and splendid and the bills are matching it.' This was 'building in faith'; but the contractors were sympathetic and payments, somehow, were always met on time, though finances have remained precarious ever since. By early 1967 the overall budget stood at £480,000; but by June a team of staff had been appointed, the building commissioned, and the first patients were beginning to arrive. By the opening day, 24 July 1967, all debts had been cleared.

An article published soon after the opening, in the *British Hospital Journal and Social Service Review* amounts to a prospectus for St Christopher's. The hospice 'will try to fill the gap that exists in both research and teaching concerning the care of patients dying of cancer and those needing skilled relief in other long-term illnesses and their relatives' (Saunders 1967b: 2127). The hospice contained fifty-four inpatient beds, an outpatient clinic and also sixteen beds available for the long-term needs of staff themselves and their families. There would be an emphasis on providing continuity of care for those able to return home and there were plans for a domiciliary service. Relatives' involvement in care would be encouraged. Research on pain, developed at St Joseph's, would be extended. The hospice was to be 'a religious foundation of very open character', and there was a sense that the whole endeavour amounted to an elaborate pilot scheme which could have extremely far-reaching implications.

Indeed, Cicely Saunders and others around her, even before the opening of St Christopher's, had developed a sense that this was a project far greater than building a single new hospice, taxing though that may have proved. In early 1967 an American colleague wrote from New York:

> I think you should realize that you have two obligations. One is to continue your work which you are doing in the development of your own center at St Christopher's, and the other is to teach the world what you have learned.

At the end of the year, Dr Herman Feifel, the distinguished psychologist, writing with congratulations from Los Angeles put it more succinctly: 'May it bring comfort and solace to many – may it galvanize many others to follow your path.'

So it was that the practical accomplishment was about more than St Christopher's Hospice alone. A nascent movement (Clark 1998*b*) was now in evidence which in order to flourish and grow would continue to need from Cicely Saunders enormous levels of personal energy, commitment, and resilience.

Personal changes

By 1958 it was already ten years since the death of David Tasma, whose final days had been such a source of motivation to Cicely Saunders. He was and remains St Christopher's 'founding patient', the inspiration for what was to follow: a man who felt he had achieved so little in life and yet for whom the manner of his dying resulted in so much.

In the early 1960s, however, there were other personal losses which had a profound effect. In particular there was Antoni Michniewicz, another Pole, cared for at St Joseph's Hospice. Shirley du Boulay (1994) has described how deeply happy Cicely Saunders was with Antoni during their months together, even as he was dying. When he died, however, there was an experience of complete heartbreak. Moreover it was a sorrow which was only shared with a very few close friends. And through it all she continued to work and to plan for St Christopher's. During the following months another precious patient and friend also died. This was 'Mrs G', whom she had known for seven years, all of them spent in hospital suffering from quadriplegia and then blindness. In March 1961 *Nursing Times* published Cicely Saunders' account of 'Mrs G', with an accompanying note from the editor stating:

> Because this is the most remarkable and inspiring account of a patient we have ever read, we are devoting four pages to it. If we believe that those who suffer most have most to give, then Mrs G's influence will extend far beyond those who had the privilege of caring for her (Saunders 1961: 394).

Finally, in June 1961 came the death of Cicely Saunders' own father, Gordon Saunders. He had been ill for some time, but her grief was further complicated by what seemed unfair terms in his will.

It was a painful triad of losses and one of its most obvious manifestations was anger; so much so that she briefly sought psychiatric help. As she remarked later: 'I got my bereavements muddled up.' Yet we see at this time two remarkable and contrasting dimensions to Cicely Saunders' life. In the external world she was a mass of energy, organizing tirelessly, lobbying and cajoling at a crucial early phase of St Christopher's development. Internally she was experiencing the most profound sorrows, yearnings, and resentments – for things lost, for hopes dashed, for circumstances never achieved.

These two apparently distinct elements can be seen to meet on one crucial area of common ground: that of religion and Cicely Saunders' own Christian faith. For it is here that we see the confluence of the public and the private, some accommodation between activity in the world and the strivings of the spirit; a mental system in which to forge the means to overcome grief and to create something from it.

Following a rather dramatic religious experience in the 1940s, Cicely Saunders had moved in Christian evangelical circles for several years. Yet she also found herself at ease in the Roman Catholic ambience of St Joseph's. She was inclined to worship intently and to read widely. From the outset, therefore, her personal beliefs and ideas about religion were absolutely central to her plans for St Christopher's. It is through the evolving sense of a personal *calling* that we see this most visibly. It is strongly evidenced in her early correspondence about the idea of St Christopher's, where many passages make reference to a sense of being drawn by God to this work. Within a few years it was as if the *whole project* had taken on a sense of something predetermined and meant to be: some part of a greater purpose.

Characteristically, however, there was to be no straightforward and simplistic blueprint. The precise character of St Christopher's religious status required careful consideration. This constitutes a crucial dimension of this formative decade and one which was to have profound effects on the developments which followed. Under the influence of liberal theologians and inspired by the new religious communities which had been established at Taizé, Grandchamp, and elsewhere, one conception of St Christopher's was as a community dedicated to the care of the dying and with its own rule or order. Such a community would no doubt have provided very special care for those admitted to it; but it would not have offered a platform for the wider aim – to influence and promote terminal care in general. Imperceptibly, therefore, the idea of St Christopher's as a religious community, in the strong sense, was modulated (Clark 2001). Undoubtedly, St Christopher's became an organization of Christian motivation; but in opting for a strategy of practical action in the world, rather than an ethic of caring located outside it, Cicely Saunders and her colleagues gave birth to an idea capable of wide adaptation and development across cultures and settings.

It is quite clear from a reading of the letters which follow that during these years leading up to 1967 the hospice movement was already in formation. The opening of St Christopher's in July of that year can now be seen, not as the start of the modern hospice initiative, but as the culmination of a project which made that initiative possible. For it was in these years, to use the words of Michel Foucault, that 'the conditions of possibility' for the hospice movement were created. Although by 1967 the term 'hospice movement' had not yet appeared in the lexicon of terminal care, nevertheless its foundations were firmly established. In the decade after 1958, between the ages of forty and fifty, Cicely Saunders had undertaken a remarkable personal project. Harnessing her own faith, her private sorrows, her professional skills, and her indomitable energies, she had gathered around her the support of friends and colleagues who, with her, made St Christopher's Hospice possible. With that, a far wider vision could also be realized.

References

Clark, D. (1998*a*) An annotated bibliography of the publications of Cicely Saunders – 1: 1958–67. *Palliative Medicine,* **12**: 181–93.

Clark, D. (1998*b*) Originating a movement: Cicely Saunders and the development of St Christopher's Hospice, 1957–67. *Mortality,* **3**(1): 43–63.

Clark, D. (1999) 'Total pain', disciplinary power and the body in the work of Cicely Saunders, 1958–67. *Social Science and Medicine,* **49**: 727–36.

Clark, D. (2001) Religion, medicine, and community in the early origins of St Christopher's Hospice. *Journal of Palliative Medicine,* **4**(3): 353–60.

du Boulay, S. (1984) *Cicely Saunders: The founder of the modern hospice movement.* London: Hodder and Stoughton.

Saunders, C. (1958) Dying of cancer. *St Thomas's Hospital Gazette,* **56**(2): 37–47.

Saunders, C. (1960*a*) The management of patients in the terminal stage. In *Cancer,* Vol. 6 (ed. R. Raven). London: Butterworth, pp. 403–17.

Saunders, C. (1960*b*) *Care of the dying.* London: Nursing Times reprint.

Saunders, C. (1961) A patient. *Nursing Times,* 31 March: 394–7.

Saunders, C. (1963*a*) The treatment of intractable pain in terminal cancer. *Proceedings of the Royal Society of Medicine,* **56**(3), March: 195–7.

Saunders, C. (1963*b*) Distress in dying. Letter. *British Medical Journal,* **ii**: 746.

Saunders, C. (1965) The last stages of life. *American Journal of Nursing,* **65**: 70–5.

Saunders, C. (1966) The care of the dying. *Guy's Hospital Gazette,* **80**, 19 March: 136–42.

Saunders, C. (1967*a*) *The management of terminal illness.* London: Hospital Medicine Publications.

Saunders, C. (1967*b*) St Christopher's Hospice. *British Hospital Journal and Social Service Review,* **LXXVII**: 2127–30.

Letters, 1959–1967

Peggy Nuttall

Nursing Times, London

26 May 1959 At long last here are four articles for you.[1] I had to re-write them and found it took me much longer than I expected. There are, as you say, quite a lot of corrections in them at the moment, but as I felt that you well might want to change a few things I have left them as they are. I have found in writing them that the religious aspect will keep breaking through as I do feel that this cannot be left out of this kind of work. If you think, however, that it is too insistent I will do something about it. The length of the articles is rather varied but it just came out that way.

I wondered whether an introductory one might perhaps start with a consideration of euthanasia? I know that this is not the responsibility of nurses but in view of the fact that it has been discussed fairly recently in the press I thought it might make the best introduction. This, of course, is taking a good deal of heart searching to write and at present I am tending to bring it in as just one aspect of the whole problem of pain and trying to deal very briefly with that in one paragraph (!) and going on from there to introduce the whole subject of the dying. My whole point being that firstly euthanasia is wrong, and secondly it should be unnecessary if terminal cancer patients are properly cared for. I will be guided by you if you do not think this is a good idea and I will send you a draft as soon as I can. The last one that is to be done is the one on mental suffering which is also getting beaten into shape at the moment.

I am sorry to be so long but I have been a bit pressed for time and also I keep finding out new things in this work all the time. Incidentally, is there any question of copyright in these articles because I might try and write a book one day about this subject?

Dr J. R. Heller

National Cancer Institute, Maryland, USA

12 June 1959 Thank you very much for your letter of May 26th. I was most interested in your comments and references; I have read one article by Dr Sutherland[2] and will get hold of the others.

I quite agree with you that it is difficult to define the situation out of context with the care of terminal patients generally. From my own experience so far I think that it is not ideal to nurse the long-term chronic sick patients and senile cases in the same ward as terminal cancer patients. The latter are so often in a younger age group and their problems are not by any means the same. "Terminal Hospitals" that I know in London are all established for the care of patients with a prognosis of three months or under. Their turnover is therefore a relatively quick one and we receive patients who are, as it were, pre-selected as having problems of pain or of some social nature. I find that my most difficult cases come in the 40–60

---

[1] Part of a series of six articles on care of the dying, commissioned by Peggy Nuttall, editor of *Nursing Times*, and which first appeared in 1959; they were later published in a set as C. Saunders, *Care of the dying* (London: Nursing Times reprint, 1960).

[2] Probably A. M. Sutherland, Psychological impact of cancer and its therapy, *Medical Clinics of North America*, **40** (1956): 705.

age group. It continues to impress me that the nursing staff and, perhaps to a lesser extent, the doctors become experts and are rarely, if ever, defeated by the patient's pain or other distress. I am becoming more and more convinced that institutions of this kind are the best places for a very large number of these patients.

I have not any reprints to send you on this topic at the moment but am waiting to receive some from a chapter I wrote in Mr Raven's book "Cancer",[3] and a series that is shortly coming out in the Nursing Times. I will send you these when I have them.

Brigadier H. L. Glyn Hughes

London

22 July 1959 I would be most interested and grateful to have your opinion about the scheme[4] I enclose, and would greatly appreciate an opportunity to come and discuss it with you. I know that you now have a view over this whole situation which no-one else can have,[5] and that you probably have your own plans afoot, but the enclosed is an attempt to sketch out a pattern which has come to me as I have been working at St Luke's and St Joseph's during the last months. I have always had in mind that I might try and start a work of this kind myself and lately I have felt impelled to begin planning.

As you will see I have tried to plan something on the lines of St Joseph's because I think that in many ways it is an ideal set up, and because I think that it has something to give to the staff as well as the patients. Also I would like some of the emphasis to be on the professional and middle class patients who I am sure are often the ones who suffer most as they grow old and ill. In particular, there is lamentably little provision for nurses themselves. You will also see that I have tried to tuck in a few young chronics, partly because I have one patient whom I must take with me wherever I go (both her husband and her mother want to come and work, and very good they would be too!). But partly because I believe that this scheme might be an answer for a small group.

I have only roughly sketched out something about finance. I am truly not asking for money, and in any case remember that you said that was not your job, but again I am hoping that you can advise me about it.

I am quite aware that one person cannot expect to do much on her own, but this problem has been on my mind for a long time and somehow it seems to me that the time has come to try and do some practical planning and to find the people who would want to help.

---

3 This appeared as C. Saunders, The management of patients in the terminal stage, in *Cancer*, Vol. 6 (ed. R. Raven) (London: Butterworth, 1960), pp. 403–17.

4 She is referring here to a ten-page document entitled *The scheme* in which Cicely Saunders set out some of the detail of her idea for a home for dying people. The home would contain sixty beds, a description is given of the ward layout, decoration, and organization, and there are guidelines about staffing levels and associated capital and revenue costs. Contractual arrangements with the National Health Service are anticipated, but the home would otherwise be independent in order to maintain 'freedom of thought and action'. The home would reflect the values and beliefs of a religious community.

5 Dr Glyn Hughes, at the request of the Gulbenkian Foundation, was just finalizing his report on terminal care facilities in Britain: H. L. Glyn Hughes, *Peace at the last. A survey of terminal care in the United Kingdom* (London: Galouste Gulbenkian Foundation, 1960).

Incidentally, I had just written a series of articles on this type of nursing for the Nursing Times and was hoping they might stir up some interest when the printing strike got in first.

I do hope that you have quite recovered from your accident and are keeping well. I very much look forward to the chance of meeting you again.

Jack Wallace[6]

London

29 October 1959 I am afraid that it is a very long time since I saw you but I have heard from time to time from Miss Packer and others who have met you. I hope that both you and Lucy[7] are well. Now I am writing for your help.

I think that you know that I have been interested in the problems of the dying for a number of years and qualified with that work in mind. For the past year I have had a Fellowship here[8] and have been working in two of the Homes which only take in patients who are actually dying of cancer. It has been infinitely interesting and rewarding both from the medical and the spiritual point of view.

Now I am being impelled to get down to some practical planning of a new foundation for such patients and I enclose a scheme with which I am trying to get interest and eventually money. I am afraid that at the moment the "we" throughout is editorial (or even royal!) but I am gradually meeting people who would be prepared to be either Trustees or be on a Board of Reference. Recently I have had a long talk with John Stott,[9] and he thought that I had reached the stage of going into the legal implications of forming a Trust, making it a really Christian foundation, and doing some degree of tying up so that it didn't get into the hands of cranks or non-Christians in years to come etc. We both thought that you would be the person to consult about this and I would be most grateful if I could come and see you sometime about it.

I am convinced that this is a great need, and that many people would help once we are really organized, and once it is not just an individualistic affair. One rich Trust is interested, I think, I have had encouragement from someone in King Edward's Hospital Fund, and I do believe that the Lord means something of this kind to come to pass.

I move about most days and am often difficult to catch. I am, however, at home most evenings, at Ambassador 7450, if you would like to ring up to arrange a meeting.

With kind regards to Lucy and yourself

---

6 An evangelical Christian friend and a lawyer, Jack Wallace (d. 1980) was a source of enormous support and encouragement to Cicely Saunders, particularly in these early days of the St Christopher's initiative and before the appointment of Lord Thurlow as its Chairman.

7 Lucy Wallace, his wife.

8 St Mary's Hospital, Department of Pharmacology.

9 The Vicar of All Soul's Church, Langham Place, London, where Cicely Saunders was then a member.

Jack Wallace

London

26 November 1959 It was very nice indeed to discuss "St Christopher's Hospice"[10] with you last week. Thank you very much indeed for offering to be a Trustee, – there is no-one I would rather have.

Since I saw you I have written to Dr Brinton, the neurologist at St Mary's about whom I spoke, and he has indicated that he admires the project very much, and says he is grateful for the chance of taking part in it but he does not feel he can make up his mind without "a bit of subconscious digestion". He feels doubtful whether he would be able to justify my selection, – from a real humility about spiritual things, – but I am sure we can get over that one. There still remains the problem of his other commitments. However, I do feel fairly hopeful of his finally accepting.

As soon as I have any other news I will let you know.

Dr L. Colebrook[11]

Farnham Royal, Buckinghamshire

8 December 1959 Thank you very much for your letter. I am rather contrite because I have been meaning to write to you and send you the [Nursing Times] articles ever since they came out. But I have been terribly busy. I had no idea they would reach such a large audience, and they seem to have aroused a considerable amount of interest, – enough to convince me once again that this is a problem which needs tackling.

About the sentence you mention. – What I was trying to bring out, is the importance of knowing each patient and their reaction to their pain and/or discomfort. In the old days we were taught that in nursing pneumonia or typhoid patients one had to lift every effort off their shoulders and even think for them. I think the care of the dying calls for something rather more individual. We have to try to watch what a patient's disease is meaning to him, and never let him get overwhelmed by it. I do not claim that none of my patients suffers any pain or distress at all, but only that I try and keep it within their own personal limits of endurance. So much of this is done by the nursing staff, and consists of individual and careful nursing. The '90%' would, I hope, say to you at any time of day or night that they are pretty comfortable. The other day I took a Ward Round of students at St Joseph's. I told them about some of the patients outside the wards, and then let them loose to chat to anybody, confident that nobody would let me down by saying that they had been miserable or in agony ever since they had been there. None of them did.

---

[10] A first reference to the hospice by name – eight years before opening.

[11] Leonard Colebrook, FRS (1883–1967), the bacteriologist and a supporter, at the end of his life, of the Euthanasia Society. In a letter to Cicely Saunders of 4 December 1959 he congratulated her on her articles in the *Nursing Times*, all of which he had read. He did, however, ask her to explain the four words italicized in the following sentence: 'We can relieve the suffering of 90% of the patients and bring it *within their diminished compass* where we cannot relieve it entirely'. He was also surprised that she had reproached the Euthanasia Society for producing no data about the suffering of the terminally ill (though he acknowledged this to be true), stating that this had been the reason he had contacted her in the first place.

I think that really the most constructive thing I could do for you would be to take you, and your wife if she would like to come, round St Joseph's. I really would like to do this as it is so hard to talk about people in the abstract.

I did not reproach the Euthanasia Society for not having produced any data, – it was merely a statement of fact, which of course I knew just because you had got in touch with me. It was probably rather mean, but was a useful piece of information to have acquired! Seriously though, I do feel strongly that yours is not the answer. We can relieve suffering if we will put our minds and hearts to it. It is just because so few people do, that pathetic cases exist. You will not find them in the Terminal Homes, but rather in General and Chronic Wards, or in their own homes.

I am happy to say I have at last acquired a secretary,[12] and she is catching up fast with all my statistics. I will indeed let you have my findings of the past year when I have got them tabulated. I am left with the conviction that there is a great need for Terminal Homes, that there is much to be done in this field generally, but that no experience of illness is ever wasted but can always be transformed into something of eternal value, and often to something of joy here, and that it is an infinitely worthwhile work. I am enclosing a Scheme for a Home we hope and intend to found – (I find an increasing number of people interested in it). I am very interested to hear what you think of it.

With kind regards to you and your wife.

Brigadier Glyn Hughes

London

28 January 1960 I am afraid it is a very long time since I last wrote, but a good deal seems to have been happening.

I would very much like to see you again sometime and I wonder whether you and your wife might like to come to dinner one evening. I'm afraid I live up rather a lot of stairs, but if you feel strong enough I would very much like you to come. Perhaps you could ring me up and we could arrange something.

I have been brooding over your report from time to time, and I have made a few queries and a few corrections of merely a drafting nature, but I am sure that you have probably done all this yourself by this time. I would like to say though, that having been through it several times, I am even more impressed by the magnitude of the task and find it more fascinating than ever. I also find that as I go through, your pattern and layout are much more evident and easy to follow. I wonder how far you have got now. I very much look forward to seeing the finished product, and if you are still at the drafting stage I would very much enjoy a discussion about it like we had before.

When I was reading through, I was struck by some of the remarks which fit in with things which I have discovered at St Joseph's over this past year. I have just done a summary of the work on about the first 340 patients, and I am enclosing for you copies of some of the tables which we have made and some comments on symptoms, and the kind of things which we find the most difficult to control. Most of it is self-explanatory. I am interested to see what you said about senile-confused, because we find that we get a great many who are confused

---

[12] Jenny Powley.

in various ways; you will see from the figures how many it amounts to. I am summarising and analysing the St Luke's figures at the moment, but I have included the data of the 'Length of Stay' because it is very much the same pattern as that at St Joseph's, and also as what you found at the Hostel of God. The figures of the 'Unsatisfactory' group are of course based on very subjective assessments and probably based on the fact of whether I happened to come in the ward on a day when one of these patients was particularly noisy or miserable. Doctor Stewart[13] of course is interested in the groups about whom we could do more. You I think will be interested in the number of patients who came in too late. You will find a separate table giving a few brief details of this whole unsatisfactory group. They are I'm afraid in alphabetical order in the copy which you have, as I have not got one under the proper groupings at the moment. I hope that if you are interested you can find your way about them. It would be an awfully interesting survey to go round visiting the homes of the patients who came in too late, and find why this happened. You will see there were a few patients who I felt we could have done better with pain, and I have also included a copy of something I have just sent off to a friend of mine who is just beginning his first house job. He wanted to know something about my "findings". Having written this I now think that I had probably better settle down to polishing it up and producing it as a sort of 'Hints for Housemen', because this is by no means the first time I have been asked for suggestions. I have actually taken two or three teaching rounds of students at St Joseph's and one of the consultants at St Thomas's says he is going to bring his firm round regularly. Certainly, as you say, this is a great gap in teaching at the moment. As you can see I have said nothing epoch-making whatsoever, except that people who have worked in general and chronic wards do seem to think it is rather epoch-making that every one of our patients looks peaceful, contented and free from pain, whenever they come round the Hospice. I do not pretend for a moment that that is my work, above all it is that of the Sister, but they do need quite a lot of guidance in the matter of drugs, and they after all are far more experienced than the average ward sister.

Of course, most of the work is just the good nursing. And I would add one comment to your remarks about the need for nursing as good as that needed by acute patients. I think one should add that it is very repetitive nursing, that you need skilled and experienced supervision, and that you do need good numbers in the wards, but I think I would add that a lot of the work can be done by assistant or untrained nurses, incidentally I find that they are often much better than nurses in training, but I don't think we need to say that.

I cannot tell you how much I enjoy working at St Joseph's, and, of course, my own plans for a Home are very much based on the set-up there. I am making some slight progress in that direction at the moment and am trying to find people who would like to be Trustees and am trying to draw up Terms of Trust for discussion with them and to get all this part settled before we start asking for money. I think that it is very important to be certain at this stage what we are really trying to do, and how we really want to do it. Of course, again, I am looking forward to discussing it with you.

---

[13] Dr (later Professor) Harold Stewart, CBE (d. 2001). A tennis-playing acquaintance of Cicely Saunders' father, he had invited her to conduct research with him, after she qualified in medicine, at St Mary's Hospital, Department of Pharmacology. The research was funded by the Sir Halley Stewart Trust, of which he was a trustee. Conducted mainly at St Joseph's Hospice, it was concerned with pain in terminally ill patients.

Pam Bright is coming to dinner with me next week and I am very much looking forward to discussing her book with her. She is obviously a superlative nurse as well as a most pleasing writer. I am so glad that I have met her. Thank you very much for introducing us.

I am enclosing also a booklet which has just come out of my series in the Nursing Times. I don't expect that you really want to plod through it all but I would very much like you to have it.

I do hope that we will be meeting again sometime soon.

With kind regards to you both

The Right Reverend the Lord Bishop of Stepney[14]

London

9 February 1960 It was a very great privilege and pleasure to join in Mr B's confirmation service at St Joseph's a little time ago, and I very much enjoyed meeting you at that time.

I am writing to know whether I could come and see you and ask for your help and advice. I have been interested in the problem of the care of the dying for a long time, and believe that I was led by God to read medicine in order to do this work. He has seemed to me, of late, to be calling me to try and found another work rather similar to that which is going on at St Joseph's. I am enclosing a Scheme which I have drawn up about this, and some of us have been thinking and praying about it while I have been trying to gather up as trustees people who would be suitable to advise on the various aspects of the work. I have now reached a rather difficult stage. I am very anxious that this work should be a Church of England one, and that it should be broadly based in the Church. I have been a member of All Souls' Church, Langham Place, for some years and therefore know a considerable number of evangelical churchmen, but I have also been greatly helped by people of a very different approach and I am much impressed by their work with dying patients. I very badly want somehow to bring these two groups together, and it is here that I need advice and guidance. The whole thing seems so far beyond my capacity, both spiritually and practically, but yet I believe that it is the way that we are being led so far. I would not call myself a definite Evangelical but just a member of the Church of England, I suppose I do approach this matter from that point of view yet I do find it most helpful working with people of different churchmanship and would not be without it.

I am sure that this kind of thing must have been attempted before by those better qualified than I am, and that you will know about it. I will not bother you with further details of where we have reached so far but hope that you may perhaps be able to give me an opportunity of discussing it all with you, and I hope that perhaps this will be the next way through which Our Lord will speak to us.

I am also enclosing a reprint of the series of articles I was asked to write for the 'Nursing Times'. I'm afraid some of it is rather technical and would not interest you, but I thought perhaps as you had been round St Joseph's that you might be interested to see it. This work is one in which we meet people in great need, but meet so many to whom the Lord has been

---

14 Evered Lunt (1901–82) was the local Bishop to St Joseph's Hospice, Hackney, at this time and was soon to become an important source of spiritual counsel to Cicely Saunders herself.

drawing close and who are most responsive to our attempts at helping spiritually. I do long for our Church to do more of it.

I know how extremely busy you are, but have been encouraged to write to you by Mr Shergold and Mr Winter[15] and would be most grateful for your help.

Dr J. R. Heller

National Cancer Institute, Maryland, USA

10 February 1960 I am afraid it is a very long time since I had your helpful letter at the end of May last year in which you said you would appreciate any reprints I might have on the subject of the care of patients dying of cancer. Everything was very held up by our printing strike and I have only just received the two which I now enclose, with my compliments.

Since I wrote to you in June, I have continued to work with this type of patient and have become more and more convinced that there is a great need in this country at least for more accommodation for them, and for more teaching on this aspect of medicine. When I wrote to you I said that I felt that it was not ideal to mix long-term chronic sick patients in the same wards as terminal cancer patients. I am not now quite so convinced of this, or at least I think that there is a place for Homes which would welcome both classes of people. A small group of us are trying to make plans for such an institution. This idea owes a great deal to the Home of 156 beds, in which I am working at present. I wonder if anything of this nature exists in the United States, or if you could suggest anywhere I could find out about it.

You will see from my reprints that they were both written before I had had time to collect and analyse figures about my patients' pain and other symptoms, and their relief. My figures now include some 500 patients, and although I have not yet done a controlled clinical trial of any individual drug, I am going to try and write this up as "clinical observations" in this field.

It is difficult to sort one's way through the mass of literature on new analgesics and tranquillisers, and so I have been trying to establish a simple regimen which could be followed by any general practitioner or intern. I would be most interested in your comments and criticism.

Dr L. Colebrook

Farnham Royal, Buckinghamshire

25 February 1960 We all very much enjoyed meeting you when you came round St Joseph's. I do hope we didn't bully you too much! We shall be very pleased for you to bring your wife any time, and also any other members of the [Euthanasia] Society who would like to come. Reverend Mother herself will be away for the next month as she has gone out to see about equipping a new hospital which the Sisters are going to run in Northern Rhodesia. I think it would be a pity if they missed her.

I thought you would be interested to hear that Mrs V the patient with a fungating cancer who was having morphine gr. i four times a day when you saw her, and who had been on

---

[15] Both chaplains at St Joseph's.

morphine since April of last year, died just under a fortnight after you saw her. Later in the week in which you did see her, she suddenly went downhill for no very obvious reason. She once needed a slightly increased dose of morphine, but after that the pain receded. We never cut down morphine quickly under these circumstances, lest patients should suffer from the withdrawal syndrome, but I am quite sure that the pain did what it so often does – disappears spontaneously for the last few days. She was very peaceful; I think realised what was happening but was quite unafraid. She slipped quietly into unconsciousness about twenty-four hours before she actually died. We miss her very much, but remember her with nothing but admiration and gratitude. Mr M, the cheerful bus conductor who was so very short of breath, but otherwise looked fairly well, has been getting up quite a lot since you saw him, and I am letting him go home this weekend. I only hope he comes back sober! He realises what is happening and he just badly wants to go out to see his home again, and we are very willing to let him do so as his wife is prepared to cope knowing she can bring him back right away if there is any trouble.

I will let you have a summary of my figures when I can get it completed for you, giving the figures of symptoms and of the type of treatment given, and the patients whom I felt were unsatisfactory for one reason or another. I would be very interested to read your pamphlet about euthanasia when you finally publish it.

With kind regards to you and your wife

Dr Hugh de Wardener[16]

St Thomas's Hospital, London

1 March 1960 I thought you might be interested to read this record of a conversation I had with Mrs G[17] the other day. When she was so ill and so unhappy last year, I used to say to the nurses that this wasn't her and that I was quite sure that she would have no memory of it afterwards, should she recover. I don't know whether I really believed it myself, but I am very glad to have this record; I think it shows that all the unhappiness has gone past recall however hard you try to make her remember. I think it is also interesting to see how, although she remembers that she had pain, it hadn't got much reality for her; she talks about it very impersonally and it doesn't really worry her.

I have just acquired a portable tape-recorder, which is obviously going to be the most tremendous help. Mrs G knew that I had it there but of course couldn't see the microphone, and I think forgot that she was being recorded while we were talking. I do find, however, that even when people can see it they still forget it and go on as if it were not there. The trouble is that I have not always got the machine with me when my patients suddenly start making absolutely splendid remarks. I wish I had had it the other day when I took the chairman of the Euthanasia Society round St Joseph's. I might have paid my patients to say all the things that they did to him! He wrote me an extremely nice letter afterwards, saying

---

16 Dr de Wardener had a specialist interest in kidney problems; for a time Cicely Saunders had been one of his housemen. Mrs G (see below, footnote 17) had been under his care.

17 This very special patient had been admitted to hospital in 1953 and was cared for by Cicely Saunders over a period of seven years until her death. A full account of Mrs G and her experiences later appeared in C. Saunders, A patient, *Nursing Times* (31 March 1961): 394–7.

that if all patients could die in places like that, there would be no work for the Society to do. A little while, and I shall have the Society working to produce Terminal Homes rather than to produce a Bill which will obviously never get through Parliament anyway.

Dr Olive Wyon[18]

Cambridge

4 March 1960 You will not know my name, unless by any chance Sister Penelope of Wantage[19] has mentioned me to you in a recent letter. I wrote to her asking her advice about something and she gave me your name as somebody who might be able to help.

I am a doctor of medicine, having read this rather late in life after training first as a nurse and then as an almoner. I read medicine because I was so interested and challenged by the problems of patients dying of cancer, and have for the past twelve years had in mind the hope that I might be led to found a new Home for these patients. I am now working with them, as I have a clinical research Fellowship, and spend my time at St Joseph's Hospice – a small hospital of 156 beds – run by the Irish Sisters of Charity in Hackney. I am enclosing a reprint of some articles which I wrote for the 'Nursing Times' at their request last year, and which contain something of what I have learnt there so far. I am also enclosing a scheme for a Home which I am trying to plan for at the moment. A small group of us have gathered together to think and pray about it, and I am very fortunate in the contacts that I have had with people in the nursing and medical worlds, who can help; but we have a very long way to go yet.

The problem about which I wrote to Sister Penelope, is the question of the 'Community' which some people seem to see envisaged in my plan. I am tremendously impressed by the love and care which the Irish Sisters of Charity give to our patients, – something more than an ordinary group of professional women could ever give, I think. But I was not really thinking of anything nearly so definite as a real new Community, I think I was using the term in a much less technical way. I asked Sister Penelope whether I was attempting the impossible to hope that a secular group of people without any kind of rule would be able to hold together and give the feeling of security, which I want so much to help our patients. I am a member of the Church of England, and have belonged to a most helpful evangelical church ever since I was converted about thirteen or fourteen years ago. But I have also learnt a great deal from the writings of Sister Penelope and others, and find that I have to try and learn and take from all branches of the Church. I have seen both groups of people help these particular patients, in their different ways, and very badly want to draw together these people in this Home. So I am really faced with two problems. On the spiritual side, I know that the spiritual work is of paramount importance and while it goes hand in hand all the time with our medical work, it is the only lasting help that we can give to our people.

---

[18] Olive Wyon (1881–1966) the respected theologian and translator, at this time retired and living in Cambridge and soon to become an important source of advice to Cicely Saunders on new religious communities: see O. Wyon, *Living springs. New religious movements in Western Europe* (London: SCM Press, 1963).

[19] It was at Wantage, with the Anglican nuns of St Mary the Virgin, that Cicely Saunders had undertaken a private retreat at the Mother House the previous year, 1959, and there that she had sought to clarify the sense of calling to her work with the dying.

They are tremendously responsive, – it is as if they say 'You have taken away my pain; I will listen to whatever you have to say'. I feel that the work should be a definitely Church of England one rather than interdenominational and that it must be widely based in the Church, and not just in one wing. Then the other problem is this question of a Community of those who work there. I think myself that this matter should be held in abeyance; I may have adumbrated it in my scheme, but I had not been thinking of going any further than pray for the right people to come, and wait for the leading of the Spirit should He want us to draw together more definitely. My medical problems, and those of raising money are formidable enough, but I think the spiritual side is the all-important one, and that is what I would very much like to discuss with you if you feel you could spare me some time.

Sister Penelope, in her letter to me, feels that people that are to work together must make specific undertakings of some sort, and must know clearly who is responsible for what and what their powers are, and that there must be some provision for getting rid of people. She mentions the French Community at Grandchamp,[20] and then goes on to tell me about you and your knowledge of them. I expect that weekends are probably difficult for you; they are the only times when it is possible for me to come up to Cambridge. Is there any chance of my seeing you on the evening of Saturday, 12th March, or any time on Sunday, 13th, or during the weekend of March 26–27th?

I bought 'Consider Him'[21] last week, and would like to thank you very much for what I have read so far.

Christopher Saunders[22]

Little Wilbraham, Cambridgeshire

4 March 1960 I have been meaning to send you a copy of the enclosed ever since I had it typed out. It really is exceedingly helpful and has been very well received by the other people who have been thinking about these plans with me. One person who made an extremely favourable comment on it, is Miss Edwards – the Director of the Division of Nursing of King Edward's Hospital Fund, a consultant to WHO on nursing organisation, – a very competent judge of such things. I have drawn a rough chart, and perhaps by the time this letter gets typed I shall have a rather more elegant one which I could enclose as well. I can't do it today because I'm flat on my beastly back; not for long I'm sure.

I did very much enjoy our time with you. I think the family is most excellent; Philip the Fearless, extremely intelligent and very charming, and Kate, not on her best but even so a

---

20 More detail on the Grandchamp Community in Switzerland appears in Cicely Saunders' letter to Jack Wallace of 16 March 1960, p. 26–7. The community is described by Olive Wyon (*Living springs*, pp. 68–75) as having informal beginnings among a group of ecumenically oriented women in 1931. The sisters adopted the Rule of Taizé in 1953 and later opened 'fraternities' in France, Switzerland, North Africa, the Middle East, and Latin America.

21 A recent book by Olive Wyon, published by SCM Press, London.

22 Cicely Saunders' youngest brother (b. 1926) and a management consultant trained at Harvard Business School. He gave considerable advice on organizational issues in these early days of planning.

very high-class baby. I think Mummy enjoyed it very much; I must try and bring her again. She is better than she was, but still not really too good. I'm afraid I've not had time to be very helpful myself as I have been a bit hard pressed lately.

I was very pleased indeed with Daddy when I was out there last weekend. He was round the garden, and we also went out for a short trip to look at some property! He manages the stairs really very well, and although he does puff and blow a bit he always did at the best of times. I don't think he will ever get back quite where he was however, but he has got a very fine constitution for someone of his age, and he probably will surprise his doctors yet.

I have written to my old tutor at Oxford, who is much in sympathy with my aims and objects and am sending her your memorandum, asking if she can make suggestions for further reading on this subject. It is her line, and although she is very elderly now she has a very acute mind and I think might be helpful. I'm meeting the organiser of a thing you may have heard of called Christian Team Work, next week. This is organised by my solicitor friend, Jack Wallace, who spends his life – as a solicitor should, I think – pointing out snags and trying to pin me down and hold me down etc. The head almoner of St Thomas's has said that she will certainly give her name and all she can in the way of advice and help and time. The ex-Matron, – very interested and extremely helpful over dinner with Miss Edwards the other night, but not quite ready to give her name as yet, anyway. She is too busy at the moment to feel that she can do much, and I don't think likes to put her name to anything where she is not going to be able to contribute something practical. However, we shall see. The question of a Community I think rather goes into abeyance. Actually, I always had it in abeyance myself, it was prodded into discussion by one or two people who read my original scheme, but even so I am quietly accumulating knowledge and thought about this. I am hoping to come up to Cambridge sometime soon to meet a wise old woman who lives there – by name Dr Olive Wyon. If I do come, perhaps I shall be able to combine it with a call on you and Shirley again, which would be very nice.

In the meantime, many thanks for doing this for me. It has been extremely helpful; I shall be on to you for your help again I know.

Jack Wallace

London

14 March 1960 Thank you very much for arranging the meeting on Thursday. I enjoyed it very much and thought it was very helpful. I got I think "the full treatment", and we went on until just about 3.0 pm. I am enclosing a copy of a letter I have written to Bruce Reed:[23] I hope that I have reported him correctly; I have just given what I remember of what he said, very briefly, and have not for the most part added my own answers or comments.

I don't think I agree with him about the formation of a Community first and foremost, and I certainly don't agree with him about his method of going about it, for example, writing a letter in the Press. I have already heard from one or two cranks because of my articles, and I think I would be swamped with them. So far the Lord has sent me quite a few people who have seen something of this vision. One or two you haven't met, and the others that you have. I'm sure that if He really wants someone like me to be in some way the founder of

---

[23] A consultant in Christian charitable work, met through Jack Wallace.

something as important as a new type of work or Order, then He will be very definite in sending people with the same feeling and burden. I would much rather leave it to Him, and go on with the things which so far I do see more clearly. I have always been very lucky in having very definite guidance; – perhaps I'm spoilt, and cannot really expect it to continue. Our strongest line in getting money eventually, will be a question of research for treatment of pain for patients with cancer, or in carrying out a new and successful course of treatment, but of course, above all I know that if we are meant to do this then the money will come.

I am off to see Dr Wyon tomorrow. Meantime I am busier than ever at St Joseph's. I have been asked to give a lecture to the whole Medical School at St Thomas's in a few months' time, and also to take a round of Bart's students in the near future. So whether I like it or not, I am deeply entangled in the medical teaching side of this work, and that does seem to me to be a definite leading.

In a little while I think I will be getting more dogmatic and stop asking advice, but I do pray that that will be of the Lord and not just of me.

With kindest regards to Lucy

Dr T. J. Deeley
Hammersmith Hospital
London

15 March 1960 I have not sent Mr M[24] up for his radiotherapy treatment for the last two or three weeks because he has really not been well enough to cope with the journey. I am afraid that it looks unlikely that he will be fit to come and see you again. He is developing ascites and is very slowly going downhill.

Thank you very much for seeing him again and treating him; it has made a great difference to his acceptance of his condition. I do not know if it is due to the radiotherapy or to the regular Brompton Mixture with a slightly increased dose of morphia, but he assures me that he has no pain, except mild pain on the lateral side of his right arm from time to time.

Jack Wallace
London

16 March 1960 I am sorry to unload yet another lengthy letter on you but I think that as you have got yourself entangled with this work you will have to bear with it, as my spiritual odyssey is so much tied up with this whole project, – or perhaps we ought to say vice versa. And as by now you will probably have heard Bruce Reed's side of the matter I think I would like to try and tell you something about my visit to Dr Wyon last Sunday, because that visit

---

[24] A reference to Antoni Michniewicz, the Polish patient at St Joseph's to whom Cicely Saunders became deeply attached and about whom she first spoke publicly in a 1977 BBC television programme: see C. Saunders, A window in your home, in *The light of experience* (London: BBC, 1977), pp. 100–5. For a further account see Chapter 8 of S. du Boulay, *Cicely Saunders. The founder of the modern hospice movement* (London, Hodder and Stoughton, 1984). Antoni Michniewicz died on 15 August 1960.

seemed to me to produce a really strong ray of light into what has been a rather cloudy and difficult situation. I don't know how much you know about her, – quite probably more than I do, – but she started life as a Congregationalist, she was Principal of a Women's Theological College in Edinburgh for some time, she is a Doctor of Divinity, has obviously done a great deal of lecturing and writing, – for example she gave the St Giles Lectures in the Cathedral in Edinburgh in 1958, she has been on the Cambridge Pastorate and she is one of the visiting lecturers for CMS. She is in her seventies. She has been an Anglican for some long time but although she now goes to the Franciscan Church in Cambridge she is not on the electoral roll because she feels she cannot do that because she knows that they do not approve of people going to Communion Services in other denominations and she herself could not feel it was right to stop doing so. I'm sure she has done other things of which I do not know at present. A delightful person with a great sense of humour and a very nice woman.

We spent two and a half hours talking on Sunday, and discussed the whole problem from a variety of angles. She felt in the first place that this was a very important 'concern'. Recently a friend of hers was in hospital and came out with a great burden for the patients she had seen in the ward dying in loneliness and with no-one to help them spiritually. She had tried to help a girl with a cerebral tumour who had been moved into a side-ward, and who had been asking for her, but had not been allowed to go and see her because she was just another patient. Dr Wyon saw this as a very important medical problem and a real need. She saw it as something that could be, and should be approached from the medical angle as a problem in its own right, although at the same time she saw how the medical and spiritual were intermingled. But she did say that she thought the thing to do was to go ahead on the medical and administrative side, even while the spiritual side was not fully sorted out. I think she really thought that one could have as trustees a number of people who had a lot to give medically and yet were not very definite spiritually; she did not think this would spoil the whole work for the future but thought that it was inevitable with a work of this nature.

She saw the theological or spiritual problem both from my personal angle and from the angle of the work as a whole. She said that she could see that I was in a difficult 'transitional' stage; she knew that I was deeply grateful to the IVF[25] and to All Souls, but could see that I was 'bursting out of my chrysalis', not wanting to lose what I had been given but searching for something more that I knew I needed and which I knew was important. She said that I must go on feeling my way and probing every available source of help, saying that I could find my place as the Holy Spirit led me. She knew that my friends would find it hard to pin me down and to see what I was really getting at, but not to worry. She thought that the Bishop of Stepney was the ideal person to help, both personally and talking of the project as a whole. She knows him very well and thinks that apart from the fact that he is the ideal person, the fact that I am working in his diocese is a strong lead to seeking his help. She was very interested in this question of 'community', and in fact she is writing a book on this sort of thing at the moment. She has a great knowledge of communities as a whole, she tried her vocation at the Anglo-Catholic Sisterhood at Truro many years ago, and has friends at Malvern and Wantage and other communities and has also been staying

---

25 The Inter-Varsity Fellowship of Protestant students to which the various university Christian Unions were affiliated.

at several Protestant communities on the Continent and knows a good deal about the new movement of secular communities which is going on in the Roman Catholic Church as well. She talked at length about the French-Swiss Calvinist Sisterhood at Grandchamp where she has stayed several times. This was started by a social worker who felt a great call to a life of prayer when she was immersed in her practical work. She gave this up and went away to pray. She was joined by two others and then by quite a large number. They have a connection with a community of men over the French Border who have helped them in various ways. They have started an Order in the sense that members take the usual three vows (not until they are over thirty years old), live a common life and have a large number of associates. They started with a life of prayer, but have been led more and more into practical work, and people flock to them for advice and help. In particular a large number of nurses have come to them asking for spiritual help in their particular work. Small numbers have gone out from the Community to start new Houses, for example, there are three in a working-class district of Paris, living in a disused Mission Hall. One of them works full-time in a factory to support the three of them. The others spend their time in prayer and in answering an increasing number of calls for help from their neighbours who come to them for spiritual advice as well as other kinds of help. Another group is starting in Uruguay, this is led by a woman in her forties who is only an associate member of the community. This Order found that they felt a great need for some form of liturgical prayer, and with the help of some of the brothers of the neighbouring Order have made up their own liturgy. Dr Wyon says that this is extremely interesting, as of course they come from a tradition which does not have anything of this nature. She also says that they are finding an increased emphasis on the importance of Eucharist worship; they are feeling their way towards this at the moment. The Mother Superior is now in her seventies, and Dr Wyon urged me to go out and stay there and meet her and other senior members of the Community (all of whom fortunately speak English fairly well) as soon as I could go. I am writing to them asking if I could go later on this summer.

Dr Wyon thought that our work was the kind that would need something of this background for those carrying it on, but she feels that it would certainly have to be a pioneer effort and on very unusual lines. But she said that this is the kind of thing that many people are feeling called to start all over the Protestant world at present, not only among Protestants, it is happening as well among Catholics. It seems to be one of the ways in which the Holy Spirit is working today. She says we should go on thinking and praying about and following up any line that we saw, any opening that was given to us, and felt that the pattern would finally be shown. She knew that we could not hurry and did not seem to think that it mattered that the medical side might go far ahead before we saw our way clearly in this discussion.

I found her immensely encouraging and I do hope that you will get something of our discussion from this letter. She wants me to keep in touch with her and let her know what happens, and I am immensely grateful to her for her help. It was interesting that a lot of what she said answered questions raised by Bruce Reed. She gave me the impression of somebody who was deeply spiritual and had a most unusual grasp of a great width of spiritual experience. She was encouraging on all counts and not destructive at all. I felt that she really knew this subject, indeed that in some ways it was one of her subjects, and that she also understood and sympathised with my own personal problems and was helpful here as well.

I hope that you will see this as a leading, as I do, both to go ahead on the medical and secular side and to continue to pray in confidence about the spiritual side.

The Mother Superior
Communauté de Grandchamp, Switzerland

30 March 1960 I have been given your name by Dr Olive Wyon of Cambridge as someone who may perhaps be able to help me. I have thought for a number of years that God was calling me to try and found a Home for patients dying of cancer, and while I was discussing this with Dr Wyon recently, she thought that I should write to you and ask if I might come and see you about it.

I have been a nurse and a hospital almoner and have been interested in the problem of dying patients for some twelve years, and qualified as a doctor of medicine in order to do this work. At present, I am working in a Home run by Roman Catholic nuns, for a mixed group of patients including some forty-five who are in the last stages of cancer. I am a member of the Church of England myself and have a Research Fellowship under St Mary's Hospital, London. I have worked in the past in secular Homes of this nature and am very impressed by the extra love and care which in many cases the nuns are able to give over and above what is usually given by the ordinary nurse. I am very anxious indeed that my own Home should have something of this, and while I am going ahead with plans on the administrative and medical side, I am trying to find out all I can about the possibilities of living in a community and of founding the work in communal as well as private prayer. I feel extremely hesitant about this but am trying to follow any lead that I believe the Holy Spirit gives me. Dr Wyon was exceedingly helpful and I would like to follow her advice and come and see you if that is possible. I would be able to take a week or ten days' holiday some time in the late summer, and would fit in with any time which you could offer me as far as possible.

I am enclosing a copy of some articles I was asked to write for the 'Nursing Times', and also the first draft of my own plans, should you have time to look through them. I am sorry that my French is not good, but I understand from Dr Wyon that you and other members of the Community do read and speak English. If I am going to be able to come I will try and improve my French before I do so!

I do not know how the dying are cared for in your country, but we see them so often here in pain, and in great loneliness, and I feel a burden for them in both ways. Our medical work has been most encouraging and we can practically always relieve pain and distress. I am also finding a wonderful response to spiritual things, and if God does mean us to found a new Home, we want very much that both sides should be kept in mind.

Christopher Saunders
Little Wilbraham, Cambridgeshire

5 April 1960 I think that I am beginning to get the pattern of the administration of my place sorted out, and I think I have now got to discuss and finalise the terms of trust with the small group who will be the actual trustees or legal owners of the Home. I wonder whether you would join us? As a matter of fact I nearly asked you at the very beginning and mentioned it to Daddy. He immediately said "O, no, you want to have the big names" and I tucked the matter back into my subconscious. However, I now think that the big names will not actually be the ones who draw up the terms of trust, but the ones who join in once the aims and so on have been defined. The actual defining should be, I think, the work of a small group in whom I have complete confidence. At the moment these consist of: Jack Wallace, (my solicitor friend) Madge Drake,[26] Rosetta Burch,[27] Miss Read, Head almoner at St Thomas's, Miss Edwards, probably, Director of the Division of Nursing of King Edward's Hospital Fund, and now I would like to add you, please, if I may.

I know that you are very busy and I know that you do not know much about the actual medical side of this, but you do know a lot about administration and organisation, and also I like you. Will you join us? This is not necessarily going to mean a tremendous amount of work, but it will mean meeting fairly soon to discuss the terms of trust and to get them into a form which we can then present to Counsel for his opinion. I understand that getting yourself approved as a Charity by the Inland Revenue takes a long time, and I'm sure that I ought to get ahead with it even where other matters are still under discussion. Someone wants to leave me some money at the moment and as I am not yet a Trust it obviously has to go to St Mary's, and the work for the dying under them. But it is stimulating me to get ahead. As it seems the time has come.

There have been various developments since I saw you last, but really too long to write about. I will tell you when I see you and send you all the relevant literature if you do think you could join us, at least during the present stage.

Jack Wallace

London

28 June 1960 Here is something in the nature of another progress report. I saw Rosetta and Martin Burch on Sunday evening and told Rosetta about my most helpful time with the Bishop of Stepney. She thought he sounded an ideal person for an adviser and a visitor, and very happy to hear that he was interested in the project. Martin gave me some very helpful hints on approaching the Charity we have been thinking of, and which perhaps shall be nameless.

I have arranged to meet the architect who did the new wing at St Joseph's at that Hospital in about two weeks time. We are going to go round and talk about the sort of thing I have in mind, and he is going to give me a draft estimate which will be sufficient for us to have some idea of cost etc for our coming approaches to Charities. Miss Edwards has been ill almost ever since we met and so hasn't been able to do anything about estimates via the King's Fund, but I think this should be adequate for our purpose.

---

[26] A family friend, who ran a convalescent home in Barnstaple, met through Rosetta Burch.

[27] A social worker, whom Cicely Saunders had first met whilst they were both still in training as lady almoners, in 1945.

I have also spoken to Miss Read who says that she thinks that the time is now ripe for her to have a word with Sir Donald Allen[28] and she is going to do this within the next two weeks before she goes on holiday, and she is going to ask him if he would see us some time at the end of July or the beginning of August. I told her about the Bishop and how helpful and interested he was and she was delighted. She thought it was a good idea to get estimates from the architect and seemed to be happy about the way things were going.

I have not heard anything from Lord Amulree[29] since I wrote to him about three weeks ago. I am not altogether surprised as he obviously is an exceedingly busy person. Miss Read also tells me that although he is helpful with advice on his own lines he is not really able now to undertake anything very demanding, so I am not awfully hopeful that we shall collect him as one of our names even though he has been on a committee of St Columba's,[30] a similar Home, in the past. We still lack a second doctor, and I am not sure what we can do about this. However, I am sure that the right person will turn up eventually. Miss Read, incidentally, also thought that Sir Donald himself might be helpful in suggesting people who would be interested in this kind of project; he is obviously an exceedingly important person with whom to get on well! Meanwhile work at St Joseph's continues unabated. I have one or two particularly responsive patients recently, who are always the greatest joy, although I do long to go and do a follow-up afterwards and see how they are getting on.

With best wishes to you and to Lucy

PS   I have just received the enclosed[31] from two Sisters who used to work at St Columba's and now run their own Nursing Home; also a copy of their covering letter. I need not tell you how pleased I was to get it.

Christopher Saunders

Little Wilbraham, Cambridgeshire

19 July 1960 I'm sorry I never write, but I am very glad indeed to hear that Shirley is so much better and also that you have such a very exciting holiday about to begin. I hope you have a really excellent time. I must say I envy you for I would simply love to see St Sophia and some of the other mosaics. I have a book of Byzantine painting and mosaic and there are some perfectly beautiful things which came out of the Church of Kahriehdjami.

If you have time before you go away I enclose a few things to bring you more or less up to date with what is going on. I was very fortunate to get an introduction to Sir Donald Allen, the Secretary of the City Parochial Foundation, via Miss Read the head almoner at St Thomas's and one of my Working Committee. I enclose a copy of a summary of the

---

[28] Sir Donald Allen, of the City Parochial Foundation, is described by du Boulay as 'the spider in the middle of the web – he knew everybody in the world of fund-raising' (du Boulay, *Cicely Saunders*, p. 122).

[29] The geriatrician, later Vice-President and President of St Christopher's.

[30] St Columba's Hospital had first been founded in London as a *Friedenheim*, or home of peace for the dying, in 1885. It was renamed St Columba's in 1915, integrated into the National Health Service after 1948, and closed in 1981.

[31] See letters to Christopher Saunders, 30 August 1960, p. 34, and to Revd David Rudall, 7 January 1964, p. 65.

interview which I dictated that evening, and I was encouraged by it and even more by the fact that he wrote that same day to Miss Read about the project. Going on from there, I got on to my solicitor and got him to arrange a conference with Counsel who has been sitting on the Terms of Trust for two months already. We went to see him yesterday afternoon and I think he now knows exactly what I want and will get on with it. I thought it would be very much easier all round if I could see him and explain exactly what I wanted rather than leave him just with the Terms of Trust as Jack had drafted them. Counsel thinks that probably the best thing would be for us to form a guaranteed company. When I get his draft I am sending it to Sir Donald Allen and will also be showing it to George Booth.[32]

All this made me want to be very certain about the religious foundation and so I got in touch with the Bishop of Stepney again. (I think I told you that I had two and a half hours with him about a month ago and how exceedingly helpful and interested he was.) Anyway, I did, and he also wrote me a letter saying that if he could be of service to me he would gladly do so.) Anyway, I saw the Bishop again on Friday afternoon. We sat at the back of St Lawrence Church Jewry for about an hour, and shouted at each other above a practising organist. He, in his turn, thinks that he would like to consult with the Bishop of London, as this will probably be in his diocese and was going to bring the matter up at the Staff Meeting yesterday. I gave him a very brief summary of our plans and so on, to take with him, should the opportunity arise to bring it up, and I thought you would like to see a copy of that, which I also enclose.

There was a Report published on Terminal Care in the United Kingdom for the Gulbenkian Trust about ten days ago; you may have seen it reported in the 'Times'. I had to do the review for the 'Nursing Times' this last week. Dr Glyn Hughes who wrote it has been my connection with the Gulbenkian Trust, whom I think I probably mentioned to you before. He came to dinner with me last week. I gather from him that he has never met any of the trustees and has really no entrée into their deliberations or recommendations at all. I did have another line on the Gulbenkian Trust via someone else, and he also told me last week that at the moment they are not thinking of doing much more than their work on the Arts, Libraries, etc. I think probably what will happen will be that they will see what repercussions there are from this Report and act accordingly. Anyway, I don't think there is anything more one can do about this at the moment, but I have a very good introduction to somebody whom I think will be extremely helpful, but which will not actually take place until October.

Canon Max Warren of the Church Missionary Society has been very helpful, and I think is very interested in this project. He is going away himself at the end of August for about four or five months, but he has done some good work for me in the meantime. I will let you know about that later when I see what comes of it.

Altogether I am not displeased with the way things are going. I did like Sir Donald Allen and I was very pleased indeed with what he said, but I would not like it to be thought that I imagined I had any promise from him even should the religious basis be within his terms of reference.[33] He really said that this was the kind of project in which they were interested

---

[32] An estate agent in Cicely Saunders' father's office at John D. Wood and Co., London.

[33] The City Parochial Foundation would not support uni-denominational projects and this, after much heart-searching, was a strong factor in the decision which determined that St Christopher's Hospice would be an interdenominational Christian foundation, rather than one based in a particular wing of the Church of England.

and that he would like to see my Terms of Trust when they came back from Counsel. He has not turned us down right away but I have no right to say that I am expecting help, or anything like that. But I know that if you should happen to meet someone who knew him, that you would appreciate all this.

I think that we have a spiritual director and a very great ally in the Bishop of Stepney, and I personally would very much like to ask him if he would be the first Visitor when the Home actually gets going. He has given me a good tough book on the Nicene Creed to be reading at the moment, by way of personal homework. I am finding it, on the whole, very helpful.

I continue to enjoy the work over at St Joseph's immensely and have had some particularly rewarding patients recently. We have started a Controlled Clinical Trial and I have been doing some teaching, so altogether I have quite a fair amount on my plate at present. But on top of this I am seeing someone from the BBC on Friday, who wants to write a book on Chronics, I am going to introduce him to some patients, and who is also considering possibly making some sort of documentary programme with me on these sort of subjects. That is very much in the blue and a difficult thing to decide on as it is full of tricky questions of etiquette, coping with relations, etc etc. Anyway, enough of this, I hope you have a lovely holiday.

The Right Reverend the Lord Bishop Bloom[34]

c/o "Meeting Point", BBC Television Centre, London

25 July 1960 I would like to say how much I enjoyed the programme 'Meeting Point' tonight, and to say how much I agreed with what you said about the importance of preparing for death.

I have worked with patients dying of cancer over the past twelve years as a nurse, an almoner and as a doctor, and exclusively with these patients over the past two years so that I have known several hundreds of people during that time. I do not agree with Miss Wright that patients do not know and are better not told and do not ask for spiritual help. Our experience is that many do realise at the end that they are dying, even when they do not ask and are not told, and they are able to accept the fact peacefully and quietly. I do not like to take the initiative in telling patients myself, but I find that because I go round on my own, and because I am not in a great hurry and am therefore able to get to know my patients personally that they very frequently do ask me questions. I think that the most important thing there is that we must listen to what the question is, and try and hear what is behind the actual words used. I am quite sure that the people who really ask, want to know and should be told and are very much better in every way for being told. I find too that, as a doctor, I get the first opportunity to try and help them spiritually. Of course, I call in the Chaplain wherever I can. This is not quite so automatic as it is in some hospitals as we are a Roman Catholic foundation although the majority of our patients are not Roman Catholic, but the Church of England Chaplain does not call as a routine to see everyone. There is no

---

34 This letter, stimulated by his television appearance, led to a long association with Archbishop Anthony Bloom of the Russian Orthodox Church, who later became a Vice-President of St Christopher's.

difficulty whatever put in the way of his coming should a patient, or should I ask him to come.

I would like to make one point which did not come up in the talk tonight, and that is that patients are often able to make very great spiritual progress in a very short space of time when they are dying. I very often find patients, almost invariably those who realise that they are dying, who turn to God apparently for the first time in their lives and who come to the most wonderful assurance and understanding and peace.

I do not know whether you would be interested to see the enclosed booklet which consists of some articles which I wrote for the 'Nursing Times' at their request last year. I am hopeful eventually to found another Home for these patients, and am therefore intensely interested in anything to do with them. If you have written anything about it yourself or could suggest anything else that I could read, or anyone else whom I could see I would be most grateful.

Sister Françoise
Communauté de Grandchamp, Switzerland

9 August 1960 Thank you very much indeed for your most kind letter which was a great comfort and help to me. It is very good to know that you understand and also that you will be praying for us. I will be remembering you as well.

My patient[35] is still alive and indeed has rallied a little over the past two weeks. He is being very good indeed, but I am all the more certain that I could not have arranged to leave at this stage.

I do very much want to come to Grandchamp some time; perhaps when I know that I am free I could write again, and there might be a possibility of coming in the next month or two. I am particularly anxious to come because we are drawing up the legal documents for the foundation of a Home for the dying, and the question of the religious basis, whether it should be definitely Church of England or a more interdenominational one, is under discussion and the final decision rests with me, and I have not yet really seen God's way through, and I have been hoping particularly that He will help me to part of the answer at any rate while I am having a time of quietness and prayer while I am with you.

With every good wish and prayer for your work.

Christopher Saunders
Little Wilbraham, Cambridgeshire

30 August 1960 I am enclosing the Memorandum produced by our Counsel, Mr James Freeman, and also the copies of the comments I have received so far from other members of the Working Committee. I have not made much in the way of comment myself so far, partly because I wanted to hear what everyone thought about it and partly because I just haven't been able to get down to it.

---

[35] A reference to Antoni Michniewicz, to stay with whom in his final days, Cicely Saunders had postponed her planned visit to Grandchamp that summer.

I am sorry I was rather brief with you when you asked me something about St Christopher's when I saw you at The Chase the other day. The trouble was that there was somebody for whom I care terribly dying at St Joseph's at that moment,[36] and the only thing I wanted was to get back to help him safely through, and I couldn't really think about anything else. He did die in immense peace when I was there with him the next day and the whole thing does fit perfectly into its own place, but it hasn't made it awfully easy to think about other things either then or now. However, we are beginning to tick over slowly once more.

I am still not completely happy about the religious foundation, although I think that Rosetta as usual has put her finger on the important points. I am waiting to talk to the Bishop of Stepney again; he has been on holiday all this month but will be back shortly. I also agree with what George Booth says, although what makes me particularly anxious about this all the way through is that I have watched both St Luke's and St Columba's starting off with the right spirit and the right people and then gradually changing in character. I enclose a copy of the Prayer Letter written by two sisters who tried to carry on after the Home was moved in 1957. I won't bother you with the whole story of how the Matron, and Assistant Matron have retired after having no consideration at all given to their feelings about the choice of the new building etc, nor the fact that the £70,000 given by other people for rebuilding were really swallowed up by the machinations of the Hospital Management Committee. I hear the same sort of thing from the one really Christian Sister who is now left at St Luke's.

The other question about the religious foundation is whether we should be in some way Church of England or more interdenominational. If we are the latter it will make it very much easier for us to get money from Sir Donald Allen who really is one of the major givers of charitable funds at the moment in London. I am so anxious not to be weighed by this that I probably am stepping too far backwards in the other direction. What I would love is to be able to do something like the Church of South India, but that is hardly possible here! One thing though I would note is that he has been quite able to give to the Mayflower Trust which is an undenominational work with a Church of England chapel attached, I think we could do that, but I very much prefer something that is 'inter' rather than 'un-'. I think there is a great difference between the highest and the lowest common factor.

You may prefer to ring me up about all this; I am in most evenings and shall be delighted to hear from you.

I thought both of you looked as if you had had a bit of a journey but had benefited from your holiday. I do hope Shirley goes on from strength to strength. It would be lovely to come up and see you sometime, I wonder if it would be a good idea to bring Mummy some weekend, although of course if we do we don't have so long to talk. I think really Saturday is a better day for travelling than Sunday at the moment, but I don't know how good that is for you.

I was very lucky in meeting somebody from the North East Metropolitan Regional Board the other day at St Joseph's and at the same time Brigadier Glyn Hughes who has just done a Report on terminal care in the United Kingdom. I am enclosing a copy of that for you because it won't take you very long to read and I do think it does show you a little

---

[36] Antoni Michniewicz.

bit of what is going on at the moment. I have tucked in a copy of my own review of it which I did for the 'Nursing Times'; it was well written up in the 'Times', 'Telegraph' and 'Manchester Guardian', but so far the medical journals have treated it with lofty uncon-cern. At least I have not been able to find anything about it in them and I think this is rather indicative of the medical profession's attitude to this problem and why it remains such a problem. Incidentally, did you hear that Mr C died at home in rather distressing circum-stances, his own doctor being quite unable to get him into any hospital in the district at all. I think it brought home to Daddy and the rest of John D Wood what a problem this is at the moment.

Many thanks for your interest. I am sorry I have been lying a bit low; it would be very nice to hear from you again.

Sister Françoise

Communauté de Grandchamp, Switzerland

30 August 1960 Thank you for your letter of 25th August, and also for so kindly sending me the notes of the Retreat. I will be using them in my times of prayer over the next few days. It is very wonderful to me that you should take such an interest in me and in our work, and it is the greatest encouragement. It is a work full of joy, but one so often feels helpless before the sorrow and problems of one's patients and in great need of the interest and above all the prayers of others.

It is particularly kind of you to remember my patient so faithfully; he is now in the presence of his Saviour and I know that your prayers with others helped to make his end the holy and peaceful one that it was. The words of Isaiah 55:12 were true for him "For you shall go out with joy and be led forth with peace." I was there most of his last two days; from the physical point of view it was wonderfully easy and quiet and he kept his complete clarity of mind until an hour before he died and his faith and trust were never clouded. He was a Roman Catholic and the hospital where I work is run by Roman Catholic nuns, but we truly found that we were one in Christ Jesus. One of the nuns once said to me "he lights up like a candle when you talk to him of Our Lord" and I know that that was so. It is a measure of the impression he made that not one of the nuns thinks that he is in Purgatory but safe with the Saviour whom he loves. His daughter was with him at the end and was greatly comforted by seeing all this, for her mother had died in pain and distress and she had been so frightened that this last bit would be hard for him too.

Now I do not know what I will be able to do about a holiday for another doctor is away now and then my secretary will be away herself. It rather looks as if it will be October before I can be free, and even then I am not quite certain how things will be going. However, I am sure that I will have the chance to come and see you one day and am very greatly looking forward to it.

As a thank offering for the Lord's working in all this and for your share in it I have asked my Bank to send you something towards the work of your Community which I would have given you should I have been able to come.

With my thanks and prayers

Dr L. Colebrook

Farnham Royal, Buckinghamshire

1 September 1960 Dr Exton Smith[37] has recently sent me the draft of his paper about terminal illness with the copy of your comments. I have only just started getting down to reading this properly and have not yet got many comments of my own to make.

I am writing, however, to say I was so sorry to see that you have been so unfortunate as to break your leg. I do hope that it is mending well and that you are quite fit by now.

I expect you have also seen Brigadier Glyn Hughes' Report to the Gulbenkian Foundation – 'Peace at the Last'. I think that this Report came out at a rather opportune moment for my own plans and applications, although actually he does call for admission of patients to general hospitals and to tie up between chronic and general hospitals, rather than the establishment of further terminal units. I do think, however, that such a unit would be a very great help in showing others a possible unit for future planning. He certainly shows how bad conditions are in very many places, and I think there is no doubt about that.

I still remain convinced that what we need are more 'St Joseph's' and am plodding on with my own plans. We are getting the legal side tied up at the moment and are beginning to make applications to one or two of the Trusts. We have a long way to go yet but I have also got the architect who did the new wing at St Joseph's to do me some sketch plans as sort of visual aids, and also so that we can get fairly accurate estimates as to the size of site we shall need and the amount of money we shall have to raise. Both are pretty formidable I can tell you!

You may be interested to know that Mr N had most of the summer at home and has just come back to me with, I think, cardiac involvement. It may, however, just be an intercurrent coronary and I may yet get him back into circulation once more. It is interesting that his chest X-ray has not altered at all since last January. I was fortunate in being able to discharge another patient 'cured' for the time-being, and to get Mr N in when he suddenly became an emergency; otherwise, of course, the only way in which I could produce a bed out of the blue would be to go over to your principles, and I do not think there is much likelihood of that. I still feel strongly that we should not take such a step, but I still feel equally strongly that we have a very great responsibility to do more for those whose end is not 'as gentle as we would wish'.

Please remember me most kindly to Mrs Colebrook. I do not suppose that you could possibly climb my stairs, but it would be so nice if you could come and have a meal with me sometime. Anyway, I will look forward to meeting you again somewhere.

---

[37] Dr A. N. Exton Smith, a physician at London's Whittington Hospital; his paper (which appeared as A. N. Exton Smith, Terminal illness in the aged, *The Lancet,* 5 August 1961: 305–8) reported observations on a series of 220 hospital patients, aged 60–101 years.

Dr A. N. Exton Smith

London

2 September 1960 Thank you very much for sending me your Report of the results of your survey on terminal illness. I was very interested indeed to see it because it fills up part of the general picture which my experience does not cover at present.

I was very interested too to see Dr Colebrook's comments and I would very much like the opportunity of meeting again and discussing the matter. Perhaps you would get in touch with me as you suggest, some time in the near future. The best place to get me is St Joseph's Hospice (Telephone No AMHerst 0861); I am there all day Monday, Wednesday and Friday and usually on Thursday afternoon as well.

By way of a few introductory comments I would say that your experience about the pain of your patients with cancer does bear out mine, in that it is not the older age-group who gets severe pain. I will assess my figures for the over-sixties and let you have the numbers if you would be interested; I think that it would certainly come out something like a quarter or even less and I can hardly think of any patients over 75 who have had severe pain at all. I notice that Dr Colebrook points out that there are none of the ear, nose and throat or spinal lesions among your group. I would not agree with him actually that it is the ENT patients who get a lot of pain, I usually find that that is easily controlled. Carcinoma of cervix I think is the most difficult both from the point of view of pain and of general distress; and I think that carcinoma of breast with bone secondaries probably comes second to that. In both these groups it is the patients between 40 and 60 yrs. who tax our skill.

I was very interested in your comments about the patient's mental state and awareness of dying. I would heartily endorse your comment that 'in a busy hospital ward there is lack of opportunity of getting to know the patients'. I think the opportunity to do this is the answer to most mental distress and often to organic pain and discomfort and is one of the strong points in favour of having more Homes such as St Joseph's.

Of course, Dr Colebrook comments on the numbers who expressed a wish to die and I do agree with him that we still have a lot to do to help terminal patients, but expressing a wish to die does not necessarily mean that one would ask for euthanasia should the opportunity be offered. Many of us feel the 'death wish' from time to time when life gets a bit much for us, and I remember in the programme on euthanasia, which you may have seen in 'Lifeline' in April, 1959, the doctor who was also a patient said how he had periods of wanting to die followed by much braver ones when he knew that he had to accept and cope with what had happened to him, and he goes on to say when he is asked whether he ought to resist this feeling – 'I feel that it should be resisted and that eventually, by prayer, communication, that for most people there will be a way back and some sort of relief, or recompense for what one has had to give up.' From my experience in knowing a number of patients pretty well I would say that that is not just his feeling but that of many others as well.

However, I think if I start talking about that I shall go on much too long and I had better wait until we have a chance to meet. I will leave it to you to telephone or write when you have got time.

Dr K. J. Rustomjee[38]

Colombo, Ceylon

16 November 1960 It was a great pleasure to see you when you came round St Joseph's and I do hope that you saw all that you wanted to see during your time with us. I was very interested in what you said about the Homes you had seen elsewhere and, of course, in what you told me of your own plans. I am afraid that you will find, as we do in this country, that it is difficult to find enough people to keep a really adequate staff of the right kind. I do feel strongly myself that some kind of religious vocation among at least a number of the staff is really essential if the patients are to be given all the help they need and if the staff themselves are to be able to carry on with this kind of work all the time.

I think that both doctors and nurses have to reorientate their thinking and realise that they are not aiming at cure, but at comfort of all kinds. If your patients are being helped spiritually and find acceptance and strength then you are seeing successes and this work is not depressing, at least, you can always see your way through depression. Our patients are almost all splendid in one way or another, but I think that the ones who both suffer the most and achieve the most are the more intelligent ones. Certainly there is a great satisfaction in caring for the less intelligent who so often have a capacity for so much affection, but I think I would find it hard myself if I did not have at least a sprinkling of patients with a deeper insight and more capacity for thinking about and discussing their problems.

I do hope that you will be able to found your Home in the near future because it does sound as if it is very greatly needed. I think that patients with lesions of the oro-pharynx are a particularly needy group, although we do not have very many of them ourselves at any one time. I do hope you will let me know what happens, and I would be grateful for any reports you may publish about your progress.

I am enclosing two reprints. I know that there is rather a lot of repetition but I thought that possibly they might be of interest to you. I am also enclosing a list of the main diagnoses, and some of the symptoms, for the first group of patients whose notes I have summarised. I thought that the incidence of pain etc in the different age groups might be of interest too. This is only the beginnings of a thesis I hope to write on this whole question of their management and treatment and all the needs which we are meeting in England at present.

I shall look forward to hearing about your progress.

Dr Olive Wyon

Cambridge

6 December 1960 It was so nice to hear of you from Stephen Smalley[39] the other day, and I hope that perhaps I will be able to come up and see him next term and that you will be able to spare me some time again then.

---

[38] Dr Rustomjee was President and Chairman of the Ceylon Cancer Society from 1951. Following his visit to St Joseph's Hospice, Hackney, in 1960 where he met Cicely Saunders for the first time, he provided various introductions for her in the USA. His work led to the opening of the Bandaranaike Memorial Home for terminally ill cancer patients in Colombo, Ceylon, on 19 November 1962.

[39] A friend of Cicely Saunders and later Dean of Chester.

Quite a lot of things have happened since I saw you, and of course, I continue working with my dying patients all day and every day as well. I had very nice letters indeed from Grandchamp, but unfortunately, although I arranged to go there in August I had to cancel it. I had a patient who became a very special friend and after being with us for many months he died just as I would have been in Switzerland. I realised that this would happen about a fortnight before I was due to go. I could not have left him, and he died in wonderful faith and peace, and I know it was right to have stayed. I am still hoping to go, however, and am going to try and arrange something in the late spring. I am all the more anxious to go as they were so understanding and so nice when I had to write to them about this.

I have seen the Bishop of Stepney several times since I saw you, and he has been the greatest possible help to me as I have been trying to sort out my own problems and the religious basis of the Home at the same time. We have decided that it shall be an inter-denominational foundation, although we will have something in the documents stating as firmly as we can that it must be carried out as a Christian work as well as a medical one. The chapel will be open for all denominations to use, although we hope to have a regular Church of England Communion Service and, of course, most of the people working and the majority of the patients will be Church of England, in any case. I found that I just couldn't think it was right to be exclusive. First of all, I could not be exclusively evangelical and thought that perhaps it would therefore have to be Anglican to keep it safe from heresy or secularisation. But then it didn't seem right to be that either, and in our legal Memorandum stands the statement "There shall be a chapel available for Christian worship", and I do not think that really we could be much broader than that! I only pray that the Holy Spirit will keep it as His work. I do not think that we can tie things down more nor ensure that it will.

I met Mrs Max Warren at the Valedictory Service of a friend of mine in the CMS and thence went to dinner with her and Canon Warren. I had a most stimulating evening with him, and in turn had an introduction with Sir Kenneth Grubb.[40] He was most helpful and has been round St Joseph's with me and is at the moment perusing our Memorandum, and may I hope be able to give us some support. He will certainly give us advice and introductions which will be very valuable indeed.

Stephen told me of the people you had suggested who might be interested. I now have a small working committee and we are meeting on Wednesday this week and I will tell them of your suggestions, – thank you very much. Someone had mentioned the Dean of Westminster to me before, and I certainly had him in the back of my mind. Our immediate problem at the moment, is that we have to send in an official appeal to a very wealthy Trust in the early part of the New Year and although we already have the help and blessing of the Bishop of Stepney we are very thin on the medical side. It is not easy to find people who really care about this problem nor indeed eminent doctors who are also real Christians. This is not going to be an easy thing for which to make a public appeal and so we are going to be rather dependent on the Trusts, and they will all tend to say "Why has this not been done by the Health Service?" and probably not even read through our appeal unless they see the name of someone they know in the medical world who has obviously approved of it and given his name to it. This is not to say that I am letting the medical side come upper-

---

40 Sir Kenneth Grubb was President of the Church Missionary Society and became a constant source of guidance and advice to Cicely Saunders as the plans for St Christopher's unfolded.

most but just that I am trying to follow up the different leadings as they are given, and this seems to be the immediate problem.

The work at St. Joseph's continues to be very rewarding and often very encouraging. There is an exceedingly nice Church of England chaplain coming now who does "referred work only". This is rather forced on us by circumstances but we find actually that it is a very effective way of using his rather limited time. We were both in despair with a patient the other day and I rang the Bishop of Stepney who came over himself to see her. It was wonderful to have him, and wonderful to have the opportunity of discussing her problems and our problems in general with him. We have now had two visits from him within a year, and I think we are the only hospital in the diocese which has had such an honour!

It does not seem to have been right to think very much more along the lines of a Community for this Home at the moment. I think if we are going to be drawn together more closely in this work, that it will happen when we get there. Anyway, there has not been any further leading in that direction so far. I do not think that it is just because I am lazy (although I am), but one seems to have to cope with one aspect of this whole problem at a time. Probably this is because one only has energy after usual work to cope with that much. Also being bereaved oneself does take up a very great deal of one's emotions and therefore 'drive', but, of course, teaches one more than anything else about this problem and the Lord's answer to every bit of it.

I do hope that I will see you again, and in the not too distant future.

With best wishes, and many thanks for your interest

The Right Reverend the Lord Bishop of Stepney
London

13 January 1961 The plans for St Christopher's Hospice are going along slowly but I hope steadily. We are in the process of forming a company limited by guarantee, and the Inland Revenue have said that they will consider us as a charity. We are sending our appeal in to The City Parochial Foundation this month but have not yet got our final appeal printed for sending to the other Trusts who may be interested. I am enclosing a draft of the Memorandum and also of the précis, because I would like you to see them and especially the parts which refer to the spiritual side of the work. I think I told you that I was very fortunate in being given an introduction to Sir Kenneth Grubb, and he most kindly came round St Joseph's with me and has been very helpful with various suggestions. He introduced me to Lord Taylor and I had a most helpful interview with the two of them just before Christmas. I was extremely encouraged that Lord Taylor was quite convinced by the end that this project would come about and is prepared to help us in various ways although, unfortunately, not to take on any position in the company itself.[41] He suggested to me that it was really time for me to see the Bishop of Southwark as I wish to work in South London, in his diocese. Several people, including Dr Olive Wyon, have also suggested that I should see the Dean of Westminster who they think is also likely to be interested in such a project. Do you agree that the time has come to approach them? I do not want to bother

---

41 Cicely Saunders was at this time rather unsuccessfully scouring the House of Lords for a peer who would take on the role of Chairman of the organizing committee for St Christopher's.

important people unnecessarily, but I myself would very much like to see them and discuss it. Could I also say that I am having your help and blessing?

I spoke to your secretary yesterday morning about Mrs W and I expect that she will have told you that she is, physically, considerably better; in fact, rather remarkably so. She is mentally much less disturbed than when you saw her, and is also, I believe, showing some glimmers of response to spiritual things. Anyway, she does truly pray the prayer which you taught her and does not have to be reminded every time I see her.

I am going to give a talk in Cambridge in the near future, and I hope very much that I might see Dr Wyon again then. I only wish that it were as easy to find important people in the medical world who are interested in this problem as it is to find such Christians.

Soeur Geneviève

Communauté de Grandchamp, Switzerland

9 February 1961 Thank you very much for your letter of the 1st February and also for the list of Retreats for this year.

I have spoken to the other doctors at the hospital and it will be convenient for everybody for me to go away in June, so I would like therefore to come as you suggest on 8th June and stay a little while after the Retreat. I will let you know exactly how long nearer the time, if I may.

I am very glad indeed to see that this Retreat will be in English and also that it will be in silence. I feel such great need to have time to listen to God.

I am hoping while I am in Switzerland that I may possibly arrange to see Dr Paul Tournier[42] whose books you may know. I believe he is still practising in Geneva and I am going to try and find out his address through the publishers so that I can write and ask if it will be possible to see him. I am wondering also whether I could perhaps see one of the Deaconess Hospitals where nursing is so completely a vocation. I would think of doing both these things after the Retreat and after perhaps a day or two longer with you. I do not want to do anything in a hurry but thought that this would be an opportunity to see these people while I was in the country. I do not know if by any chance you know either Dr Tournier or a Deaconess Hospital which is fairly near Grandchamp.

Please do not worry to answer this if you do not know. I seem to take up such a lot of your time with correspondence already.

Remembering you and your work in prayer.

---

[42] Paul Tournier (1891–1986) was a general practitioner in Geneva, Switzerland, for nearly fifty years and sought to practise what he called 'the medicine of the person'. Famously, he wrote to all his patients in 1937 stating that henceforth he would go beyond their physical disorders to the deeper problems of the whole personality. Soon afterwards he wrote his first book, *Médecine de la personne* (Neuchâtel and Paris: Delachaux et Niestlé), which appeared in English as *The healing of persons* (London: Collins, 1966). His many subsequent books were widely translated and published around the world. His book, *A doctor's casebook in the light of the Bible* (London: SCM Press, 1964), was referred to by Cicely Saunders in her early publications.

Jack Wallace

London

28 February 1961 Thank you for your letter and the draft minutes for a meeting of St Christopher's Hospice Limited.

I am not quite sure whether we are really ready for this because we are still so short of personnel. I have not got anybody in mind for the Chairman or the Secretary and surely it would not be right just to appoint one of ourselves for a limited period only. However, if you do think we should perhaps you would let me know and I will organise at least one of the others to come along for a meeting with you and Mr Marsh.

I had a letter yesterday from Lord Limerick. I wrote to him originally on the 24th January and when I received no reply I found out how to get hold of his secretary and wrote to him again at his home address. I think that the first must have gone astray as apparently he is always very punctilious. He wrote back to say that he really could not give any practical help because he and his wife already supported a Home for the Dying for very many years and cannot extend their rather numerous commitments.

I also gathered from his letter that he had not read "Care of the Dying"[43] because he also obviously thought that I was advocating euthanasia! I have written to him today saying that I am sorry that he cannot help us as I, of course, understand, but also making it clear that this is diametrically opposed to what I do think, because, although I am sure he will never think or speak of me again, I would not like someone like him to have such a very false impression.

I am now not quite certain whom to tackle next. I had the enclosed letter from Sir Kenneth Grubb on 6th February, which of course fits in with what Lord Taylor said himself about Lord Amory, but I am not at all sure whether there is any chance of his being interested if he has just taken over the Medical Research Council, and also I would like to know more about his position as a Christian. What do you think about all this?

The Bishop of Stepney is, of course, frightfully busy because it's Lent. I wrote to him quite a long time ago and I have spoken to his secretary twice since then about our matters. She is going to ask him if there is a chance of his seeing me sometime in the not too distant future. I want to ask him to be Visitor to St Christopher's – a step which I think would be agreeable to all of you, and also his advice about possibly approaching the Dean of Westminster.

I have heard nothing more from Dr Boucher of the Ministry of Health who said he would like to come round St Joseph's at some stage. I can't very well prod him again.

Mr Graham, of the Elderly Invalids' Fund, whom I think would be helpful in knowing the right people is coming round next week. His visit was postponed because he was ill.

I know that Sir Donald Allen's Committee has had my Memorandum in front of them but I do not know when the relevant Committee meeting will be taking place.

I have just finished preparing a paper to read to The Royal Society of Health and at the moment am preparing my lecture to St Thomas's on 16th March. This is rather an honour and comes as part of a very high-powered series from outside speakers, so preparation takes every available moment. It may, however, lead to something that is helpful to St Christopher's, and so I am praying that it will be guided to that end if it is right.

....

[43] The pamphlet version of the *Nursing Times* articles cited above.

I think you should probably know that I have finally decided to leave All Souls and join a church a bit nearer to me. I think John Stott and I parted very sadly and I don't think I can really explain what led me to do this at the end of a long letter. Please believe me when I say that while I am most truly grateful for all I have been given at All Souls, I was quite convinced that the Lord meant me to take this step and it has certainly not been done in a hurry.

I wonder if you heard anything from your friend, the headmaster? I had rather a wonderful time with a young doctor who was up in St Thomas's for treatment, and who was in very much the same position. I was exceedingly grateful for the opportunity of meeting him and of seeing so many of his problems just fade away. I was so grateful for being allowed to see something that had been given to us, being used.

PS   I am really very pleased that Lord Limerick has refused without further discussion. I was not at all happy about asking somebody who would not be likely to do this work as a spiritual one, as you know, but was really unable to do anything else in view of the help I had been given by Sir Kenneth Grubb and Lord Taylor. I knew that the Lord would step [in] and prevent this being done and although it has held us up I am sure that the right person will be produced at the right time.

Dr K. J. Rustomjee

Colombo, Ceylon

13 April 1961 Thank you so much for your letter of 30th March and your good wishes for Easter. I was very busy at the time as my father is ill with heart failure and I was helping to look after him. Fortunately I had a week's holiday in any case so had time to spare. I am glad to say that he is improving slowly and I am able to make an occasional visit as he lives quite near London.

All the same, I did have a little time to think about Easter itself and to rejoice.

Thank you too for all the things you have sent me – the report of your tour and the story of the Cancer Society and also the photographs. I was so interested to see one of your wife and also of the Annual General Meeting. You seem to be getting on apace with your Terminal Home and I do hope that you will be able to open as soon as you hope.

My own plans seem to be going much more slowly than yours but we seem to be making progress. I am sure this is the most difficult stage and one must not be disheartened by the number of people who say 'What a splendid idea' and also 'I'm quite sure you will get what you want' but who will not actually do anything about it themselves!

I was able to send my patient from Ceylon home from St Joseph's as she was so much better and her granddaughter was able to have her. Perhaps she will come back to us when she gets more ill once more. St Joseph's goes on very much the same as usual and is looking very beautiful at the moment with tulips and flowering trees and shrubs coming out in the courtyard. I am sorry for you in all your heat. Our patients find that very hard to bear and ours is nothing compared to yours of course.

Dr Olive Wyon

Cambridge

15 May 1961 I am enclosing the booklet of prayers written by the Lithuanian girls which impresses me so much, although of course I am not used to some of their ways of approach. But I think their acceptance and charity are really wonderful and I have found it most helpful and inspiring.

I am all set to go out to Grandchamp on 7th June and am greatly looking forward to it. My father has been very ill and I had real fears that I might not be able to go after all, but he is improving slowly all the time, and at the moment it seems that it will be quite all right for me to go.

Things have been moving slowly for some time and I did not really know which way to step next. Now, suddenly things are opening out. I was asked to speak at the Royal Society of Health Congress at Blackpool, and while I was there met two extremely important people in the Ministry of Health and also the County Medical Officer of the LCC. I was talking about the personal aspects of looking after patients dying of cancer, and they seemed to be really interested in the subject and I had long discussions with them. Since then, Dr Scott of the LCC has spoken to the Secretary of the Trust from whom I am hoping very much to have my first funds, and could not have committed himself more, both to his interest and support and also to promising as far as he can maintenance to patients in due course. He has also introduced me to the head of the Welfare Department of the LCC and I am going round one of their Homes with him as soon as we both have a free day. One of the deputy secretaries in the Ministry of Health, Dame Enid Russell-Smith, also told me that they might be able to help in finding a site. As it happens I have heard of a hospital that is closing, and have written to her about this, and she writes back to say that she is consulting with her colleagues about it and will let me know. She and Dr Scott both write extremely kindly, and both said that although there was a formidable uphill task ahead they believed that this Home we are planning would come about.

I was very interested indeed that Dr Scott asked about the question of some form of community for St Christopher's, saying, "What is going to happen when you go?". I do not think myself that it is only when I go because I am quite certain it is not a thing to be carried on one person's shoulders, and certainly not in a spiritual sphere. He was interested when I told him that I was going to Grandchamp, and I was glad that he was immediately beginning to think of it in these sort of terms. I think that he is probably the answer to our prayer for another doctor who would be both interested in the work and have some importance in the world outside. That he should immediately talk of the spiritual side of the work made me very happy.

I am most happy in my new church and finding that a lot of questions are being answered and problems sorted out. I am hoping very much to see the Bishop of Stepney again before I go to Switzerland, especially now that things seem to be beginning to move on the practical level.

I hope it will not be too long before I can come up to Cambridge again. I did so enjoy our day together and hope perhaps we may repeat it, or something like it.

Soeur Geneviève

Communauté de Grandchamp, Switzerland

14 July 1961 I enclose a copy of the Memorial Service we had for my father[44] in which we tried to show our trust in the Lord's love and forgiveness and in the strength of His resurrection, and also our love and gratitude for my father. This of course was not the ordinary burial service which had already taken place privately. I am sending it to you because the whole service was so full of trust and joyfulness and we were really uplifted and we knew that this was by your prayers and those of our other friends. Thank you all so much.

Since I have been back one or two things have happened that make me think that perhaps there will be openings in the way of money and a possible site within the next few months. Everything seems to be very safely held and guided and I am just waiting to see what develops. I feel much quieter in my heart about the spiritual side, and my visit to you even though it was so short was such a help there. I have talked with the Bishop of Stepney and with two of my friends who have prayed for this work for a long time, and they all feel that it is God's will that we should go ahead as practical openings occur and trust the Lord Himself to draw together those for whom the main care will be the spiritual side of the work and to show us the pattern there in His own time. I saw the Bishop this week and he was very certain and encouraging about this.

In the meantime, we see continual evidence of Our Lord's working at St Joseph's Hospice. I have several younger patients at the moment, one of them recently widowed, who will be leaving a daughter of only fifteen-and-a-half. She is not bitter, but she feels so very lost and in darkness and finds it hard indeed to trust in God's love. The Church of England chaplain has spent a lot of time with her and it is wonderful to see how much more peaceful she is, and how light is beginning to dawn in her darkness. The same sort of thing is happening with other patients and I never stop being grateful to God for giving me this work and for letting me be here while He is working out the future and our own plans. It does give one so much confidence about work with the dying when we see Him working in this kind of situation all the time.

Please remember me to everyone and especially to Soeur Gilberte. I am very much looking forward to my next visit to you and remember you very often.

Professor William Bennett Bean

State University of Iowa, USA

22 August 1961 I am very interested in the problems of dying patients, particularly those dying of cancer, and I am at present carrying out research under this Department into the relief of their physical and mental distress.

As no doubt you know, it is very difficult to find anything in the medical literature on this subject although I think that the "Care of the Aged, the Dying and the Dead" by Worcester of Harvard, remains the best thing that has been written.[45] In the course of correspondence

---

[44] Gordon Saunders, born 1889, died 18 June 1961.

[45] Dr Alfred Worcester, professor of hygiene at Harvard Medical School in the early years of the twentieth century, supporter of nursing reform, and author of essays on *Care of the aged, the dying and the dead* (Springfield, Ill.: Thomas, 1940).

with Professor Dr Hans Heinrich Berg of Hamburg, he mentioned to me a book by Professor Bean of Iowa University, who I think must have been your father. The title of the book is "Caritas medici" but he did not give me any further information. I wonder if you could possibly give me further details and let me know whether it is still available. I am unable to trace it through our Royal Society of Medicine Library.

If by any chance you are interested in this subject yourself I would be very grateful indeed if you could let me know anything you have written or know of as we are anxious to do what we can to try to fill a gap which exists in this country, both in the way of provision for these patients and in teaching.

Sir Kenneth Grubb

Downton, Wiltshire

17 October 1961 An official letter from the City Parochial Foundation arrived this weekend and I am delighted to be able to tell you that Sir Donald Allen writes as follows:-

> "With reference to our many conversations and to the correspondence which has passed between us in the above matter I have now to inform you that the Trustees will be prepared to earmark from their surplus income during the five years 1961/65 the sum of £50,000 and to make this available when satisfactory assurances are received that the Hospice will be established."

This is most wonderful news and has given us a splendid start. Unfortunately our Chairman, Mr Jack Wallace, is exceedingly ill in hospital at the moment, although he is at last making improvement and I believe will be back at work within a few months. Dr Harold Stewart, the head of my Department at St Mary's, has offered to be acting Vice Chairman for the time being and I think one of the next steps will be to enlarge the Committee. I am very grateful for your help on that line already and I will let you know what happens.

In the meantime my next step is to discuss plans with Dr Albertine Winner of the Ministry of Health who has been exceedingly encouraging in her interest in the project.

Soeur Geneviève

Communauté de Grandchamp, Switzerland

24 October 1961 It is a long time since I wrote to you but I have remembered you very often both in prayer for your work and also in gratefulness for all that you gave me while I was with you and continue to give with your prayers. It is the greatest help to me to remember Grandchamp in the midst of a rather busy life, both to think of its peace and prayer continually going on, and also to remember the quietness and nearness to Our Lord which in spite of everything found me while I was with you.

I am very happy to be able to tell you that I do believe that the way is beginning to open up for us here and there. Firstly, several people in the last week or two have told me that they were wondering whether God was calling them into some such work as we are envisaging. They are people who are prepared to pray and work quietly towards that end, knowing that it is unlikely that the actual Home could possibly be opened for another three or four years. One of them is of great importance in the world of nursing and is feeling particularly strongly that the future of nursing in England may well lie in some forms of nursing orders as general professional nursing is becoming more and more exercised over questions of salary and status and still there is a crisis in nursing with ever decreasing numbers. This particular person tells me that she has really only been a committed and definite Christian for the past 18 months or so. As a matter of fact I had held back from asking her if she would be interested in working with us about two years ago, just because I was not certain that she would be in sympathy with that side of the work. It did not seem right to me at the time to have an open discussion about it and now it seems that things have been quietly unfolding without my having done anything other than to continue to pray that God will send us the right people in His time. I quote this as just an example of what seems to be beginning to happen.

I am also very glad to tell you that the trust on whom I have been waiting for the past year have just let me know that they have earmarked £50,000 for us. This is a most wonderful gift and not only does it give us a financial start but also will give confidence as we appeal to other people in due course. It means also that I can now go and discuss our plans with the sort of people in public life who I will have to interest and among whom I hope we will find one or two who can help us on the business side. That is going to be an essential part of the project which is of necessity rather a large one.

I am very fortunate in that I will be meeting the Bishop of Stepney, our spiritual adviser so far in this work, later this week. He has visited St Joseph's Hospice where I am now working and has been the greatest help and encouragement to me personally ever since I began to try and make plans. I am also meeting Dr Wyon early next month. As you probably know she has been very busy coping with illness in her own family since she returned from America. I am very much looking forward to seeing her. All the time my work with our dying patients continues. I am very happy to be able to tell you that the young mother for whom I asked you especially to pray is still with us, and there is even a chance that she may be able to go home for a little while with her young daughter. Her physical condition has improved considerably and her mental and spiritual state very much more so. She has been full of faith and patience while she has been with us and I think that although such a long illness is very hard indeed to endure yet it has helped her immensely to see how steady and faithful her daughter has been. The problem of trying to help the young mothers who are leaving their children whether they yet realise it or not, remains one of my most pressing ones. I have two others with me at the moment. One of my biggest problems is to know how to organise my own life so that I do not get so busy that I cannot be helpful to anyone. I am continually being asked to write or to lecture and although I believe strongly that it is important to do this and to try and help others to see the opportunities and rewards of this work and the needs of the dying yet one can get so swamped with that sort of thing that the patients who one has to care for day by day suffer. Father Gibberd[46] introduced me to the Vicar of a church quite near where I live and I now go there and am given much support and help.

I know that you remember us continually and I cannot thank you enough for that. The people who are beginning to come forward as being interested in the work are of different denominations and also are very different branches of the Church of England so that

---

[46] Whilst at Grandchamp the previous year she had made her confession to Father Gibberd.

prayer for unity will be very much a part of our work and the support we need. May I let you know how things go on and I hope very much that I will be able to come out again next year and meet you all again and pray with you.

Sue Ryder

Cavendish, Suffolk

12 March 1962 I am enclosing a cheque for the work of the Ryder Cheshire Foundation[47] and would be grateful if you would direct it towards the work that you are doing in Poland. I would very much like to have your news letter and also any other information that you have about the work in Poland.

Your homes in Poland interest me very much and especially any that you may have now for patients suffering from incurable cancer. I am carrying out research among this particular group of patients myself at the moment and in particular we are working with drugs used for pain and all the other discomforts of such illness. I am afraid that much suffering must go unrelieved in Poland because of the shortage of hospitals and supplies and as I have had several friends and patients from Poland who have impressed me deeply I have always hoped that possibly some of the work we were doing might be of help one day to their countrymen.

I do not expect that anything we are doing could really be of help to your work in Poland at present but if there is any way in which you are interested or which you think could be relevant I would so much like to know.

Sister Alexa

Diaconessenhuis, Naarden, Holland

12 March 1962 Thank you very much for your letter before Christmas. I am afraid you are a much better correspondent than I am and I hope you will excuse a typed letter.

Thank you so much for all your enquiries and good wishes. My mother has really been very much happier and more settled since my father's death – I am not quite sure whether I told you that they had been separated for many years – I think that now she knows that all misunderstandings are at an end so far as he is concerned it is much easier for her. She is well settled with someone to look after her and will probably join me eventually when we start our own work. In the meantime however all is well.

The work itself goes on. I am not quite so busy at St Joseph's Hospice where I have been working, for I have just a slightly smaller number of patients all the time. However, it keeps me busy enough and added to it I seem to do a great deal of lecturing and discussing and teaching all the various problems that come up with incurable illness and the care of the dying. I enjoy all this very much but it does take time.

---

[47] Sue Ryder (d. 2000), who had married the philanthropist, Leonard Cheshire (d. 1992), was conducting extensive charitable work in Poland at this time. Later in the year she was joined on a visit by Cicely Saunders, who supplied a quantity of pain-relieving drugs for use in Polish hospitals. For more on the life and work of Sue Ryder, see her autobiography *And the morrow is theirs* (Bristol: The Burleigh Press, 1975).

At the same time we go on with our plans. On the practical side we now have the promise of money and are waiting to hear from another charitable company whether they may perhaps take on nearly all the rest of the finances. That would be wonderful but I am not expecting this until it actually happens, if it does. I have to go on waiting patiently and of course their committee has a great deal of work to do before they finally decide. At the same time I was approached by a teaching hospital to go down and talk to various members of their medical committee. I have now spoken to the Board of Governors and others and I think that it looks as if they are going to be interested in our having a friendly liaison with them and they, I think, will help us in acquiring a site near to them. Of course the most important side is the spiritual foundation and the way we will run this home when we finally build it. Here everything is more intangible but people are being called to pray for us and a few are thinking of coming to work and I believe just a few of them really with a true vocation.

But enough of my news. I was very interested in everything that you said about yourself and so glad that the operation went so well. You seem to have had a very short convalescence. I was also interested in all you said about the community and as I see from your letter you were expecting your mother to leave in February. Probably the decisions have been made. I do hope that you were clearly shown what to do. I wonder what will happen and whether you will see clearly what you have to do.

I saw Soeur Genevieve less than a week before she died. I met her daughter in England just before she went out to be with her and the family and the doctor asked me if I would go out to see her which I duly did. It was lovely to see her just at that time although she was, of course, very weak and ill and in considerable pain at times. We had a short time together on three separate occasions and I will never forget the things she said and the things we were able to share, mostly without words. I stayed in the deaconess hospital where she was a patient for two nights and spent a long time with the deaconesses and then I had just one night at Grandchamp and met and talked to the Sisters. It was lovely to see them and to share both their grief and their comfort.

Father Gibberd has been out there recently and I have spoken to him on the telephone since then. He tells me that they are managing very well and he sounded happy about the community and its future. I do not know whether I will get there in the summer. I think it is not likely that I will go for the retreat that he is leading.

I wonder whether we will meet there again. I do hope so. In the meantime I will remember you and all your decisions.

With my best wishes for your future.

Dr Albertine Winner[48]

Ministry of Health, London

22 March 1962 I understand from your secretary that you have been away for a few days, I do hope that this was a break and not just work. I have not forgotten what you told me and I do hope that everything was kept safely.

---

[48] Dame Albertine Winner (1907–88); at this time England's Deputy Chief Medical Officer, though later she became Deputy Medical Director at St Christopher's Hospice, and subsequently Chairman of its Council.

I was just ringing to let you know, in case you have not heard from Dr Cooksey, that the King's College Hospital interviews seem to have really gone very well. They were exceedingly nice to me and I had a most kind letter from Lord Normanby of which I enclose a copy. Since then he has telephoned me to say they will have to wait until their meeting at the end of April as there has to be a meeting of the Development Committee first before they can finally suggest a specific site.[49]

I am going down to King's again to talk over the actual details of the possible site or sites with Mr Banks, the House Governor tomorrow morning, I have not felt that I was in a position to be at all critical about what we were going to be offered but now the matter has been approved in principle he has kindly suggested I should come down and talk to him before the Development Committee actually meets. I am not quite certain whether there really is a suitable site available a bit further away from the hospital but I must admit if there were I think I would choose that rather than the one just below their own planned extension on Denmark Hill. With the new long term road planning there is obviously going to be a great deal of traffic along there, there would be no room at all for any kind of extension, and also although I know the present committee only want a friendly kind of liaison and quite understand our feelings about being independent yet one does have the feeling that, in say twenty years time, our nearness to the hospital might make us feel a little bit like Naboth.

I am well aware what a very great help it is to us that King's should have taken such an interest and given us such support and I do not think we will be in a position to say 'no' to anything that we are offered. However I am very grateful for the opportunity for further discussion before the committee actually meets because I understand that they have not got any definite plans in mind themselves for these sites.

I am still waiting to hear from the Drapers. I am not getting impatient because I know it takes a City Company a very long time to consider such things and obviously they must have other proposals to discuss. I have of course let them know about King's because it does give us a great deal more status and respectability.

The Priest in Charge

St Andrew's Bobola Polish Church, London

28 August 1962 I was moved to come to your church last Sunday morning because I was so impressed by the BBC programme, 'The Black Madonna' and by the singing at Czestochowa. I am neither a Roman Catholic nor a Pole, but I have had strong personal ties with several Poles and have cared for them at St Joseph's Hospice, Hackney, where I am one of the doctors. Among them was one who impressed me very deeply by his faith and courage.

I would like to thank you for the service and also to say how beautiful and inspiring I found your church. I go regularly to my own church, an Anglican one, but I hope that I may sometimes come again and join as much as I can in your worship of our same Lord.

[49] She is referring here to discussions, not realized, that St Christopher's might be built on land owned by King's College Hospital.

Would you please also allow me to bring a friend to take one or two coloured slides of your church? I am going to lecture in America next year about the work at St Joseph's and the care of people who are dying of cancer and will be taking slides of our building and some of our patients there. The Risen Christ in your church so perfectly expresses his victory and compassionate love in all our sufferings that I would very much like to include this also when I speak to various church groups and seminaries. Would you agree to my doing this?

The Reverend Almon R. Pepper

Department of Christian Social Relations, New York, USA

12 December 1962 It is now rather a long time since the Reverend Benjamin Holmes[50] wrote to you about my prospective visit to the United States but there have been a number of problems to sort out at this end. I apologise for the delay and the concern it has caused you. I think Mr Holmes told you I was going to Poland for a short visit and I have just returned. I feel more able to plan my trip to the States.

Another reason for the delay was that I was rather overwhelmed by the suggestions which Mr Holmes passed on to me. I have been given a grant from the Hospital where I did my nursing training, St Thomas's, London, to find out what I can about the care of terminal patients in the States and I am really going over to try to learn and not to teach. I would, however, be very glad to meet anyone interested, either in the medical or pastoral field and if I were asked to give a few lectures I would be glad to do so.

Your suggestion of setting up small groups for discussion interests me very much indeed but I had hoped that it would be on the understanding that I am here primarily to learn from you.

Plans for the trip have not been finalised but I am expecting to fly to New York at the end of March and to stay in the States for two months in all. I think the first month would be in and around New York and the second making my way in various steps across the States to finish with a short holiday and rest with a friend in British Columbia before flying home directly from there. The only thing that I have so far arranged definitely is a lecture at the General Theological Seminary in New York on April 24, as I had a very nice letter from Professor Carper asking me to meet their Senior Class. I will be lecturing at Yale University Medical School but the date for this has not yet been fixed.

My other visits still remain to be arranged. I am hoping to see a number of places in New York and also to visit Harvard, Washington and other centres. I am waiting at the moment to hear from the American Cancer Society as I wrote some time ago and have not yet had a reply.

[50] The Reverend Benjamin Holmes, an Episcopalian priest based in Saratoga Springs, New York, had visited Cicely Saunders at St Joseph's Hospice, Hackney, in 1961. He encouraged her to come to the United States and subsequently made various introductions, including the one referred to here. Almon Pepper (d. 1973) was Director of the Department of Christian Social Relations, Protestant Episcopal Church, New York; later he became a Vice-President of St Christopher's and attended the opening ceremony in 1967. These early American contacts led to a ground-breaking visit to the USA by Cicely Saunders in 1963, during which she made extensive and enduring links with a wide variety of individuals engaged in the care of the dying.

I am not sure whether you will think it is better to leave arrangements until I arrive or whether you would like to make more detailed suggestions at this stage. I do not want to overcrowd my programme so that I am unable to assimilate anything except superficially, but I do want to use the time to best advantage. My experience in doing this sort of thing is at the moment limited to my short trip to Warsaw and I do not want to be too ambitious.

Sister Alexa

Utrecht, Holland

30 January 1963 Thank you very much indeed for your long letter, I was very interested to hear all your news and thank you for telling me all about it. You seem to have come a long way since you wrote to me last time. I am very glad that your year at the Deaconess Hospital went so well, as of course it must have done from what you tell me. I am sorry, however, to hear that your next step is being held up by your health and I do hope that the University Hospital will quickly find what is the matter and be able to help.

It is wonderful to think of your going to Grandchamp and also that you should be going with a companion and I pray that this will not have to be postponed for very long. I heard recently from Sister Gilberte who takes such a personal interest in St Christopher's, our hoped for hospice. She sounded well and was just off to St Moritz for a holiday. I am so grateful that we have her prayers so continually and I love getting her letters.

Our own plans move very slowly but we had a meeting of a group of people who are interested in coming to work with us and who are praying for the plans and also for my patients at St Joseph's in the meantime. This took place in the summer and was led for us by the Bishop of Stepney who is our Spiritual Adviser. It was a wonderful day and a great encouragement. We are meeting again on March 17th and I think there will be more of us this time. We may also have news of a site and a grant of money by that time. I think that we are nearer this than we have ever been before. It is not that we have actually had our application turned down but just that people have taken so many months to make up their minds. It does look, however, as if we are making a step forward and I am sure that when it happens it will be the right time and that we will know that.

In the meantime, I am still working with my same patients and doing more and more lecturing and am also writing when I can manage to fit it in. There is a great deal of interest in the problems of these patients and I believe that because the matter has been brought out and discussed that perhaps there will be patients better cared for in places very far distant from St Christopher's and that after all is part of the work.

I am going over to the United States for a two months' visit in the spring to see what work they are doing over there although I do not think that I will probably find anything better than we have in Europe. I have also just had a short visit to Poland which was most fascinating and inspiring, it certainly made me realise how fortunate we are over here, and also what a tremendous part a Church can still play even under a Socialist Government.

I will let you know if anything really important happens to us, but in the meantime, I will be remembering you and hope that I will hear the good news that you have arrived safe and well at Grandchamp.

Mother Mary Paula

Culver City, California, USA

20 February 1963 I know that you will rejoice with me to hear that King Edward's Hospital Fund have given us a splendid grant. They have allowed us up to £30,000 for a site and we had already found a suitable one for £27,000 and have gone ahead and made an offer subject to Town Planning Permission. We had already applied for that in faith while the King's Fund were considering our application and the final decision will be made on March 14th. It is a suitable place down in South East London and near Transport and also with quite a lot of open space near.

This means that we will at last get going although, of course, we have a great deal of money to raise and a great many things to do but it is a start and it will get things going at last.

I was so glad to have your letter but I am very sorry that I will not be seeing you when I come to California. However, I think you must be longing to get back to Dublin. It sounds difficult to manage and I have certainly remembered you as we all have at St Joseph's. I will keep a note of the addresses that you gave me and will call and see them. I am getting very excited about my trip but it has gone a little bit into the background during the last few days while I have been rejoicing over our good fortune for St Christopher's Hospice.

I hope I will be in Ireland again before so very long and I will look forward to seeing you then.

Dr Herman Feifel[51]

University of Southern California School of Medicine, USA

27 February 1963 I have been meaning for a long time to write and tell you how very interested I was in your book "The Meaning of Death". Like you, I have found it very difficult to find any literature on this subject and it is my major interest. I have worked with these patients as a nurse, as a medical social worker and have now qualified as a doctor in order to continue in this field. For the past four and a half years I have held a Clinical Research Fellowship in the Department of Pharmacology, St Mary's Hospital Medical School and have been caring for some 50 patients with terminal cancer in a hospice for patients with chronic and terminal illnesses in the East End of London. This Fellowship was originally given to investigate the treatment of pain and other distress but of course you cannot begin to try to help a patient's pain without trying to look after the whole person and from the beginning this has meant a very broad approach to the whole problem or at least as I myself am capable of making it.

The stimulus that has made me finally write to you is that I have now been given a travelling scholarship from my old nursing school at St Thomas's (where I also read medicine) and I am coming over to the United States on March 27th for nine weeks in all. I have various introductions and people to see and will be giving a few lectures while I am over. At the

---

51 Herman Feifel (b. 1915), chief psychologist at the Veteran's Administration in Los Angeles and author of key early works on aspects of death and dying. The letter refers to his book *The meaning of death* (New York: McGraw Hill, 1959). Herman Feifel and Cicely Saunders were to meet frequently and maintain a regular correspondence in subsequent years.

moment the only ones that are arranged are at Yale University School of Medicine and the Medical Society of New Haven and at the General Theological Seminary in New York but I am meeting the Reverend Almon Pepper of the Episcopal Church as soon as I arrive and also various doctors in New York and my programme will not be arranged in detail until then.

I am intending to come over to California in May and I wonder whether there is any chance of my meeting you. I would appreciate the opportunity of some discussion of these problems very much indeed. I am sending by second class airmail three reprints which may show you a little bit of the work that we are trying to do. The booklet of course was originally written for nurses and I think that probably fundamentally that is still very much part of my approach to the situation.

If you are able to meet me, I would be very grateful and if you could also tell me of any one else who would be interested to hear something of our experience and, more important, have something to teach us, and if there are any homes similar to that in which I work, to which you could give me an introduction, I would be very glad.

We are at present very much involved in trying to start another hospice similar to that in which I am working. This has been my aim for a number of years and now at last we have just been given a splendid grant by King Edward's Hospital Fund for London which will enable us to buy a site and other charitable trusts have promised, or are going to promise, us money which will enable us to begin building in the very near future. All this makes it all the more important for me to see any similar work that I can find and to learn what I can from the approach of other people.

I hope possibly that I may meet one or two of the other contributors to your book while I am on the Eastern side of the United States as I have read other works of theirs already and been very interested in them.

Dr Herman Feifel

Los Angeles, USA

17 June 1963 Thank you for your letter of May 27th which was waiting for me when I got home. The remainder of my stay was just as good as the rest and I think that the Rancho Los Amigos was one of the very best places that I went to and Dr Brown put on the most wonderful programme for me in San Francisco.[52] California must certainly be visited again and I think that this will happen somehow.

I am enclosing a reprint of the session at the Royal Society of Medicine[53] as I thought you might be interested to see it although, of course, it is more on the physical rather than the mental distress of our patients.

[52] She had been introduced in 1963 by Herman Feifel to the social anthropologist and writer on healthcare organization, Dr Esther Lucile Brown. They subsequently corresponded in detail. Dr Brown introduced her in turn to the imaginative nursing and attention to detail which was a feature of care at Rancho Los Amigos Hospital, in California.

[53] This appeared as C. Saunders, The treatment of intractable pain in terminal cancer, *Proceedings of the Royal Society of Medicine*, **56**(3), (1963): 195–7.

I just got back in time to sign the contract for our site. There had been complications which had to be dealt with by the lawyers but it now seems to be all in order and so we have gone ahead. I have been down to see it of course and it has an extremely happy atmosphere which is quite tangible when you go there. I am sure that it is going to be a good place to work at and pray that it will be a good place to come to. We will be in the throes of raising money and getting plans done now but I will let you know how things go on and also if I manage to get anything else in writing, I will send it along to you.

Thank you again for all the efforts you made to make my stay in California so profitable and enjoyable.

Dr Esther Lucile Brown

San Francisco, USA

4 July 1963 I have enjoyed your two books[54] so much and am now going through them in more detail because I see that I will want to quote them often. Writing a report on my trip is being somewhat arduous but interesting, though difficult to sandwich in with patients, lectures and the latest developments of St Christopher's Hospice.

I am also getting some further reprints done of articles for you. I have run out of everything and am getting a few redone (not that there are all that many anyway). But I will send them along to you in due course.

My noble colleagues carried on while I was away, rather glad I was out of the country I think, as Town Planning Permission being granted, some further and quite unexpected snag appeared and had to be dealt with by the lawyers as fast as possible, and we nearly lost the site even at that stage. However, all is well, and I signed the contract the other day, and it really is ours. Now it merely remains to raise a fantastic sum of money, build it, fill it with the right staff and put it firmly on the right foundations in every way! But I know now, that it is really 'meant' to happen and that I have to find a pattern that is really there for the finding.

When I met your secretary she told me that she was coming back to England this summer. Please remind her that she promised to get in touch with me, because if she is interested I would so much like to show her St Joseph's, and if by any chance she wanted a job for a while, I am without anyone at the moment except for part-time in the evenings and am slowly going mad, doing my own typing, so perhaps we could get together. It probably isn't really the sort of thing she wants, but I thought that there just might be a possibility.

I cannot tell you how much I have enjoyed getting back to my own patients once more. But taking on some 45, many of whom I had never seen before, getting all the problems which had been saved up for me at once, made me realize that they are quite a burden. But a very possible burden and a very rewarding one, when you are really working as a community (or a 'peer group'?). We are getting on with the plans of St Christopher's at the moment, and the whole thing must be planned with this in mind, as you say.

---

54 Probably E. L. Brown, *Newer dimensions of patient care,* Part 1: *The use of the physical and social environment for therapeutic purposes* (New York, Russell Sage Foundation, 1961) and E. L. Brown, *Newer dimensions of patient care,* Part 2: *Improving staff motivation and competence* (New York, Russell Sage Foundation, 1962).

Tomorrow I lunch with the people who gave us the site and some others who may help with the building. I will let you know how we go on.

Edna Rossiter

Shaughnessy Hospital, Vancouver, British Columbia

17 July 1963 At long last I have some Reprints which I am sending as I thought they might interest you. The Symposium at the Royal Society of Medicine was very interesting and I was very pleased that it aroused a lot of interest in our particular problem.

I am glad to tell you that I just got back in time to sign the contract for the site and now the money has been handed over and it is really ours. It was a very good coincidence that the day after the money order was actually handed to the previous owners, I had arranged to take the Bishop of Stepney, our Spiritual Adviser or Visitor, down to the site so that we could have a little private blessing and dedication of it. He is just the right person for this kind of thing and told me that he thought it was really an "apostolic occasion". Now there is a great deal of money to raise but I am sure that it will go ahead.

The photographs that I took the evening I was with you have really come out very well and as soon as I can spare the slides from showing them to various people, I will have some prints made and send them to you. It was the most lovely evening and I did so enjoy it.

Professor I. N. Mensh

University of California, Los Angeles, USA

16 August 1963 When you so kindly saw me at rather short notice in May you were most helpful in enabling me to go to Rancho Los Amigos Hospital and we also had an interesting discussion about writings on the care of patients dying of cancer, and their psychological as well as their medical problems. I was very grateful for your interest and I hope that perhaps I will get back to California again one day and not be in quite such a rush next time. I think now that I know something more of the people who are really interested in this field it will make it much easier. I did, however, find my trip extremely profitable and satisfying and am, as you see, still catching up with thinking of all the people whom I met.

I am now enclosing some reprints about the work which I have been trying to do, which I thought might interest you. The major work is of course the thesis on the five years' care of these patients, which now includes 1,000 analysed records. This is a very unwieldy amount of material to handle, and of course as I am trying to talk about intangible things as well as about the drugs and the dosages and the methods we use, I am not finding it easy to get this into a form which will be adequate and really presentable. However, in spite of all the other demands this is getting on slowly.

I think I mentioned to you that we are now founding another institution for these patients. We have been given a grant by King Edward's Hospital Fund for London, which has enabled us to buy a very suitable site and now we have to go ahead and build. At the present moment we are expanding our Council of Management and drawing up detailed plans from estimates so that the major Building Fund Appeal can go ahead. We have been promised monies which will enable us to start once they are released, but we have to be just one step further on before this will be so. I am more than ever convinced that there is a real place for such small units, not only for patients with terminal cancer, but also to include some with other long term illnesses and frail and elderly relations of the staff. This last group is included both to acquire the right stable staff, but also to give something of the feeling of community which is so extremely important in work of this kind, both for the patients and for the staff themselves. This project will have a close connection with two London Teaching Hospitals and also with the facilities in the community, because while we need the informality of the small unit, we also need very much not to be in any kind of backwater.

Although I did not see any completely comparable institution in the USA, you can imagine that the trip produced a great deal of information and many stimulating ideas, often just as stimulating if I disagreed as if I agreed.

Thank you again for your interest and help. I hope that maybe we will meet again one day.

Soeur Gilberte

Grandchamp, Switzerland

21 August 1963 You may just possibly be seeing a friend of mine in the near future, Colonel Hubert Madge and his family are staying near Taizé for their holiday at the moment and may go over to Grandchamp during that time. They are great friends of mine and there is just a possibility that he might help us in the work for St Christopher's Hospice. This is not at all definite and he is thinking about it while he is on holiday and we are having further discussions on his return. It would be wonderful if he could come to help us but I know that the Lord will show us both what is the right plan and send the right person in due course.

I have been trying to see how I could plan a visit to you but it does still seem very uncertain. I wonder if you could let me know when you would have a Retreat which you think would be specially suited for me to come to. I would obviously prefer it when there was a leader who at least speaks some English but I think my French is up to somebody who talks slowly for the actual addresses.

The plans, as usual, go on slowly. We had many complications in getting the site but it really is ours now, and it has a lovely peaceful feeling to it. The day after it was really ours, the Bishop of Stepney came down with me and blessed and dedicated it to the work. This was a very quiet and private moment but had a feeling of absolute rightness about it.

We have many practical things to think of but in the meantime the group of people interested in St Christopher's are getting to know each other better. I am very pleased that one or two of them are now writing to each other. We will be meeting as a whole again on October 19th. The Bishop will be there to lead us once more and I hope that the Russian Orthodox Archbishop, Anthony Bloom, who has agreed to come on to our Council, will also be able to come for a short time. He of course is a very busy person but has had St Christopher's in his prayers for a long time.

The problems of the distress of the dying have been discussed recently both in the Medical Press and also in The Times. We are hoping very much that we can publish letters about the work we are trying to do and if this does happen it would seem to be a wonderful well timed moment but the conviction that God is guiding in the details as well as in the foundations remains very quiet and certain.

I hope you will have some holiday and perhaps get to St Moritz as usual. I often think of the peace of Grandchamp although I know that, like the peace at St Joseph's, it is never just without cost.

With love to you all at the Community and with my prayers,

Dr Eric Wilkes

Baslow, Derbyshire

12 September 1963 Many thanks for your letter. I am fascinated to hear that you are going to try and start some kind of hospice in your part of the world.[55] I will certainly collect up a set of slides for you and send them on in due course. In the meantime however I would dearly love to know a little more about this because of course I am bursting with ideas about beginning such institutions!

If in any way I could be a help to you I would gladly meet for a discussion if you should think that this would be profitable.

Our own plans are going fairly well at the moment and if you would be interested I would send you a memorandum of our aims and the progress so far. The King's Fund are being extremely helpful and having their imprimatur is a tremendous advantage to us.

Dr M. Sloan

National Institutes of Health, Bethesda, Maryland, USA

7 October 1963 This is just to let you know that I have rather diffidently sent you a copy of the Report[56] about my tour in the United States which I wrote for the people who so kindly gave me the money to make it possible. As you will see it is written rather informally and is not an attempt to cover all the ground but rather to bring out a few of the questions that I think were discussed most profitably from my own point of view. I have certainly found now that I am back how exceedingly valuable it all was. I find this both while I am working with patients at St Joseph's and also as we go ahead with planning St Christopher's Hospice. I will also enclose a Memorandum about the latter which sums up what we are trying to do and also give some idea of the progress so far. At the moment we are engaged in getting the detailed plans at a stage ready for discussion for the experts at the King Edward's Hospital Fund and also trying to be ready to answer all the questions we may expect from the people who we hope will give us money. This is an exciting stage and it is marvellous to go down and see our own site, and to imagine what it is going to be like eventually.

I was delighted to meet Dr Clare Ryder when she stopped in London for a weekend on her way to the Gerontological Congress. I had a delightful afternoon when she came to

[55] At this time working as a GP in rural Derbyshire, Eric Wilkes (b. 1920) later went on to become Professor of Community Medicine at the University of Sheffield and to found St Luke's Hospice in the city in 1971.

[56] On returning from the USA in 1963, Cicely Saunders wrote a detailed 37-page report of her eight-week coast-to-coast visit and went to considerable trouble in distributing it to those whom she had met during her time there.

St Joseph's and found it extremely interesting to discuss a little bit of the work with her. I do hope that if you are ever in London you may perhaps have a chance of doing the same, as I would particularly enjoy taking you round and continuing our discussion.

With every hope of meeting you again sometime.

_____

Sister Alexa

Communauté de Grandchamp, Switzerland

8 October 1963 I must apologise first of all that I have not written to you since you sent me your change of address with the good news that you have been able to join the Community at Grandchamp. I am very glad indeed that the way has opened for you to do this and I hope that all goes well now.

The enclosed memorandum about St Christopher's will tell you more or less the stage we have now reached. There have been a few developments since I wrote it but I am not yet sure when we will be able to launch the appeal for money. The next meeting of all those interested is going to be rather larger than before because it is going to include some people who are rather helping us from outside rather than from inside. I think that probably we will start planning for a week-end retreat for those who are really committed to the work and so there will be an inner circle as well as the whole group of people who are interested. It is very apparent that the work is becoming more and more that of a group than of one person and of course this is absolutely essential and is probably the reason why the developments have been rather slow up till now.

I think I told you in my last letter that I was going out to the United States for a visit of two months. I thoroughly enjoyed every moment of this and worked very hard indeed visiting eighteen hospitals and innumerable people. Everyone was extremely kind and hospitable and very generous of their information as well as of their time.

My next trip abroad is going to be a short holiday in Holland. I am going out with my mother just for a week to Amsterdam from the 28th October. She has one or two friends out there and so I would be able to leave her alone for the odd day or two. If there is anywhere or anybody that you feel that I really ought to see while I am there I would be most grateful if you had time to drop me a line about it. You will know how easy it is to get to places from Amsterdam but I believe that somewhere like Utrecht would only take a short while. I have actually had a letter for a reprint of one of my articles from a doctor in Utrecht who obviously speaks English and I believe that Dr Buytendijk is still the Professor of Psychology at the University there. His book on pain was absolutely fascinating and a real enlightenment for me. I hesitate to ask such an important person whether I could see them but am very tempted to do this. You will be able to tell me whether people in Holland are as willing to give time to casual visitors as they are in the USA. I have never been so importunate in all my life and found that it has paid a very good dividend.

I heard recently from Soeur Gilberte from Taizé. I am very glad to know that she has remembered us so constantly. I had hoped when I wrote to her that I might possibly be able to try and find my way out for a retreat but I think that I will have to leave that until next year at least. I hope that I will get the list of retreats from Grandchamp in due course. I do very much want to come again and hope that I will manage it next year.

Dr Mason F. Lord

Baltimore City Hospital, Maryland, USA

8 October 1963 I do not know whether you will ever have time to plod through this but I am sending you a copy of my report of my tour in the United States and also one or two reprints about the work we have been doing. I am rather diffident about doing this in view of what you told me about your 'conference' and 'report' when you first began working in Baltimore. I hope you will forgive me for my comments about your own work which impressed me very much and I was interested in the difference between that and the intensive programmes. As I turn to the latter I think to myself I was all the more pleased to see what you were doing.

I am also enclosing a memorandum about St Christopher's Hospice which has now reached the stage as you will see of having a site and while we enlarge the Council, gather in some well known Vice-Presidents, we are getting the plans done with the architect so they can be discussed by the experts at King Edward's Hospital Fund and have, as it were, their imprimatur when we make our Building Fund appeal. When we finally have St Christopher's open and working I hope that maybe there will be some real tie in with the work of the local doctors and I am particularly glad to have Brigadier Glyn-Hughes on the Council as he is Director of a large General Practitioners' Centre nearby. I know that we are doing this on a small scale but I am quite certain that we could not have anything larger. The development in the future will I hope be in teaching and in either inspiring other work or in expanding ourselves in other places. Anyway, at the moment I have the formidable proposition of raising at least £250,000 and that will probably keep me busy for some little time to come.

I do not know whether you ever find yourself in England, but if you do I do hope you will come and see us either at St Joseph's or, after the next two or three years, at St Christopher's.

I heard of you the other day from Mrs Sainsbury who I think sat next to you at a dinner party when she was over with her husband a few months ago. She gave me some very good advice about raising money which I hope to be able to take in the near future.

With very good wishes for your own work and if you do write any reports or articles about it I would be most grateful for reprints.

The Right Reverend the Lord Bishop of Stepney

London

17 October 1963 It was very good indeed to see you the other day and I thought that we were able to gather up a tremendous lot in the time we had. I have so often noticed that the things that are necessary somehow pack into the time that is available and it never seems to matter very much when that time seems rather short. Thank you very much for sending me away feeling so safe.

I am looking forward very much indeed to Saturday morning at Riddell House.[57] I have suggested to everyone that we should meet at 10.30 but there are one or two people who say

---

[57] This meeting would have been one of a regular series of 'St Christopher's Days' at which friends and supporters of the hospice came together for the exchange of ideas, news, and plans.

that they may be a little bit late. I think that the first few minutes in any case will be used in our meeting again. I am saying this because I also want to emphasise that you must not let it be a rush for you and that if you are going to be a little later than 10.30 that will be very all right by us.

It has occurred to me that it might be a very good idea if quite a number of us were reading the same books for Advent and Lent. This came to my mind as I have been re-reading Olive Wyon's book on Prayer. If you think that this is a good idea I would rather like to bring a dozen copies of that and of her book 'The Grace of the Passion' and just suggest that people should read these if they care to. She will not be with us unfortunately so this does make it rather a good opportunity to suggest them. I do not know however what you will think about this and if you don't think it a good idea it won't matter because I will certainly use them up as Christmas presents. I won't put them out until you come and I have had a word with you about it. This is by no means a directive to people but I think that it might help us to know a little bit more about what the others are thinking and these two books have been such a tremendous help to me that I would like to share them. One or two people have already been given them and read them and thought that this might be a good idea. I am sorry I had not thought of it in time to have discussed it with you before.

The Archbishop is hoping to come for the morning and the Chaplain of St Thomas's Mr Skues should be there also. The other new member of Council, the Reverend Alfred Barton of whom I told you is hoping to be there for the whole day.

As I think I told you there will be a few new people there, two very keen Christian nurses who are hoping to come on to the staff but who have not been able to come before because they work down in Plymouth, and also two people from King Edward's Hospital Fund, in their personal capacity of course, who have been interested in the project for a long time now and also I hope Dr Albertine Winner of the Ministry of Health – otherwise the group will be very much the same as before with one or two absentees unfortunately but approximately the same number or perhaps rather more. I will have a copy of the plans and the architect is coming in the afternoon but I do not think that these additions will make very much difference to the sort of things we will want to talk about.

Professor F. J. J. Buytendijk

Professor of Psychology, University of Utrecht, Holland

17 October 1963 Your book on pain was one of the most exciting things I have read since I started five years ago trying to do research on the control of pain among patients with terminal cancer.[58] I am coming over to Holland for a week's holiday on the 28th October and will be staying at the Hotel Poort von Cleeve in Amsterdam. If you speak English as I am afraid I have no Dutch, and if you have any time that you could spare me I would be very grateful indeed of any opportunity to come over and discuss some of these problems with you. I am enclosing a number of reprints of articles I have written about the work we are

---

[58] It was first published as F. J. J. Buytendijk, *Over de Pijn* (Utrecht: 1943) and appeared in English as *Pain: its modes and functions* (trans. Eda O'Sheil) (London: Hutchinson, 1961). F. J. J. Buytendijk (1887–1974) completed his medical studies in 1909 and later wrote widely on philosophical anthropology and had an international reputation as a phenomenological scholar; his book on pain was translated from the Dutch into German, French, English, and Italian.

trying to do. You will understand that I do not often find people who are in the same field or who have a similar approach to these problems and that any chance of meeting you would be a very great honour to me but I will quite understand if it is not possible for you to arrange it at rather short notice.

Marty Herrmann[59]
New York, USA

14 November 1963 Very many thanks for your letter which came while I was away on holiday. I am glad that you have kept well and have no more trouble with your back. I hope it will continue to behave. I am sure that you are as busy as usual.

I did send a copy of the Report to Mrs Rabinowitz at the same time as I sent yours. Very good luck to you in your attempt to get some money from them for Cancer Care. I am afraid I have got rather short of copies as I seem to have more of a demand for them than I expected and have not really got one to spare for Mrs Michaels and do hope that you will be able to share yours. I was obviously rather pessimistic in thinking of the number of people who would want to see it.

I have just had my 'summer holiday' which actually had very much better weather than many people had who took it at a more orthodox time. We had lovely autumn colourings in the Cotswolds and I also had a very exciting week in Amsterdam with lots of lovely pictures to look at. I think I found the Van Goghs more exciting than anything else.

We are getting all the things lined up for answering the questions when making our Building Fund Appeal so I have not got very many exciting news for you. We have though just been granted time for the Appeal in the 'Week's Good Cause' on the BBC next February. This is a very good thing both for raising money and also for getting the project known, so I hope that we will have everything lined up to answer all the questions by the time that happens.

The Revd A. E. Barton
Cottisford Rectory, Northamptonshire

31 December 1963 This is just to send you a copy of the suggested script for our Appeal. The BBC were very definite that I should do this myself and as I had taken a rough script with me to get some idea of the amount of information we could get into four and a half minutes they have seen and already approved it. I have now had to discuss it with the BMA and Medical Defence Union as there is always the problem of a doctor being accused of advertising. So long as I am not billed as 'Doctor' but just as my own name without prefix they do not think that there is any danger.

I wanted all the Council to see this in case they had other suggestions and although I do not want to change too much it is not irrevocable and so I would be very glad of your comments. It is a little bit on the long side but if I go fairly fast I will probably get it all in although we may perhaps have to cut the odd sentence to do so.

---

[59] Supporter of the organization Cancer Care, Inc. in New York, whose lifelong friendship with Cicely Saunders began in 1963.

Our search for a secretary has so far been unsuccessful but I am going to talk to the Reverend Robert J Connell of Methodist Homes for the Aged on Thursday. I had to get in touch with him to refer about an applicant. Said applicant was not suitable but I am going to meet Mr Connell on Thursday and he may have someone up his sleeve. He may also be a suitable person to keep in touch with as you probably know the Methodist Homes for the Aged is a very sizeable body now and has a great deal of experience of that sort of work and very similar to ours in many ways. He sounds extremely nice on the telephone and I did wonder whether possibly he might be our non-conformist for whom we have been rather vaguely searching.

With all good wishes for 1964 and looking forward to seeing you on January 15th Council meeting.

Florence Wald[60]
School of Nursing, Yale University, Connecticut, USA

31 December 1963 Thank you so much for sending me the abstracts of studies completed by your Masters students last year. I have not had time to do more than glance through them but I am very glad to find myself on your mailing list and I know I will find them very interesting.

I am sending you a copy of my report of my tour in the USA as you may perhaps be interested to read this in return. As you will see it is written rather informally just for the people who were kind enough to give me the money and I have only been able to hint at some of the things I learnt while I was there. I would be interested in any comments about it should you have time but I realise that this could be difficult for you.

I am also enclosing a memorandum about the work which we are planning and about which I told you. I have made some progress since I wrote it and I have every hope of having got enough money during this coming year to be able to go straight ahead when the detailed plans are ready which will be in some seven months time. Perhaps I am being over-optimistic but one day I know I'll be writing to let you know that we have laid the foundation stone.

I hope very much that I will be coming back to the USA again and perhaps will have the pleasure of meeting you once more. I so much enjoyed my time in the School of Nursing and only wish that it could have been longer.

With greetings to everyone that I met then.

Robert G. Twycross[61]
Oxford

6 January 1964 Thank you for your letter of 5th January. I am so sorry to be a nuisance, but since I wrote to you I have had a request to speak to the British Postgraduate Medical

---

60 Dean of nursing at Yale University, where she first met Cicely Saunders in 1963, leading to a life-long friendship and professional association.

61 Robert Twycross, later a leading figure in the world of palliative care and at this time still a medical student, had first met Cicely Saunders in the previous year, 1963. In 1964 he founded the Radcliffe Christian Medical Society at Oxford simply to have a pretext for inviting her to give a lecture there.

Federation on the 1st May, and I wonder if I could after all change my date with you to either the 15th or the 22nd May. It would be a rush for me to get down to you after giving the other talk, and also I do not like to do two important things in one afternoon if I can avoid it.

I am sorry to ask you to change, but as it is so far ahead I do hope that this will be equally good for you.

Before I actually choose the title I wonder if you would let me know whether this is to be an SCM meeting mainly for members or whether it is an open meeting, also whether you want the spiritual side of the work stressed, or whether you consider it should be a clearly medical talk. Obviously I would mention the spiritual side, but the emphasis can vary considerably. Could you also let me know whether you think it would be suitable to show some colour transparencies of the patients. These are not to show painful lesions but to show the look on the patients' faces, and in my experience they really do contribute a great deal to a talk and in some part at least take the place of an actual round. If this is difficult I would quite understand or if you think that they would not be suitable, but I find usually they are quite illuminating.

The Reverend David Rudall

Stroud, Gloucestershire

7 January 1964 My friends Miss Howlett and Miss Birchett late of St Columba's Hospital have suggested that I should write to you and I hope that you will forgive me for bothering you.

I am very anxious to learn what I can of the history of St Columba's and I understand that you collected up a considerable amount of data and were going to write this story. If you have anything in print or any notes that you could possibly spare me I would be so grateful if you could at least let me look at them. I will certainly promise to return anything that you want back.

The reason for this is that I have had a request for something of the histories of all the various Homes for patients with terminal cancer in London from a psychiatrist I met in Holland who is very interested in this problem. I have been interested in it myself for many years and am actually in the process of founding another Home at the moment. I have all the original reports of St Luke's Hospital in Bayswater and this is a most inspiring story and indeed one of the things which has stimulated me into trying to do this myself. Anything that you could possibly send me about St Columba's would be of very great interest and help to me.

Professor Dr F. J. J. Buytendijk

Psychologisch Laboratorium, Utrecht, Holland

16 January 1964 I am enclosing what I have been able to find of the early histories of three of the "Homes for the Dying" in London. As you will see it all happened within a very short space of time and it looks as if the letter to the "Times" which formed the initial move for the Hostel of God might very possibly have been seen by Dr Howard Barrett and inspired him to think again of his own hopes of founding a similar home.

There is another Home founded by an evangelical Christian lady at about the same time. The Home itself has no records of its founding now as it has been taken over by the Health Service. The late Matron has put me in touch with someone who was going to try and write a history but I have not had any reply to my letter to him so it looks as if I am not going to be fortunate there.

I have just copied out things from the first reports as I thought you would be interested in the attitude and way of writing as well as in the actual story. Dr Howard Barrett had a great gift for writing and I have read through all his reports during the twenty or more years during which he was Medical Superintendent. They make fascinating reading to me with great interest in the patient as an individual person.

We are just about in the position to launch our Building Fund Appeal and I am fortunate in having a short broadcast as the Week's Good Cause on the 16th February. I hope from then on interest and also money will come our way and that when our detailed plans are completed late in the summer we will be in a position to go straight ahead.

With best wishes for 1964.

Miss Peggy Harding

Bristol

30 January 1964 Thank you so much for your letter and also for sending on the £1 and enchanting letter from Miss Curle.[62] I have written directly to her of course and as she is in the area not too far away from the future site perhaps one day I will have the chance of seeing her.

I am so glad that you are rather better and hope that you will be able to take on the visiting tour you mentioned.

Perhaps we may possibly meet when you come up to London after Easter.

Dr Esther Lucile Brown

San Francisco, USA

2 March 1964 I was very grateful to you for your card and I hope that all is well with you. I am writing now to ask your advice on something as I think you are probably one of the people most able to give me the information I want.

St Christopher's is making good progress and I am enclosing a brochure which we managed to get ready in time for the launching of our Building Fund Appeal which started with a broadcast on our BBC Home Service as the "Week's Good Cause" on 16th February and as you know one of the things I want very much to continue is the research we have been doing and of course I want to develop it further. The other day I had occasion to be talking with Sir George Godber the Chief Medical Officer of our Ministry of Health and I told him that I was hoping very much that I would be able to send a nurse over to the States

---

[62] Peggy Harding was the editor of a magazine (*The Road*) published by The Fellowship of the Road ('a society for sick and handicapped folk'), which first began in 1948. Cicely Saunders supported the Society and came to know some of its members as close friends. Miss Curle, referred to here, gave regular small donations to the St Christopher's cause in the early days and was visited by Cicely Saunders at her home in Croydon. She died in the hospice in the 1970s.

to learn the methods of analgesic trials and observations which Dr Paddock has developed from the work of Drs Houde and Wallenstein at Memorial Hospital. He was very interested and immediately said that he was sure he could help us to get a WHO grant when I could find the nurse. Well, I think I have now done this because one of the people who particularly wanted to come and work with us is very keen to do this. I think she will be a most suitable person. She was the Ward Sister who looked after my patient "Mrs G" who I think you will remember from one of the reprints I must have sent you. Anyway, she is an exceedingly nice person of about my own age who was a Ward Sister for 12 years and has now been working in administration for some three or four years. She is very anxious to get back nearer to patients again and would be the ideal person for the job of which I am thinking.

I think we want to have just one nurse who has this responsibility at St Christopher's and has not the responsibility of running a ward. Not only do I want to do analgesic trials but I do want to do some basic nursing research. Doreen Norton whose report on geriatric nursing research you may have read is going to continue her work and I hope that we will have a connection with her but on the whole we will be breaking fresh ground and I think Verena Weist is someone who could do this. She is not the type of nurse who would have got her "Masters" but she is a very able and exceedingly nice person who is outstanding as a Ward Sister and who always enjoyed not only all the personal contacts with the patients but also the technical side and efficient organisation.[63]

I am writing to Dr Paddock because I would very much like her to have the training in the methods of observation with his staff rather than in Memorial Hospital because I think San Francisco would be a much nicer place for her to stay and his department probably more in her line than the one at Memorial.

What I would really like to know from you would be what other centres you think she should visit while she is in the States. I would very much like to arrange something of a tour for her and make certain that she does not miss anything that is being done with real basic nursing of the kind of very ill patients that we are thinking of that is going on.

I think that the time for her tour will most likely be next spring. I have a hope in my mind that I might perhaps be able to make myself free to come over for two or three weeks to introduce her and to meet some of my own friends again. If you think there is any chance of one or two bodies asking me to lecture to them so that I would be able to afford the journey I would be very glad indeed.

All this is very far ahead I know but if we are going to apply for a WHO grant we shall have to do this early in the summer.

With very good wishes and I do hope I will be seeing you again.

Dr Olive Wyon

Cambridge

24 March 1964 Many thanks indeed for your letter. It is I who should be thanking you for coming into St Christopher's circle and to St Christopher's "Day" not the other way round.

I am afraid I had not noticed your hot water bottle until you mentioned it but I will get it packed up and posted to you under separate cover. I made the bed up with the same

---

[63] Verena Weist (later Galton) became the first Matron of St Christopher's.

sheets for my brother to stay the odd night and very carefully did not disturb it further down.

I had a lovely restful time on Sunday but unfortunately had one of these gastric bugs Sunday night and had to spend yesterday in bed. I am just about recovered and will be at St Joseph's as usual tomorrow.

I think it was an excellent "Day" and I am very happy about the way it is gradually coming together and taking shape. I think you were quite right in that it was certainly the moment for the four of us to get together and talk about some kind of statement of our aims and beliefs and I very much look forward to that session.[64] I think the discussion on the Sembal Trust revealed a lot and was profitable in its own way. It seems to me that whereas the majority of us would not agree with those who feel strongly that it would be wrong to apply for such money[65] yet what we do believe is that we should not upset these "weaker brethren" if that is what we must call them. If they are going to be offended it would be rather a sad thing for St Christopher's and I think the answer probably is that we should not apply but would not refuse if the money were offered to us. I know this is not a logical position but then I do not think that logic is the most important thing or is an inevitable presupposition for any decision.

I have asked Mowbrays to see if they can get any copies of the "Grace of the Passion" and have not heard whether they can or cannot do so. If they say they cannot I will be very grateful if you could get me eight or ten copies as I am quite certain I will use them in the future if not all at once.

I am enclosing something towards the fare and this is St Christopher's expenses and we are very glad indeed to include it as such.

Sir George Godber

Chief Medical Officer, Ministry of Health, London

16 April 1964 You will remember that when I came to talk to you about the use of Diamorphine at St Joseph's Hospice, we discussed the possibilities of doing some further research as a development from the work done already when we once get to St Christopher's Hospice. You very kindly suggested that if I could find a nurse who would like to go over and be trained as our future "Nursing Research Officer" that you would help me in obtaining a WHO grant to make this possible.

---

64 This statement came to be known as the 'Aim and Basis'. Within it St Christopher's is defined as a religious foundation based in the Christian faith. Five underlying convictions are listed: (1) all persons who serve in the hospice will give their contribution in their own way; (2) dying people must find peace and be found by God, without being subjected to special pressures; (3) 'love is the way through', given in care, thoughtfulness, prayer, and silence; (4) such service must be group work, led by the Holy Spirit, perhaps in unexpected ways; (5) the foundation must give patients a sense of security and support, which will come through faith radiating out from the chapel into every aspect of the corporate life. The 'Aim and Basis' retained considerable currency at the hospice over many years and a 'Foundation Group' reconsidered it from time to time.

65 The Sembal Trust was endowed with profits which came from gambling; eventually a decision was taken to accept the Trust's offer of a grant of £22,680 – the cost of a six-bed ward (see du Boulay, *Cicely Saunders*, p. 128).

I have now found my nurse without any very great difficulty. I was most fortunate in that a ward Sister who had been at the Waterloo Hospital for 12 years and who I knew very well there and who is now an Assistant Matron at the Lambeth Hospital has immediately responded to this suggestion. She has been waiting for some 3 or 4 years now to come and work at St Christopher's Hospice and we have never been quite certain what her niche was going to be. We are now both convinced that this is very suitable work indeed for her to learn and develop.

I have been in touch with people in the USA concerning the possibilities of her going over to see the work with analgesics with which I was so impressed when I was there myself last year. I have had an extremely nice letter from Dr Richard Paddock who is Chief of the Anaesthetics Department of the Veterans Administration Hospital in San Francisco and Chairman of the Narcotics Programme in that group. He tells me that Miss Weist would be very welcome to go and work with them for as long as we consider necessary and has also put forward some other suggestions for her visit. I have some other ideas in my mind as well although I have not yet had time to plan them all and I think that we will need to ask if we can have a grant sufficient to cover a visit of some two months in all. I am also fortunate in that I am very likely to be asked to lecture at the National League of Nursing Annual Meeting next May (1965) in San Francisco and possibly one or two other lectures as well. This would make it possible for me to pay my own way and to take Miss Weist over and to introduce her to the people with whom I want her to work. I think this will make a lot of difference to her visit and the amount that she gets from it.

I wonder if you could very kindly tell me how we should now go about applying for a WHO grant and whether you think that there is anything else that I ought to arrange before I do so. I understood from you that I have to apply early this summer and I thought I should not delay further before asking you about this.

I am very thrilled indeed at the possibility of doing this work and will have to learn a lot from them but I also think we will have to plan the work so that it will fit in with the same informal and secure atmosphere at St Joseph's which we hope will grow in St Christopher's. I think we will only do this if we have the techniques absolutely at our finger tips and I think we will only learn that on the spot.

I am particularly excited over this project and I think that Miss Weist will be the ideal person both to develop some further nursing research (possibly with some connection with Miss Doreen Norton's work) and also in developing the teaching of any nurses who will visit us. She will certainly have as much to give the American nurses as they will have to teach her.

Thank you so much for your suggestion about this and for all your interest in St Christopher's.

Dr W. J. Moon

Austin Hospital, Victoria, Australia

14 May 1964 I must write quickly to thank you very much for your long letter of 5th May.[66] I was most interested in all that you told me and particularly in that you remind me

---

[66] This was the early stages of a detailed correspondence with Walter ('Wally') Moon, later regarded as one of the pioneers of hospice care in Australia.

of Professor Frank Shaw's work with Amiphenazole and THA. I met Professor Shaw when he was over in London 1958/9 and we used Amiphenazole for some patients at St Joseph's. One thing has always struck me about his work and that is that if he had begun with the regular giving of drugs and the enthusiasm without the Amiphenazole in the first place he would probably have found that a great many patients would have responded to that alone and that he would have had a clearer picture of the actual contribution of the drug itself. We find that we do not need to use it with a great majority of our patients and reserve it for the very small number who are drowsy on the doses needed to control their pain and for those who begin to show signs of addiction (only about 2% of our 1100 patients of which I have précised notes). Much of what he achieved with morphine and Amiphenazole is of course possible with diamorphine alone but I still need to have it in reserve for such cases.

I am also very interested indeed to hear about Mrs Austin. I have just heard today, as it happens, from the Cancer Institute in Madras which was started by a small group of women social workers. I have the stories of two Homes for patients with terminal cancer in London, both of which were also founded by women and I know the House of Calvary in New York which was founded by a group of widows. Obviously this is a job that we feel strongly about and I can only think of one hospital that I know well which was started by a man. That is St Luke's Hospital in London, in Bayswater and that was founded by a Methodist doctor in 1893.

I will wait to hear your detailed comments on my reprints because I know they will be extremely valuable. At the moment I am plodding through an immense mass of material and trying to sort out a thesis for an MD. This is not because I really want to do it myself but because my department demands it of me. However, it is very good for me to sort out my ideas if only there were not so much else to do.

Lawrence LeShan[67]

Institute of Applied Biology, New York, USA

21 May 1964 I have just read your article "The World of the Patient in Severe Pain of Long Duration" in the Journal of Chronic Diseases and also two other papers of yours published previously. I am very interested indeed in all that you say and I would be very grateful for any reprints that you can spare me.

I am working among these same patients myself and I have had experience with them as a nurse and as a social worker and have spent the last 5 years in a Hospice with 50 beds devoted to those with terminal cancer who come to us with problems making home care impossible. I am enclosing three reprints about this, two of which, as you will see, are really written for nurses but will give you something of the background of what we are doing.

You will see from these how much our work endorses what you have said although we have been tackling it from a more simple and practical point of view I think. Such writings as your first article that I mentioned helped to illuminate very much the work that we find ourselves doing in the day to day care of the patients and the principles and beliefs which we have developed in doing so.

---

[67] A psychologist who at this time was engaged in his own doctoral research in terminal care.

I am trying at the moment to produce a thesis from the work done with 1100 patients which is, of course, very superficial compared to your own work but it does bring a fairly weighty body of evidence in support of our ways of management of pain.

I will be extremely interested in any comments you care to make about this work and also perhaps when I am in the States next year there maybe an opportunity to meet and discuss this work. It is an opportunity that I would appreciate very much indeed. I am expecting to be over in either April or May 1965.

Dr Benson B. Roe

University of California Medical Centre, San Francisco, USA

11 June 1964 Your paper in the Archives of Surgery – "Are Postoperative Narcotics Necessary?" is of very great interest to me and I would be most grateful if you could spare me a reprint of it. I hesitate to seem to compare my own work with yours but I am enclosing a reprint which describes what we have been trying to do in the relief of pain among patients with terminal cancer.

I do not know whether you saw the leading article in The Lancet of 4th April 1964 which reviewed your paper. They discussed it with great interest but disagreed with one comment. In it they say "Perhaps the preoperative instruction increased the proportion of placebo reactors among his patients." It seems to me that it is a pity that this term "placebo response" should be attached so definitely to the giving of a medication. It seems to me that you were getting your results from your perceptive understanding of the patients' postoperative fears and your enthusiasm and attention to detail in removing them and that the result should have been attributed to that rather than to the infrequent injections which were merely supplementary. In any case, as you say in your paper, many patients needed no medication whatever. It seems to me that by attaching so much importance to the injections or other medication itself we can so easily forget our own responsibilities as people: the most powerful factors in any situation.

In our own situation we find that we just do not have the problems of tolerance and addiction which loom so large in some situations with these patients with terminal cancer but if we started talking about placebo response to our medication or merely thought in terms of the drugs we were giving or the methods of giving them, we would give an entirely wrong emphasis. In these circumstances I have never found myself able to plan any kind of "controlled clinical trial" that could be either representative or useful.

I would be very interested indeed to hear of any similar work you have done and if you have any other reprints I would be very grateful for them.

Theodate H. Soule[68]

United Hospital Fund of New York, USA

18 June 1964 This is now just another short progress report to let you know some really very good news. The Drapers' Company, who I think I told you before had been deliberat-

---

[68] Theodate Soule, whom Cicely Saunders first met in 1963, was a consultant with the Hospital Social Services Fund of New York and subsequently a Vice-President of St Christopher's Hospice.

ing at great length as to whether they were going to help us or not, finally made up their minds and are going to give us a grant of £50,000. This is to cover the cost of the building of the Old People's wing and it means that we will include something really very nice indeed in our first stage of building. This puts up the total cost of the first stage but we still have more than one third of that cost either given or promised.

The broadcast itself did well I think and I was sent more than £5,200. Also we gathered in nearly 300 Friends of St Christopher's and a very great deal of interest particularly from the nursing profession itself.

The plans for sending my nurse over seem to be maturing. I have had very helpful letters from Dr Paddock at San Francisco and she will be able to work in the narcotics programme of the Veterans Administration there. I have also heard from Dr Claire Ryder the Associate Chief, The Care Service Division of Chronic Diseases of the Department of Health, Education and Welfare and she is going to produce some ideas for us. I have also written and am awaiting an answer from Dean Frances Reiter of the Graduate School of Nursing of the New York College of Medicine.

I would be very grateful for an introduction to the New York Hospital and I believe that a Professor Modell whose works I much admire is also working there and I would appreciate very much an opportunity of meeting him also.

It does look as if I will be able to come with Miss Weist and we are making plans for May next year but I have not yet got any lectures actually fixed although there are several possibilities.

I do not think we are going to have too much difficulty in getting a grant for her trip but it is doubtful whether I will be able to plan for more than six to eight weeks for her in all. All this is a long way ahead but we are very shortly having to apply for her grant and any detail that I can supply is obviously important although a great deal will have to be worked out nearer the time.

I do not think I ought to bother you to do anything at the moment although it is a great help to be able to quote your name and the possibility of introductions.

I will keep you informed as to St Christopher's progress and let you know any other good news. I am at the moment waiting to go and talk to the Acting Director of the Nuffield Foundation who I am glad to say took the initiative in saying he would like to see me – always a good omen when one is going to ask for money – but I know that these things always take a very long time. So we are going ahead with the working drawings in the meantime.

Lieut. General the Lord Thurlow

Etchingham, Sussex

28 July 1964 Thank you very much indeed for the most delightful lunch at the House of Lords last week. It was a great pleasure to meet you and to know that you are really interested in the problems and prospects of St Christopher's and that you will help us.[69]

---

[69] As she continued to search for a Chairman for St Christopher's, she was introduced by its treasurer, Capt T. L. Lonsdale, to Lord Thurlow, who had just retired from the army. His father had founded the Missions to Seamen, and Lord Thurlow had been a member of its Council for some years. Lord Thurlow was to serve as Chairman throughout the detailed stages of building St Christopher's and into the operational years; he continued to hold the office until his death in 1971.

Those of the Council whom I have been able to contact so far are delighted that you will accept the position of Chairman and would be able to begin the new era with a meeting at Aldermanbury House on the 17th September. So far it seems that the afternoon is better than the morning for most people and I wonder if you could make it 2.15 as you suggested. Captain Lonsdale is officially proposing your election and you will have been duly elected (by telephone) by that date.

I have also spoken to the Bishop of Stepney, who, as you know, is our Visitor and takes an extremely active interest in everything. It was not his brother that you knew and who is now at Malvern but all the same, he is delighted to hear that you are joining us.

I am enclosing a statement which sums up our thinking so far about our religious foundation. This was prepared for us for discussion by Dr Olive Wyon and was the basis of a very excellent exchange of ideas at the last St Christopher's "Day". The paragraph that I have marked, should, I think, take the place of what we have written about the foundation on the brochure so far. The rest of it is really designed to hand out to prospective staff and others really interested in St Christopher's to give some idea of our approach. I thought you would be glad to have it as an important addition to the literature which Captain Lonsdale has already sent you.

I very much look forward to your first meeting with us and to the next developments.

The Most Reverend the Lord Archbishop Anthony Bloom
London

31 July 1964 I hear of you from time to time as having given talks to the groups that I also have to address and I do take it that this means that you are well and not quite so busy. Also I hope that you will be having a good holiday.

I am enclosing a statement which we discussed at the last St Christopher's "Day" under the leadership of the Bishop. It was prepared for us by Dr Olive Wyon, who, as you know, is a Doctor of Divinity and one of our Vice-Presidents, from various things I had written about the development of the vision of St Christopher's and its basis. We had a very good discussion in the group about this. It is by no means a definitive statement at the moment and there were quite a few minor suggestions. They did feel, however, that as a whole it presented what we wanted to say very well indeed. The paragraph I have marked will, I think, find itself in the brochure, as it is so much better than the present one about the religious foundation. The rest of it is really designed to give to someone who is interested in coming to work at St Christopher's and wants to know what we really do stand for and I think it should be considered in that light. Perhaps when you are less busy and have a chance to look at it I could come and talk to you to see if you are happy about what we say and whether you have any alterations or additions to suggest. I think we will discuss it again at the next meeting which should be sometime in November and I do hope that perhaps you will be able to come then.

As I think I told you, we have been looking and praying for the right person to take over as Chairman for a very long time. I am happy to say that I think we have really been most fortunate at last. Lord Thurlow, who has just retired from the Army where he was a Lieut General, has agreed to take this on and seems really enthusiastic about it. His father founded the Missions to Seamen and he, himself has been on the Council for a very long time and taken a very great interest in it. He was introduced to us by our Treasurer, who is also

Treasurer of the Missions to Seamen and knows him well, as does one of our Vice-Presidents, Dr Annis Gillie. Both of them felt that he was absolutely the right person and when I met him I could not have agreed more. I am sure that he will care about the spiritual side of the work and may well turn out to be a great strength there. He will also be extremely good on the administrative side, make an excellent chairman I think, and be just the kind of person to make us appear more efficient and respectable in the eyes of the world. The other piece of very good fortune is that Mr Barton is going to take over as Secretary and he will, of course, have the spiritual side very much at heart. I have always hoped that he would be our chaplain at St Christopher's eventually and he wishes to deal with the secretarial and administrative side now and then combine the two when we get there. This will be a marvellous way of getting a whole time Chaplain, which would not be justified if he were doing that only and I think it is a very good combination of the two sides of the work which are so closely interwoven.

I am sorry to write at such length but I did want to get you up to date with what is happening and also to assure you that although the Council would very much like to see you at a meeting, they do appreciate how difficult it is for you. The next meeting will be on 17th September at 2.15 at Aldermanbury House, Aldermanbury Square, in Captain Lonsdale's office. This will be the first meeting at which Lord Thurlow will take over and I am, as it were, ratifying his appointment by conversation and letters with the Council during the intervening period so that he is officially Chairman from the start of the meeting. Reading through the above I realise that I have not given you a chance to vote against him but I must admit that by now you would be in a minority but of course I would listen to anything you had to say about it.

Sister Zita Marie[70]

Providence Hospital, Kansas City, Kansas, USA

13 August 1964 I have been meaning to answer your very good long letter of 14th June ever since it arrived and here I find it is two months later. I do apologise and I am most grateful to you for writing as you did and also for your continual remembrance of the work.

I am still only in the very vague planning stage of my next trip to the States as I am waiting to hear definitely whether my nurse is going to get her grant and that I can come with her. It does look however that as we are travelling across from Washington to San Francisco it might be possible to stay a night in your area. I do not mind too much about the money for a lecture at all and if you would like a talk just in your own hospital to your own staff perhaps you might be able to manage it. I am a little hesitant about suggesting it definitely at this stage but I am certainly bearing it in mind and will remember when I get down to the more detailed planning. It certainly will not be until next May so there will be plenty of time yet.

I think that the best subject for a talk would be just "The Care of the Dying" or "The Management of Pain with patients suffering with Terminal Cancer". One can then cover

---

[70] Sister Zita Marie Cotter and Cicely Saunders first met at St Vincent's Hospital, New York, in 1963, where the former was a nurse and administrator. Sister Zita Marie was among the first American visitors to St Christopher's, working there for several months soon after the opening in 1967.

the subject fairly widely under both titles and I find that probably there is not too much difference in the needs of a medical or a nursing audience and that the same talk would do for both.

I am most fascinated by all that you say, particularly about your non-discriminatory admission policy. This does not really form a problem to us as we so rarely have semi-private accommodation with patients just sharing with twos or other small numbers. Obviously it is nothing like the same problem in a general ward.

St Christopher's goes along slowly but surely. We have been most fortunate in that Lieut General Lord Thurlow, an extremely good person and very able, has retired rather early from the Army and has accepted, among other things, the Chairmanship of our Council. I have been waiting to get somebody who would give confidence to those outside but yet in no way compromise our own position as a religious foundation by a lack of interest in that side. I think we can be confident that he will care about this in the right way and he certainly seems to have been sent to us, as indeed, have all the other people who are going to work with us. I am also losing our present rather unsatisfactory secretary to the Council and instead our future Chaplain is going to take over the administrative duties at this stage and then combine them both when we get there. This will mean that he has a position rather like a Warden and as he has no responsibility for discipline among the staff I can think of no snags to this arrangement and a great many advantages, the greatest of which is the fact that he will therefore be whole time and always there when patients need him and to hold together the services in the Chapel. He is an extremely good person and the one I have always wanted to be my Chaplain because I knew he would be able to see and to help others to see the oecumenical nature of the work without in anyway losing his definiteness. So once again he is a gift to St Christopher's. And finally I must tell you that I have acquired a really beautiful statue of a kneeling woman[71] which will go in our front entrance and set the tone for the whole building. She is quite beautiful and I will send you a photograph or bring one to show you when I have it. She is going to be in memory of a very dear aunt and Godmother of mine who died just recently. We are trying to reach everybody who comes into the Hospice without as it were flying a flag or imposing upon them and the position in which they are. This particular statue somehow said what I wanted said and one day I will tell you how I found it.

I really must stop now but I am most grateful to you for your prayers and I do remember you also in mine.

Dorothy Nayer

The American Journal of Nursing, New York, USA

22 September 1964 I am in the midst of writing your article[72] and am hoping to get it done before I go away on my belated summer holiday on the 30th September. The date at which I

---

[71] By Witold Kawalec; see letter to Sister Zita Marie of 13 April 1965, p. 83.

[72] Dorothy Nayer invited Cicely Saunders to write for the *American Journal of Nursing* after reading the report of her 1963 visit. Following a characteristically detailed correspondence, the article appeared as C. Saunders, The last stages of life, *American Journal of Nursing*, **65**(3), (1965): 70–5. It had an enormous impact and prompted many American nurses to write to the author with their supportive reflections.

am taking it rather shows you what my summer has been like and so I hope perhaps you will forgive me if the article is a little late in arriving.

I am not certain whether you ever have illustrations to your articles. I am including a number of references to individual patients either giving their comments or perhaps a little of their story. The four whose photographs I enclose have one story that links them together. When the first died some five days after I took her photograph, the second remarked to me, "She didn't suffer. They don't here. I think the motto of this place is 'There shall be no pain.' – it makes you feel very safe." When she was dying in her turn two months later I took the third photograph less than twenty-four hours before she died. I think it sums up Sister's care and all the understanding nursing that she had. It was taken with her full permission to be used for lectures or for anything I liked. I only wish that I had a photograph of her waving me Good-bye that day. The final photograph was taken on the same afternoon, of the patient in the bed opposite. She was a great friend of the dying patient and said to me "Oh Doctor, I would love to have one of those. I know I won't want it for long myself, but it would be lovely to have it in her memory." She was extremely fond of her and neither of us were careless about her dying but both of us very certain that all was well. I think it emphasises how wards, like families, have to go on.

It will not alter my writing very much if I do not include these photographs but should you think that they are suitable or that they could be reproduced satisfactorily in your Journal I would be very glad to know.

In your letter of 16th June you mentioned Dr Anselm Strauss and the two articles you were hoping to publish by him later this year. I hope that you will be able to send me these as I would be most interested to read them. I had some typescripts from him when I met him for a brief afternoon session when I was in San Francisco last year. I was also given a few reprints from your own Journal when I was at Columbus Circle as you may remember. As you have had the nursing so well covered by Virginia Kasley I have not gone into that sort of detail. What I have been trying to do is to emphasise the fact that it is looking at the patient that will teach us how to care for the dying and how to find a philosophy to sustain the work. I hope this is the sort of thing you want and if it isn't you had better let me know so that I may try and do something else for you.

When you do write I wonder if you could very kindly let me know when the National League of Nurses Conference is in San Francisco next Spring. Dr Esther Lucile Browne wrote to me some months ago that the branch of San Francisco was suggesting to the central branch that they might ask me to give a talk during this conference. As my nurse seems to be going to get her travelling Fellowship to come over next year and as I want to accompany her but need to organise quite a few lectures to make this financially possible, I would be very glad at least to know that date so that I can begin fitting some other things round it. Of course, I may not be asked after all, but at least I had better make it possible to accept. If you could let me know that date therefore, I would be most grateful.

Sir Kenneth Grubb

Downton, Wiltshire

11 November 1964 This is just to send you our Newsletter and to bring you up to date with what is happening.

Lord Thurlow is proving a most excellent Chairman, and I believe we have got absolutely the right person and just at the time when we really needed him. We are almost ready to go out to tender and hope that we can go ahead to sign the contract early next year. Before we do this I hope very much we may perhaps have one more good sized grant as that would then cover the whole of the first year's building costs. We have applications in at the moment to the Nuffield Foundation and to the Sembal Trust, and both sets of Trustees will be considering them in December. We had wondered about applying to the Sembal Trust as one or two of our members were not very happy about any money made by any form of gambling. We decided that we would not take any first step ourselves, because although I do not feel very strongly about this myself, I do feel strongly about upsetting people who want to work with us. Now, however, they have intimated that they would like us to get in touch with them, the Bishop of Stepney has given me his very well considered "go ahead" and so our application is in. I am sure that this is right.

The Reverend Almon R. Pepper
Department of Christian Social Relations, New York, USA

22 December 1964 I am afraid I am rather late with my Christmas letter to you and to your colleagues but this means that I can now give you some wonderful news which came to St Christopher's Hospice within the last few days. First of all, however, may I wish you all a very happy Christmas and every good wish for 1965.

The news is really very exciting. On the 16th December we heard that a fairly new Charitable Trust, the Sembal Trust, was going to give us £22,686, the comprehensive cost of one of our six bed wards. We had hardly recovered from this when on the 18th December the Nuffield Foundation gave us a grant of £60,000 to cover the cost of our 14 bed ground floor ward. This is quite wonderful and of course, the name of the Nuffield Foundation will be extremely valuable in our next application for money. It has also come at an extremely opportune time because we are out to tender at the moment and should have replies from the builders to discuss at our next Council meeting early in February. If one is really satisfactory we will go straight ahead and sign the contract and start building.

At the same time some other plans are afoot. An extremely nice nurse, at the moment working as Assistant Matron, is going to train as our future Nursing Research Officer. I am very anxious for her to have experience with the Narcotics Programme of the Veterans Association in San Francisco and Rancho los Amigos Hospital in Los Angeles. We have got a World Health Organisation Travelling Fellowship for her and are just completing the details of her programme. I am very anxious to come over again myself at the same time, both to introduce her to the workers in San Francisco and to learn a little bit about the work there myself and also of course to meet my many friends of the last visit. At the moment the plan is that I should come over on about the 10th May and that she should join me on the 28th or so and that we should then go over to the West fairly soon after that. My own programme, will, I hope, manage to include a few lectures for which I will be paid as I will not be able to afford it otherwise. I have one or two coming along, but it did occur to me that possibly you might have some suggestions about this. Of course, I would gladly talk to people for nothing and expect I will be doing that as well but if they could include one or two dollar earners this would be a great help.

I have written to Dr Kelsey at the General Theological Seminary and I am going to write to Dr LeShan of the Program in Religion and Psychiatry at the Union Theological Seminary. We have had some correspondence because I admire his papers about the psychosomatic aspect of cancer very much indeed and I am looking forward greatly to meeting him and some of his colleagues. Apart from this I have an invitation from Dr Molly Harrower of the Temple University Medical Center to speak at the Post Graduate Center for Mental Health and I am possibly getting one through the Reverend Robert Reeves at the Columbia Presbyterian Hospital.

While I am over there it also occurs to me that I might go ahead with an application for help from the Ford Foundation. Obviously we would have to begin doing this from this end but I have found every time that the best way to get money is to go ask people for it in person and I would like to think that I was able to go ahead with this also. Perhaps you have some ideas about this?

Please give my greetings to Mrs Munroe and to everyone else I met and I greatly look forward to the possibility of meeting you again in 1965.

Dr Esther Lucile Brown

San Francisco, USA

16 February 1965 Thank you very much for your long and helpful letter of 23rd December. I have waited before answering for some of our plans to be finalised and am now able to tell you a little bit more about our dates and prospects.

I am flying to New York on 10th May and have accepted the invitation to speak at the Postgraduate Center for Mental Health on the 13th. On the 18th I speak in Yale and on the 25th I meet with the Psychiatric Department of the Massachusetts General Hospital with Professor Lindemann, Dr Weisman and others. This I am very greatly looking forward to and expect to learn a great deal from them. I am likely to stay in Boston for two or three days and I think it is likely that I shall be speaking to the medical department there and there are certainly several other people I wish to meet.

These are the only definite dates I have for lectures at the moment and I am waiting to get in touch with Dean Reiter and Miss Lucy Germain who is now in Philadelphia, from both of whom I have invitations to speak when I can fit it into my programme. Have told the department of social relations department of the Episcopal Church Center that I would be available to do one or two other talks and am trying to keep all these various people informed so that we can keep the schedule in some degree of order.

My finances are going to be rather easier than I expected as I have heard from the Executive Secretary of the Ella Lyman Cabot Trust, Professor Gordon Allport,[73] that if I write to them in March and ask for about $750, saying that it is his suggestion, the likelihood is that they will help me once again. This is marvellous and, of course, makes the whole trip more secure financially. I cannot be too grateful to them, for not only did they help me very substantially on my last trip but they also sent me a most generous gift as

---

[73] Gordon Allport (1897–1967) was also Chair of Psychology at Harvard University and the person who introduced Cicely Saunders to the work of Viktor Frankl, in particular *Man's search for meaning* (Boston: Beacon, 1962).

"seed money" for St Christopher's and it was this that paid the expenses of our brochure and is paying for its reprinting. I am really delighted to have a link with a Trust connected with Dr Richard Cabot[74] and all that his work entailed and also with Professor Allport himself, who is such a delight to meet. I am most undeservedly fortunate in the people who support us.

I think that Miss Weist will be able to come out and join me on the 22nd May and that we will leave New York for Washington on about the 31st. I am in touch with Dr Claire Ryder and I hope that she is going to do a little planning for us in and around Washington during that week. We then fly to San Francisco during the week-end of 5th June so that she could start with Dr Paddock if this suits him on the 7th, giving her a fortnight with him before she goes to Rancho for the workshop starting on the 31st. I am very anxious that she should return to San Francisco for a further week after the workshop because I think a fortnight is running it a little fine and she may well have questions that she has had time to think of after she has left them. This part of the programme, of course, rather waits on the World Health Organisation representative in Washington. We sent all the particulars of the work we wanted to do and the invitations we had had and I understand from the representative over here that they are not likely to change the programme, but of course, their word is the final one. However, I am going ahead as well as I can on the understanding that it is unlikely they will alter any plans and I have written to Dr Paddock to ask him whether this would be a suitable time for Miss Weist to work in his department. I am waiting to hear from him at the moment. There is one snag about Miss Weist's trip and that is that whereas we had originally suggested that she should leave the hospital in which she is working and start again on her return, the Matron there is extremely loath to lose her and suggested that she apply for leave. Now, however, she is finding it very difficult to give her long enough to have a little flexibility at the beginning and end of her official six weeks. I, myself, think it is a great pity to go so far and then not to have enough time to do the thing thoroughly and I also feel that it is possible that Miss Weist may have invitations that she would like to take up at the end of her official trip and I will probably be able to give her enough dollars to make this possible. However, I am seeing her Matron next week and I hope to get this dealt with then and that she will not have to rush back and will have time to do all that she should in order to prepare herself for the work we want her to do in the future. Then my own plans, once I get to San Francisco, are at the moment quite fluid. I have an invitation to Rancho and I think that the Episcopal Church may possibly suggest one or two lectures in California also. Of course I want to see everyone I saw last time and to take more time to do it. I had hoped to end my trip with a week in British Columbia with a very great friend of mine but this is remaining open at the moment because I do have other friends, actually in Los Angeles, whom I should visit and I do not want to rush my time and miss opportunities that I should be taking. Anyway, I must be back in London by the 20th June at the very latest.

It is wonderful to have the invitation to come and stay with you in San Francisco. This will be wonderful and I do hope that you will not be away because I would so much enjoy the chance of unhurried talk with you and of discussions in between whiles when I am

---

[74] Dr Richard Cabot, a physician at Massachusetts General Hospital, had founded the Ella Lyman Cabot Trust in memory of his wife. Cicely Saunders' brother Christopher had met a Cabot family member and a trustee in Devon and the Trust subsequently supported her eight-week visit to the USA in 1963.

around visiting and meeting others. When I was in New York I did go to the Loeb Center and I think it must have been Mrs Hall whom I met there and whom I liked very much. I will certainly take the chance of going to see her again.

To finish with some news of St Christopher's, we have had a very good tender from an excellent builder who will take a personal interest in the scheme and as this is the lowest of the tenders we have received we are going to accept this and should be signing the contract very shortly. It is almost exactly at the total cost suggested by our architect and quantity surveyor as reasonable and so we are really satisfied with it. We already have another Trust interested in the project and I hope very much we will be lucky again with a grant from them. I am, at the moment, investigating the possibility of making an application to the Ford Foundation and the Episcopal Center has also sent me a list of other Foundations who might be interested in work of our kind. All this is very exciting and stimulating and I can hardly believe that after so many years somebody will shortly be sticking a spade into the ground and making a start.

Dr Olive Wyon
Cambridge

2 March 1965 Thank you so much for your letter. I have been meaning to write to you for some time and now can give you a definite date for starting building! We had an excellent tender from Fairweathers who you may possibly remember. He was the "Christian" builder and the friend of Jack Wallace's. He is also an efficient builder which is equally important or more so for this. Anyway, he produced a tender for almost exactly the price that Mr Smith said it should be and with Mr Smith's ordering of bricks and steel is able to give us a starting date of 22nd March and a two year building plan. We are going to have a small ceremony for turning the first spit at 2.30 p.m. on the 22nd March. I am going to take Evered down in the car and he is going to bless and dedicate all the work but it is going to be most informal. I do not know at all whether you will think it worth while to come and I think quite honestly that it is not especially as you will be at Nottingham just before. We are not going to have a St Christopher's "Day" this spring and the next party will be for the foundation stone with the Archbishop and we will try and have the Annual General Meeting on the same day so that everyone can combine the two.

This is all very exciting and I am so grateful. I just go around continually saying thank you.

Dr Herman Feifel
Veterans Administration, Los Angeles, USA

16 March 1965 Many thanks indeed for your letter of 2nd March and for all the good work which you have already done on my behalf. It looks as if *I* will be going round like a whirling dervish as well. As usual it is always the person who has most to do who answers by return and gets on with doing things.

I have just heard from the University of Southern California School of Medicine who have suggested that I might come on the 8th June. This is really the time when I will be in San Francisco so I have written to ask whether the 15th would possibly be all right as I have just offered the earlier time to the Veterans Administration Hospital in San Francisco. Doing things at this distance is very tiresome for everybody but I am sure we will manage to sort it out eventually. The ideal plan for me would be to spend 4 or 5 days in San Francisco from the week-end of 5th June and then come to Los Angeles for the rest of my stay and direct back to London sometime towards the end of the week beginning the 14th June. I will wait till I hear definitely from the Veterans Administration and from the University of Southern California before I go further with the other places you suggested.

The WHO have now tiresomely come up with the suggestion that Miss Weist should remain on the eastern side and say that they think she can have sufficient experience there. It remains to see what they suggest and whether I will be able to pay for her to add a trip to the west to the time that they plan for her in the east.

I had an article in the American Journal of Nursing, March number which you may care to look at. It is probably easier for you to find it direct than for me to wait until my reprints come and then send you one.

With greetings and many thanks for your efforts on my behalf and looking forward to seeing you.

Dr Colin Murray Parkes

The Tavistock Clinic, London

23 March 1965 I was very interested indeed in your article on The Pastoral Care of the Bereaved in the issue of Contact of October 1964. I wonder whether you have a spare reprint of this and of any other articles that you may have written on this subject and those related to it.[75]

My interest in this subject stems from my work in the care of patients dying with terminal cancer over the past years at St Joseph's Hospice and elsewhere. We do, of course, have a great deal to do with our patients' relatives during the time that they are with us but nothing after the patient has died. It has seemed to me that I should begin to try and learn how we can be more helpful at an earlier stage in, perhaps, preventing some of the later problems. My interest in this is all the more stimulated because we are now actually starting off in the building of a new hospice in south east London and will no longer have the firm foundation of the religious community of St Joseph's and have to learn our own way of helping.

I am enclosing a booklet about the new hospice and also some reprints of my own articles to give you some idea of what we are trying to do. If there would be any chance of my meeting with you, and perhaps with Dr Bowlby with whom I understand you have been working, I would be very grateful indeed. I would come anywhere convenient to meet you and would try to do so at a time convenient to you as it is fairly easy for me to plan my own programme. I am going on holiday at the end of this week just for a week but after that I would be free for the whole of April. On the 10th May I fly to the USA and will be meeting

---

[75] This was the first contact between Cicely Saunders and the bereavement researcher and psychiatrist Colin Murray Parkes. Soon afterwards the two met, together with John Bowlby, and in the following year, whilst in the United States, Murray Parkes set out some detailed ideas about the organization of St Christopher's. He subsequently worked at the hospice on a sessional basis for many years, undertaking support work with staff and families and conducting research.

Professor Lindemann and Dr Weisman and others at Harvard as well as other people concerned with these problems and I think it is important that I should know something more of what is happening in this country before I do this.

Sister Anne-Beatrice
Communauté de Grandchamp, Switzerland

25 March 1965 Thank you very much indeed for your card and note from the Community after I sent you the second newsletter. I am enclosing the next one and I will send one direct to Soeur Gilberte at Taizé.

We are very, very glad indeed to have your prayers and as you see, I have mentioned this in the newsletter. Since that was written we have had a very good tender from a builder with the delightful name of Fairweather and building actually began last Monday, the 22nd March. The Bishop of Stepney came to dedicate and bless the whole thing and Lord Thurlow and I dug the first spit with a foot on either side of the spade. About 50 people came and we had dogs, children, workmen hammering, birds singing and a general atmosphere of informality and welcome which I hope will always be part of St Christopher's. It was so lovely that it was such an ecumenical occasion because apart from the nuns who came from St Joseph's there were several other Catholics, some Non-Conformists, a member of the Salvation Army and some who are not truly committed to any faith at the moment although much more committed than perhaps they know.

I know you will go on remembering us and I do remember you and hope one day that I will be able to find the time to come back to the peace of Grandchamp.

Barbara G. Schutt
The American Journal of Nursing, New York, USA

6 April 1965 Thank you very much for your letter of 24th March and for sending on the letter to the nurse for me.

I have another five letters by air since I wrote to you. One was from Dr Sheldon Waxenberg of Memorial Hospital whom I met when I was in the USA two years ago and I am very delighted that this has put me in touch with him again as I shall be meeting him when I come over. Three of the others were from nurses who had a particular interest in our kind of work. They had all been grieved in one way or another by what they had seen and were obviously anxious to learn more of this kind of care. One of them asked advice on how to get the proper handling of drugs across to the doctors with whom she was working. Like nurses I had met elsewhere she had become convinced of the importance of regular giving of drugs for pain at this stage of illness. One of the three has some hope of visiting England and is hopeful that possibly she might have a chance of coming to St Joseph's at some stage. They all showed a very real interest and concern about this kind of work.

The last letter was from someone in the Veterans Home in Nelson M Holderman Memorial Hospital, California who wrote me a splendid letter of encouragement and good wishes.

I am so glad that there has been a response from your readers.[76] Naturally I feel strongly about the importance of this work and would always feel satisfied if at least we had made some other people really to look at these patients and find their own way of helping them.

Once again I look forward to seeing you.

Dr Colin Murray Parkes

The Tavistock Institute of Human Relations, London

6 April 1965 I am not sure whether this is going to reach you before you leave for the USA but I must write and thank you for sending me the reprints and for your two letters. I will look forward to meeting with you and Dr Bowlby sometime in July. I expect to be back in London about the 21st June and if I do not hear from you I will get in touch when I have seen my way through the accumulation of work.

I know the article by Aldrich on "The Dying Patient's Grief".[77] I agree with a great deal of what he says and I think that some of his remarks are most helpful. I do not agree however, that it is the patient who has the most to leave who finds it the hardest to die. In my experience, the person with the fulfilled life, with many people he loves with whom he has to part finds it easier to accept the situation than the lonely rather frustrated person who feels he is leaving things unfulfilled and no-one who will remember him deeply after he has gone. This may well be, of course, because this group of people are probably more difficult with themselves and others in any case. I do agree, however, that there are very close analogies between the feelings of the patient before he dies and those who are left behind afterwards (and, of course, when they, too, are anticipating his death and are able to face it).

However, we can discuss all this when we meet.

Sister Zita Marie

Providence Hospital, Kansas City, Kansas, USA

13 April 1965 Thank you so much for your letter of 28th March. It was lovely to have such a welcoming letter and I very greatly look forward to seeing you again.

As far as I can see at the moment I should be leaving Los Angeles during the morning of the 16th June and coming straight to Kansas. I will let you know, of course, exactly which plane I am flying on and I will be very grateful if you can meet me. I will be delighted to talk with your doctors on the night of Wednesday 16th June and will do it under any title you wish although my own preference is for the very simple "The Care of the Dying". I only ask that I shall be allowed to show slides as I am talking which are ordinary Kodak 2″ × 2″ transparencies and in showing the look on our patients' faces tell far more than I can do in words.

---

[76] These letters were in response to the article in the *American Journal of Nursing*, which had just appeared.

[77] C. Knight Aldrich, The dying patient's grief, *Journal of the American Medical Association*, **184** (1963): 329–31.

I am not quite certain how long I can stay with you at the moment because a great friend of mine[78] is taking part in the exhibition of religious art in Paris which opens on the 16th June. He is likely to be in Paris for a few days and I do very much want to fly back to London via Paris so that I can see something of the exhibition. This is important for me because he is painting for our new chapel at St Christopher's and we already have several very fine works which we will be having in various places in the hospice. It is an unexpected development of our work that we should be trying to learn to express our faith and welcome patients and their relatives in this way but it is very exciting. The sculptor,[79] who has done a most beautiful kneeling figure for our entrance hall and has designed a rather stylised St Christopher for the front entrance, is also exhibiting in this exhibition and indeed our own St Christopher is going to be sent to Paris. This means, of course, that I must make every effort to try and get there and it may cut short my visit with you but I do not think I could bear to fly straight back from Los Angeles and not see you.

Dr A. Ukleja Bortkiewicz[80]
Warsaw, Poland

15 April 1965 Thank you very much for your letter and card. It was very nice to hear from you.

This is just a note to enclose a packet of Vatican stamps which I got for Yurek when I was in Rome for a short holiday just recently. I thought that this was the best present I could send you from there but I did remember you and Poland when I found the little chapel with Our Lady of Czestohowa in the crypt of St Peter's. I am also enclosing a few other stamps that he has probably got already but can always use for swaps.

I am off to the USA on the 10th May and not back in London till the 21st June.

Robert G. Twycross
Oxford

29 April 1965 Many thanks for sending me a further copy of your article and also that by Raanan Gillon.[81] I was very interested in the further correspondence and I expect it is too late to say it but you might add that whereas, as he says, I wrote in "The Care of the Dying" sometimes pain can only be controlled by keeping the patient continually asleep, we could say that this was written in 1959 and that I had done over 5 years work since then and have found that this only very occasionally need happen. You may be interested in the enclosed

---

78 A reference to the artist Marian Bohusz-Szyszko, whom she eventually married in 1980.

79 Witold Kawalec, the Polish sculptor whom she had invited to produce a work to go over the door of St Christopher's Hospice, and whose figure of the kneeling woman had already been acquired for the entrance (see footnote 71, p. 75).

80 Cicely Saunders was introduced to Dr Bortkiewicz by Sue Ryder, when visiting Poland for the first time in 1962; she is here sending stamps to Dr Bortkiewicz's son, Yurek.

81 In late 1964 and early 1965 Raanan Gillon and Robert Twycross, as medical students, were engaged in a lively debate for and against euthanasia in the columns of the *Oxford Medical School Gazette*.

copy of the table I made of the numbers of patients that I felt were unsatisfactory in that they did not die with the peace and tranquillity for which we aim. As you see this remains a fairly constant figure but the percentage of those with pain is very small as a percentage of the overall figure of $1100 - 1.09\%$.

I hope we shall continue to reduce this figure when we have St Christopher's and when we learn more about the relief of mental pain and confusion which, as you see, remains the big problem.

Incidentally, some of the alteration to figures in those transferred too late is due to the fact that now I very rarely put in the very brief notes I have of these patients into my main figures. This would then bring down the numbers of unsatisfactory from 15% to something nearer the other figure and shows how difficult it is to reduce this percentage and how determined I am to do it somehow or other.

Major General the Lord Thurlow

Etchingham, Sussex

7 May 1965 This is just to let you know that I was able to talk to the Bishop this morning about the question of the foundation stone. He was delighted with your idea of the Bishop of Rochester and felt that this would be very important to draw him in at this stage and he thought that he would be really keen to do it. The Bishop himself would be quite unable to come on the two dates suggested in June, the 22nd or the 23rd but is keeping the two in July, also the 22nd and the 23rd. Both of those are perfectly possible for him and he will not fit anything else in until he has heard again from us. I hope very much that this would work out and the Bishop did add that he thought that probably August would be an impossible month for the Bishop of Rochester who has young children and is likely to be taking his holiday then. I know also, of course, that it is not possible for you either, so let us hope that July will turn out to be possible.

Alfred Barton has got my address in the USA and my schedule there so if there is any major good fortune he can get in touch with me. A terrible catastrophe I would prefer to remain unknown to me until my return!

I will let you know how I am getting on and I expect to find that very great progress has occurred while I have been away. I seem to remember that last time my departure was a signal for a certain number of problems but for a most adequate coping with this by everybody else and in those days we had nothing like the Council we have now.

Dr Herman Feifel

Veterans Administration, Los Angeles, USA

22 June 1965 Just a note to thank you so much for meeting me, giving me lunch and getting things organised. It was a delight to see you again and I am sure that I will be back once again and we will be able to take on where we left off.

With very good wishes for your own work and I do hope you will let me know when you have written anything further and how the project develops.

My voice held out for the rest of the journey and I finished up with two delightful days in Paris and am now back and starting in at work once more.

Dr K. J. Rustomjee

Colombo, Ceylon

29 June 1965 I have just got back from another short trip to the USA and found the report of the Ceylon Cancer Society waiting for me. In it I read of your resignation and the very nice and appropriate poem that goes with it. They will, indeed, be missing you and I expect you will be missing all the work too but you have certainly earned a happy retirement and I hope very much that you will have it.

You will be glad to hear that St Christopher's is at last in building and that the foundation stone (which will be set in the wall of the ground floor entrance) will be laid by our retired Archbishop of Canterbury, Lord Fisher, on the 22nd July. I still have quite a lot of the money to raise but we had enough to start off with and it is still coming in. The builders think it will take about two years and so by this time in 1967 we will be writing to let you know that we are actually opening. I am very grateful to all the people who have helped us and for all the good wishes and interest which includes yours.

The States was very good fun again. I did rather more lecturing than I liked to do but it did mean that the whole trip was covered financially and that was a help. I met various interested people once again but unfortunately Mrs Allen was away in Europe herself and I did not see her.

I don't suppose that you will ever be in our part of the world again but if you are I do hope that you will make St Christopher's a port of call and I will, of course, let you know what happens.

Christopher Saunders

Bishop's Stortford, Hertfordshire

6 July 1965 This is just to let you know that I have received a gift of $50 which the donor would like to go towards "liquor". Next time you are in correspondence with The Wine Society I would be very glad if you would put this towards some more wine for St Christopher's bearing in mind that patients will, on the whole, prefer red wine to white. I wonder also whether there is any possibility of getting half bottles. I know they are tiresome to store but they might well be more acceptable to patients than the large ones.

I am not sure whether other sorts of liquor are a good thing to lay down and whether we would gain anything by doing so. If you think so the one I would choose is Vodka, because this has so little taste and would go very well with our various mixtures.

The Reverend Whitney Hale[82]

Boston, USA

8 July 1965 This is just a note to let you know that we are actually laying our foundation stone on the 22nd July. We are extremely lucky in that Archbishop Lord Fisher is going to

---

[82] Cicely Saunders had been introduced to Whitney Hale (1882–1969) by Eleanor Mason of the Farncombe Community in Surrey, UK, and they first met when she visited the USA in May 1965. He had been for many years rector of the Church of the Advent in Boston and was an associate of Gordon Allport, at Yale.

do it for us and I think we will have something like a hundred people on to our rather muddy and restricted site! We are putting the stone where it is going to stay in the wall of the ground floor entrance hall and the inscription will just be very simply "To the greater glory of God this stone was laid by The Most Reverend Archbishop Lord Fisher of Lambeth, GCVO, PC, DD, 22nd July 1965."

The rest of my trip to the USA was quite as hectic as the time in Boston and I finally finished up in Los Angeles with a rather brisk laryngitis caught from the children of a friend with whom I was staying. I had to do my last three lectures rather huskily directly into the microphone. However, it was immensely worthwhile because I met a great many people interested in these problems and made some extremely profitable new contacts. We also have had a wonderful legacy of $30,000 from an old man who died in St Louis at the end of May. I have not yet been able to discover how he heard of us. It is very nice to have this gift.

It was good to get back to St Joseph's and to my patients again. At the moment my biggest problem is a girl of only 33 who has very severe pain and who was extremely frightened and anxious. She is a lapsed Catholic so we have a lot to do to help her to come safely through as I am sure she will.

Two of the Sisters from the Farncombe Community are coming to our foundation stone laying but unfortunately Sister Eleanor is going to be away so I will not see her then but I hope to see her again sometime and to tell her all about my visit with you.

Florence Wald

School of Nursing, Yale University, Connecticut, USA

13 July 1965 Your very generous cheque for $100 for the consultation fee caught up with me when I was in Providence Hospital, Kansas City just before I left the USA. I was suffering from a very bad cold caught in California at the time and trying to plod through my last two lectures and I have an awful feeling that I never managed to write a note of thanks at the time. Please accept my apologies for the delay and my most grateful thanks for this help towards expenses.

Since I got back I have been fairly swamped with work but everything is going well. The foundation stone of St Christopher's Hospice is being laid by our last Archbishop of Canterbury, Archbishop Lord Fisher, on the 22nd July. This is a very exciting moment and we are particularly pleased that Dr Almon Pepper, one of our American Vice-Presidents, is going to be there and will be taking some part in the ceremony. We are going to pack about 140 people on to a muddy and not over large site and are hoping that our really terrible July weather may let up at least for that afternoon.

I have thought a lot about your suggestion of my coming over to you for a month or so sometime next year and it certainly does appeal to me very much. This will, I think, be possible because I am now gradually tailing off my commitment at St Joseph's Hospice and by that time I should be quite able to do some travelling. I think that the chance of talking with your people would be extremely valuable for our own thinking and planning for the future and that we would learn a lot from each other. I much appreciated your suggestion that this should be in some way connected with work in the Medical School and if it could be, in some way, done in a clinical setting I think it would be very much more valuable than discussions on a theoretical level. I do not know what you think about this and whether it would be at all a welcome idea to any of the doctors.

I am really going to be very glad to have more opportunity to do some writing between now and the time when St Christopher's opens. My thesis, which is a very long one, is now just about completed[83] and I want to expand this into a book and there is something else in my mind which I want to write also.

I have been told that I am likely to be asked to speak at the Student Nurses' Convention next year and also that one or two people are writing to the American Nurses Association to suggest I speak there as well. Obviously, if I were coming to you it would be nice to try and tie these together but, of course, I do not know whether the Associations will consider doing this after all. I am committed to take part in a discussion on training in the International Congress of Gerontology in Vienna on the 24th June but I believe that the Nurses Convention should be well over by then.

I have sent some more reprints to Miss Fisher, one or two of which you may not have seen already. I much enjoyed the chance of meeting her and only wish we could have had a bit longer but then perhaps we really will have an opportunity to getting down to things in the future.

Dr C. T. Stegerhoek

Berg en Bosch Hospital, Bilthoven, Holland

26 August 1965 I have just been sent your name by Mlle Leideki Galema of the Foyer Unitas whom I met in Rome when I was on holiday there before Easter. I had written to her to ask for her prayers for our project, St Christopher's Hospice and to mention how glad we were of international and interdenominational contacts.

Mlle Galema tells me that you will be in London in September and that she will suggest to you that perhaps you might be interested in getting in touch with me while you are here. I would be delighted if you would do this and would love the opportunity to meet you and to talk of what we are trying to do and to learn something of your own work. I am enclosing one or two reprints concerning what I have been able to do so far in a Roman Catholic Hospital in London and also a brochure about St Christopher's, a new foundation which is in the process of building at the moment. This will be undenominational and I hope very much will have Roman Catholic contacts as well as those with the Russian Orthodox and Non-Conformist denominations. I myself am an Anglican and so at the moment are the majority of the Council and the prospective future staff.

I have one or two contacts in Holland already including Professor Buytendijk, whose book on pain I was so tremendously impressed by when I read it some years ago. I had an opportunity for a brief talk with him when I was in Amsterdam about eighteen months ago on holiday.

If you would care to telephone me at the above number when you reach London I would love to see you. The best time is in the morning before 8.30 but I am quite often in in the evenings also. During the day you may be lucky and find me but I am often out and then there is nobody here to answer the telephone.

---

[83] Referred to at various points in the correspondence, the thesis was never in fact submitted.

The Reverend Whitney Hale

New Hampshire, USA

7 September 1965 Thank you so much for your letter of 30th August. It was very nice indeed to hear from you again. Thank you so much for remembering me when you found the paperback. I have already read it. It is very interesting I think that two or three of the small number of homes over in England and your work over there have been started by women. This is obviously something that we have to try and do something about.

Please do not feel badly about the visit in Boston. You could not have been kinder to me and I think that I had quite enough to do. I was delighted particularly to meet Dr Fletcher and after all I had two big talks to do in Harvard Medical School. My regret was that I was really so hot and exhausted the day we drove out into the country and did not enjoy the talking with the nuns sufficiently or take advantage to learn more from them.

You may please take any vicarious satisfaction in the unexpected help you like but the real gift that you gave was not so tangible as that.

I am hoping that I will be back in the States again next year. I have been invited back to Yale to spend a whole month in the Graduate School of Nursing, with I hope some work with the Medical School as well. This looks as though it will really take place and will be towards the end of April. I will mainly be working there but I may have time for a few other trips and if I do I will certainly try and get to Boston at least for a week-end and have a chance to see some people I know including, of course, you and Mrs Hale.

Today I am writing off to another Trust in the hopes of more money. Since our £10,000 from the unknown friend in St Louis things have been quiet. I am hoping very much we will be lucky this time. There is such a lot more to do.

My time at St Joseph's is coming to an end at the beginning of October when I am due to have some holiday anyway. I have been there seven years now and as they are having many more chronic sick patients and fewer dying and as I have to get some writing done as well as all the work of St Christopher's, Reverend Mother and I have decided that now is the time for us to part. I will miss very much being with patients but I feel that I do need a sabbatical after such a long time and certainly I find it very hard to write if I am not concentrating on it exclusively. I think that after my time in Yale I will certainly want to get back again one way or another and that it may well be some experience on the side of psychology. I know that it will be shown when the time comes. Certainly the end of the time at St Joseph's was shown very clearly, not least in the fact that for the first time since I have been there, the first time in this whole seven years, I find that there is not one single patient about whom I feel the kind of responsibility that makes me feel most unhappy about going away for a holiday. They will manage all right without me and this is entirely as it should be.

Soeur Gilberte

Communauté de Taizé, Taizé, France

30 September 1965 Thank you very much indeed for your letter which I could really manage myself but had some help from a friend who speaks excellent French. I hope you will manage my English in the same way.

I do feel guilty that it is such a long time since I wrote to you especially as Mrs E died about 6 weeks after I asked you to pray for her. However, better late than never. I had a very happy report about the rest of her illness both from the doctor and the Sister of the ward. Apparently she never needed to have her drugs changed after she was stabilized while I was there and from then on she kept a peacefulness and freedom from pain that was very impressive. I think that we made a very close contact in just that short time I knew her and from what I saw then I am quite certain that she had a very real faith and that she must have left very good memories with her husband and children which I hope they will always treasure and find a help. She was so young and she had had such a hard illness and had had so much cause to feel afraid that it was wonderful to feel that that fear was apparently completely taken away.

Since I wrote St Christopher's has developed a lot. I am enclosing our progress report which we presented at the Annual General Meeting and also the Service for laying the foundation stone. There were about 140 people there and we had a lovely fine afternoon in the midst of a rainy spell. There was even rain three miles away so we felt very blessed, as indeed we were. The Archbishop made the whole Service very real and also helped to make the whole afternoon itself into something of a party. I think that this is an important aspect of the work of St Christopher's because we do want to give the welcome of the good sort of home where people can relax and just be themselves and we want everyone who comes to feel like that, the relations and the other visitors as well as the patients. I believe that it is when they are quiet and their fears and physical distress is held more steady then they can start listening to Our Lord Himself.

Today is my last day working at St Joseph's Hospice. This will seem very strange after seven years there, but it is obvious that the time has come to make a move from both sides and so I am having some holiday and then I am going to get down to concentrating on writing and lecturing for the next few months. I have another trip to America in the late spring and then will try and get some work among patients to fill in the gap which will still remain before I begin work with our own patients at St Christopher's. There is a great deal to be done and, of course, the whole problem of drawing together the right staff must take more and more time and thought. I feel very diffident at calling it a kind of community. I think it has to grow a great deal further than it has so far before it could really be honoured with such a name but I do hope that we will let the Holy Spirit lead us as He wishes and that perhaps He has something in mind of this kind.

Your own work sounds wonderfully exciting and I do hope that one day I will have a chance of visiting. Perhaps next year. I keep saying this and everything keeps pressing in on me but one day I really will get back.

Dr W. J. Moon

Austin Hospital, Victoria, Australia

18 November 1965 I am feeling very guilty that I have not written to thank you for your last letter enclosing the notes on the management of malignant paraplegia which I found extremely interesting although we are not actually coping with this problem ourselves.

I also should have written to you to say that I was very pleased to see Miss Langford although unfortunately I was not able to take her round St Joseph's to meet any of our patients. She was pushed for time and I was occupied at that moment in pulling out from the hospital and only had a few patients. However, we had a very good talk and I was able to show her some photographs and give her one or two reprints.

She told me a certain amount of the news about Austin Hospital and so I already knew that you now had been reduced to 25 beds and also into the oldest ward in the hospital. This seems to me terribly typical of what one has seen happen time and again. I remember being very struck both in Montefiore Hospital and St Barnabas Hospital in New York in the way in which the patients for whom the hospital had in large part originally been founded had gradually been relegated once more into the "failure" class while what the new management considered to be the more progressive and positive work came to the fore.

I am not going to the Tokyo Conference in 1966 as I am afraid I already have three commitments abroad. I have been invited back to the Graduate School of Nursing in Yale to do some work alongside the Medical School for a month and also to take a fairly small part in both the International Congress of Gerontology in Vienna in June and the European Congress of Anaesthetists in Copenhagen in August. It is rather interesting that the problems of pain and teaching staff to care for dying patients which are the two things I am going to be talking about seem to come more easily in these settings than in a cancer conference. It rather ties in with my experience of visiting in the USA. For example, at Memorial Hospital and the Sloan Kettering Institute I had great interest and demands for discussions and so on from the psychologists and from the nurses but not from the other doctors. It is very difficult to be geared at one and the same time to a strong therapeutic drive and to see the positive side of the care of those patients who, whatever anybody may say, are regarded as failures.

I mentioned that I was moving out of St Joseph's and I have now left there and am going to spend the time between now and starting at St Christopher's when it opens in trying to get some more writing done. I also have a very constant stream of demands for lectures. For example, I have over 15 outside lectures this month. It entails dashing around the countryside and meeting a great variety of people. As I feel like you do this is rather a crusade I cannot say "No" to these but it does take one's time and makes it very difficult to settle down to writing. The thesis is at last all but complete. I just have two very small sections to polish up: one on placebos and the other on the problems of clinical trials among these patients. In due course I will send you a copy with its rather monumental list of references. Incidentally, the immense length of the references on the sections about mental pain rather indicate where my heart really is.

I hope your thesis goes faster than mine does. Perhaps you will find that having a small number of beds – and I do hope that this will only be temporary – you will have more time for this.

I was able to leave St Joseph's without a bad conscience about patients as the present Reverend Mother is moving more towards a larger number of chronic sick patients and fewer of the really distressed dying patients and although I think this is probably only a temporary move it did mean that I could leave without feeling that I was letting them down and having done seven years I suppose I was really due for a sabbatical anyway.

Dr Albertine Winner

London

18 November 1965 Just to let you know in case there is any possible chance of your coming that the "topping off" ceremony will be at 3 p.m. on Friday, 26th November. It will be very short, of course, but I am hoping to show some slides of the development of the building to the men during the course of the proceedings and we have a very fine little flag to run up. I hope very much that it will not be a day like today. However, we cannot expect perfect weather for St Christopher's every time.

This is also to let you know that I had a slightly discouraging note acknowledging our application to the Wolfson Foundation from Lt Gen Sir Harold Redman, saying that the project does not seem to him to be one that the Trustees are likely to take on. However, I am not too discouraged by this as I do know that Sir Isaac has already said to Mr Leonard Wolfson that he wishes this appeal to have very serious consideration.

I have tried to see whether I could get a personal word to Sir Stanford Cade who once was very kind to me when his daughter took me back for a drink after visiting a patient of hers in St Joseph's but I gather he is out of the country for a few days and the list of other Trustees does not encourage me too much especially to see the name of Sir Solly Zuckerman who I cannot imagine will be very interested in what we are trying to do.

However, although I do try and lay all possible trails I can to trip up any of the Trustees, I also believe at the same time that having done all we can the final issue is safely looked after.

I am so sorry you can't come on the 4th December. We are gradually getting more and more people who are really interested in working in St Christopher's and I have several new people coming this time, including I hope someone who is interested in cooking for us!

Sister Zita Marie

Providence Hospital, Kansas City, Kansas, USA

25 November 1965 Thank you so much for the copies of 'Relay' which have just reached me. It was very nice to have news of other people in your Order as well as of Providence Hospital. I hope that our own newsletter will be reaching you by surface mail in due course. We have enclosed a picture of the foundation stone laying and also a copy of the service we had then. We are so glad to know that you have been remembering us.

Building has gone almost as scheduled and we are having a small party and ceremony tomorrow for the "topping off". This is the completion of the roof of the concrete shell of the building and we will run up a flag and the warden will say a short prayer, I am going to show a few slides of the growth of the building to the men and then we will leave them with suitable supplies of beer. This is a very small party but it is the one in which the men themselves are most interested and every time I have been to the site they have been working extremely well and we thought that it would be nice to have it.

Otherwise things have been going much as usual except that I have now left St Joseph's and will only be going over there for the occasional social visit. It became apparent that at the end of my seven years there the time had come to make a move. The present Reverend Mother is really more interested in the long term chronic sick than in the dying and in any case we had fewer beds as they have further re-building to plan. It became apparent that I could fade out without feeling that I was letting down individual patients so we agreed that it was right for me to do so. This means that I now have a sort of sabbatical year in which I will try and get some writing completed as well as all the lectures which still keep being demanded. Also, of course, the responsibilities of St Christopher's are growing, there is still money to be raised and, of course, a great deal of planning to be done. I will miss patients and if the time before our opening stretches out I will get myself back to them some way or another.

I am just back from a lovely visit to Dublin where I stayed with the nuns of our Order, the Irish Sisters of Charity, and met Mother General and many of the nuns with whom I have worked at St Joseph's. This was a delightful visit and we have a really close connection with them for St Christopher's.

I am enclosing a reprint of something I wrote recently which might interest you and the address that I gave at our Annual General Meeting after the foundation stone is going to be printed in our Nursing Times today for Advent and we will be sending copies round with our next newsletter.[84]

I am always happy when I think of our links with you. The connections that St Christopher's has in different parts of the world and in different parts of the whole Christian Communion are of importance far beyond anything we can really picture I think. In the present day it seems to me tremendously important that those of us who think of medical and nursing care with the spiritual dimension should learn from each other in order to bring this before other people in ways that are relevant to their thinking.

Dr Albertine Winner

London

9 December 1965 In the past you have always said that there is no need for us to do anything about the hope of contractual arrangements at this stage but we are now beginning to get requests to put people on our waiting list for the limited number of beds for long term patients as compared to those with terminal cancer. I have always said that we do not intend to do anything about this and indeed, really cannot at present. However, it occurs to me that if we do have contractual arrangements for these patients the Regional Board will naturally want to put those on their own waiting lists to the fore. We have no official arrangement and therefore I can hardly suggest to people that when they apply they should start putting St Christopher's on their forms. However, I wonder whether the time is beginning to approach when we ought to have some preliminary conversations with Dr Fairley or with somebody from the Board about this. Obviously the first group of these patients that we have at St Christopher's are nearly as important for the whole atmosphere of the place as the staff themselves. For instance, to have somebody like Louie will make more difference than any other one person in the whole institution.

We had a very interesting St Christopher's "Day" and the question of having some kind of out patient pain clinic came up for discussion. Professor Stewart is extremely keen on this and also that it should begin from the very start so that it is part of the very image of St Christopher's. We would have space there if we give up the accommodation that I was going to have as a flat to this and I would get a flat somewhere near which might be a better idea in any case. Obviously we are going to have to think a lot about co-operation and liaison with other people outside, both hospitals and family doctors but I do not think that this would be impossible. I had a very interesting session with Dr Robbie who is running a pain clinic at the Marsden and he is getting absolutely swamped with custom. All the consultants are more than pleased to hand over to him patients with chronic pain at quite an

84 The article appeared as C. Saunders, Watch with me, *Nursing Times*, **61**(48), (1965): 1615–17.

early stage. There seems to be no question of treading on other people's toes here. They are a group of patients that everyone finds very hard to deal with. Dr Robbie in his turn says he finds that the majority are just longing for an opportunity to find a doctor who will listen to them.

I also had a very interesting conversation with Dr Jim Parkhouse of the Nuffield Department of Anaesthetics at Oxford. He has asked me if I would take part in a symposium in the European Congress of Anaesthetists in Copenhagen next August on the problems of doing clinical trials with patients with intractable pain. I can certainly talk about the problems if not so much about the successes as one would like in the doing of trials! He was very interested in the plans for St Christopher's and very anxious that any work we did with analgesics should be done in co-operation with the work that they are doing and with some kind of link. I find that he has got a nurse working as observer now and I was interested in all that he was doing. I do not know whether you have read his papers in the proceedings of the Royal Society of Medicine but he certainly can write and I would say that his work was extremely good. Anyway I was very glad to meet him and to know that he was really interested in what we want to do. I will certainly need plenty of co-operation from other people over here and I hope that between us we will find someone who wants to have a research fellowship and do all the side of statistics and so on which I certainly am never going to cope with.

Elizabeth Jacobsen

Harper's Magazine Inc., New York, USA

16 December 1965 Thank you very much indeed for sending me the reprint of Dr Cohen's article, "LSD and the Anguish of Dying". I was very interested indeed in this particularly as I had had opportunity to talk with one or two people in Stanford University when I was in the USA earlier this year about the possibility of using LSD among these patients.

I would be very grateful indeed if you would send the enclosed letter on to Dr Cohen as I would so much like to get in touch with him and his address does not appear on the article. It may be against your principles to send correspondence on to contributors and I will quite understand this but if it is possible I would like to get in touch with him. What is of particular interest to me is the fact that my patients say something of the same kind of thing about their dying as does the patient he quoted and the vast majority of the many hundreds whom I have looked after over the past years have reached their death in a spirit of quiet serenity and acceptance. This is not with the use of LSD but with other drugs which are at present available to any physician and opportunities to give time and an attempt to understand what it feels like to be so ill.

Dr Anselm Strauss

University of California Medical Center, San Francisco, USA

19 December 1965 Your book 'Awareness of Dying'[85] was sent to me airmail by someone I met when I was over in the States earlier this year. I happen to have a perfectly fearful cold

---

[85] B. Glaser and A. Strauss, *Awareness of dying* (Chicago: Aldine, 1965).

and to be penned up in my flat and so I read straight through it yesterday and am writing straight away to say how very much I enjoyed it and how helpful I found it.

I think I am certainly one of the people you mention who read it as "realistic albeit highly organised, *descriptions* of the multifaced faceted 'dying situation'". I think probably at a first reading this is inevitable as I found myself going ahead as fast as I could go so that any remarks I make are not proper criticism at all and in any case I am never very good at doing that.

I have to get over my dislike of the phrase "terminality" and the associations of the words "terminal patients" and one or two others. I think it is difficult to find another phrase but it still remains one of my unfavourite words. There are times also when I think that we do not give quite the same interpretation to the word "pretence". I think it is not just a pretence when a patient makes up or totters to the toilet and talks and acts as if things are really quite ordinary, least not in the sense in which I use the term. I do not think it is necessarily a contradiction to live life as it were on two levels at once. Both can be true in a sense without necessarily contradicting each other as so often I think truth is something that does not entail reconciling two opposites but in holding them both in some kind of a tension so, as it were sparks fly between the two.

I am interested that religion is never discussed or hardly at all under its own heading but only under the work of the chaplain. You were obviously in contact with at least one who was extremely good. I think, however, that the religious attitude or, at least the philosophy concerning life as well as death of other members of staff is extremely important and could perhaps be emphasised more. I do not mean that in most cases they would ever speak of it directly but communication with words of security based on that dimension is, I think, of immense importance in helping the patient to find his own meaning.

I am very sad that you have to take it for granted that the management of pain is sometimes so inadequate. I am not surprised from the conversations I have had in the States and I must assure you that the pattern over here is very often no better. It is sad though that you should have to talk about inevitable addiction and dependence and finally pain that is so bad that it cannot be controlled and that you should have to talk about the patient manipulating the situation himself. The handling of narcotics in this situation is largely an unknown field as far as I can see and yet in the right situation and with the right knowledge and confidence it can be handled so that the patients do remain alert as well as tranquil and free of pain. However, that is my own hobby horse or one of them.

You only mention collective involvement briefly but I do think it is extremely important. If you have the kind of feeling in a ward that can help the nurse to say to herself not "How can I help Mrs So-and-so?" but "This is such-and-such ward, such-and-such hospital and I just happen to be the one here at the moment," a very considerable amount of the strain is eased for her. One of the most important things that we will try and do at St Christopher's is to try and build up this kind of feeling and also to show its importance to those who come to us for teaching and short time experience.

I liked immensely what you said about management of space and "drift routes". I am all for having the family in as workers as far as possible and hope we shall learn more about this when we are working at St Christopher's. Incidentally, I liked everything you said about the family and recognised very much of it although we do not have some of the problems that you do as I suppose we have more of what you refer to as "non-paying captive clientele". I can assure you, however, that they are pretty independent even in our situation.

I think that one can never be completely prepared for death. However much one grieved beforehand, however much one has really accepted that it is going to happen it is different when it does so and it has always struck me how different people look when they come the day after a death to collect the death certificate and deal with clothes and other things. There is a washed-out, empty, stunned look which never really overtakes them until that moment.

You mention break-downs and scenes on various occasions and how important the nurses find it to avoid them. I am sure this is right in so far as they can have such an effect on the morale of the ward and of other patients and yet I am equally certain that to be able to break down and really cry at the moment of death or fairly soon afterwards is a very important way of beginning the difficult process of mourning and that when we are too brave we pay for it afterwards. Here is another thing to learn.

I don't really agree with you that there is less nursing skill needed in caring for the patient when the 'nothing more to be done' phase begins. Certainly there is less technical skill needed than in the increasingly complicated procedures that may come before but the true nursing of giving comfort, understanding on physical, emotional and mental levels remains as demanding as any part of a nurse's work. It is just as you say, a different orientation which some people find very difficult to make.

I am interested in your comments about the medical ideal of prolonging life as long as possible. If you can get hold of the "Lancet" of Saturday, 23rd October 1965 I think you would find what Sir Theodore Fox says in his article there 'Purposes of Medicine' is relevant. He discussed the problem of when to stop, I think very helpfully.

I was very interested in all that you said about the disclosure of diagnosis at the Veterans Hospital. I think, though, we must always draw a line between disclosing a diagnosis even if it is to the patient a fatal one and talking more directly about prognosis. You certainly bring this in when you are talking about the time factor but, so often a discussion of telling the patient the truth brings both these problems in under the same heading very confusingly and not helpfully. They are two different problems and are dealt with in different ways.

But your thesis that we should in some way or another give the patient a chance to manage his own dying and be more able to move into open awareness is of very great importance. In fact, really what we are doing is not managing the dying patients but managing terminal illness in itself in order to leave the patient as free as possible to manage this part of life, as important as any other, and often more important, and dying itself. I am more and more convinced that when we make any kind of a hand at doing this at all the great majority of patients will more than rise to the occasion. I am also convinced that there is a great deal that we can do and should be doing to make our management more compassionate and effective.

I am sorry to go on for so long but I was extremely interested in your book and delighted to know that it was safely written and published and I know that I would never be able to make that kind of approach myself and that what you do is extremely helpful to my own work.

It was so nice to see you on the two occasions when you were in London and also to meet your wife. I hope you will be back again and be seeing St Christopher's and all that we are trying to do there. I think we will have to ask you to come and stay for a few days to tell us what we are doing and what we ought to be doing better.

Dr Margaretta K. Bowers[86]

New York, USA

6 January 1966 Thank you very much indeed for sending me on the most useful papers about hypnosis in the control of intractable pain and also your own paper "Passive Submission to the Will of God". I liked that very much indeed. I do hope that you will send me anything else along this line that you may write or give me the references. I think it is something that certainly needs saying and which many people tend to get confused. I was very interested to learn a little bit more about your own work from the other paper.

Since I wrote to you I have been in touch with Dr Tarnsby and we had quite a long talk about the use of hypnosis. He was very interested in the possibility of my using it among my patients but not terribly sanguine that it would prove of wide usefulness. He thought that I could easily learn to do this and it was best that I should join one of his courses in due time. However, there is plenty of time as St Christopher's is not likely to be open until 1967 although the building goes on well.

I read the papers with great interest. The Pavlovian approach I must say I do not find particularly easy to assimilate or agree to but it was interesting. Dr Sacerdote's writings I found much more in tune with our own approach. I noted that he said to you that he would get in touch with me directly if you thought it a good idea. I do not want you to have to bother to go on as an intermediary and so I am going to write to him directly and send him one or two of my own reprints.

Obviously a great deal of what we have been doing is to treat the patients' anxiety and fear and feelings of rejection by our interest and approach and by the general atmosphere of St Joseph's. This does not take the place of drugs but certainly enabled them to be handled in such a way that they remain effective and can be used to control physical pain and, indeed, anxiety without altering the personality or over sedating them. The doctor who uses nothing but narcotics must certainly get into trouble with them but the doctor who uses them merely as part of his approach to the patient should be able to handle them over surprisingly long periods without trouble with tolerance or dependence.

I have now completed seven years of work at St Joseph's and am taking a sort of sabbatical year to try and get some writing done and to raise the rest of the money needed for St Christopher's and do all the planning concerned with its development. I am already missing patients, and I think I will have to get myself back to them somehow before St Christopher's actually opens. In the meantime however I certainly have more than enough to do and am greatly enjoying the continual new introductions interested in the various aspects of this field of work. I am very lucky indeed in the people who help us.

Thank you once again for taking such a lot of trouble about me and my affairs. I am really grateful and hope that perhaps the use of hypnosis may prove to be another piece of our armoury against the distress that brings patients to us.

With greetings for the new year.

....

[86] Cicely Saunders first met Margaretta Bowers at the Bellevue Hospital, New York, in 1963. Dr Bowers was actively involved in the International Society for Clinical and Experimental Hypnosis and made the introduction to Dr Peter Tarnsby, a member of the Society working in London.

Dr Albertine Winner

London

13 January 1966 Just a note because I rather despair of catching you on the 'phone and please you are not to bother to answer this.

It was really just to let you know that I am going to see Dr Fairley on the 21st of this month. As it happens I also had a letter from a Miss Burton-Brown who is on the Medical Advisory Committee of the Regional Board concerned saying that they were going to discuss terminal care throughout the region in the next month or two and she wondered if I could send her some information about what I thought were the best places to plan for these patients. I sent her back a fairly long memorandum saying that while I thought possibly one or two small units in their peripheral hospitals would certainly be better than having one or two beds set aside in general wards everywhere; that the main problem was having the right staff with experience and confidence and that what would be most important for their region would be to have the pioneer research and teaching unit of St Christopher's to which any other potential staff from different units could come for courses and experience. I do think that this could develop into some sort of pattern for the whole region and I look forward to hearing what Dr Fairley himself thinks about it.

We are at the moment working out plans for the out-patient Pain Clinic and I am discussing with Professor Stewart this morning, the possibility of presenting the case for it to the Sir Halley Stewart Trust who he thinks might take it on as one of their long term projects. I had a very revealing session with Dr Robbie at the Royal Marsden the other day. He had already been round St Joseph's.

We had an excellent session on the kitchens last night with Miss Midgeley who deals with these problems for Dame Dorothy Vaisey of the Friends of the Poor, but has also had a great deal of experience in different sized units rather larger than Dame Dorothy's. I think that we have got that side sorted out now. It does certainly bring things very much nearer to be dealing with something in such detail.

I have not forgotten what I suggested last time we met and I hope the idea of the Out-Patient Pain Clinic might make it more attractive to you![87]

Dr Nathan B. Eddy

National Institutes of Health, Bethesda, Maryland

28 January 1966 You will probably remember that you were very kind and gave me an opportunity for quite a long discussion with you at the Westbury Hotel when you were in London last summer. This talk was of very great help in clearing my mind about some of the possibilities of clinical research among patients with intractable and terminal pain and I look forward to the time when our new unit will be open next year and we can try to begin putting them into effect. I hope one day that I may have a chance of discussing the next stage of the work with you.

---

[87] A reference to the idea that Dr Winner might consider going to work at St Christopher's as a doctor, which she eventually did.

I was very interested to hear Dr Everett May lecture in London last week and to hear something more about the work with phenazocine and with the related compounds. He mentioned trials among patients with chronic pain and I would be very grateful if you could spare me any reprints that you have available about this. I have a copy of your reprint of the article in the Bulletin on Narcotics 1959 volume 11 page 3 and have, of course, met other contributions of yours in the literature. Anything therefore that you have on this line I would receive most gratefully as it is obviously going to be of very great help to us in the future.

You mentioned in our discussion that you might be able to send me a copy of the Minutes of the Narcotics Programme Committee meeting that also might be relevant to our work. If these are available I would be very grateful for them also. I have to make a contribution about the use of intractable pain as a testing ground for analgesics in the European Congress of Anaesthetists this summer and while I can talk with some knowledge about the snags and complications of such work I have much less to say about successful trials and would like to fill in my knowledge as much as possible before then.

I have just heard today that we have been given a grant for the new hospice for the establishment of a pain clinic and a full time worker. I know this is all starting on a very small scale but at least we have a very considerable amount of field work to begin from with the advantages of being able to concentrate on one particular group of problems which have had all too little attention and also certainly are a gap in teaching.

With kind regards to you and Mrs Eddy

Professor J. J. Bonica[88]

University of Washington, Seattle, USA

28 January 1966 I have just been reading your chapter on Drugs for the Relief of Pain in Modell's "Drugs of Choice" 1965. I am very interested indeed in this problem and have been working with a large number of patients with pain from terminal cancer. These mostly have distress of a degree severe enough, in combination with their general illness, to make admission to hospital essential. I have not been using regional blocks of any kind but our unit admits patients from other units or from home at a stage when this is not considered any longer to be a valuable contribution to their comfort and I have, therefore, been concentrating on work with opiates and their adjuvants and also on a multiphasic approach to this whole problem.

I am writing now because you gave a reference to Ripley in page 216 who you say has written an excellent dissertation on the subject of severe intractable pain which I gather from your writing includes a discussion of psychiatric techniques. You do not give the reference to this and I would be very grateful indeed if you could very kindly send it to me. At the same time I would be most grateful for any other reprints on the use of drugs or on this particular approach which you could spare me.

I am enclosing one or two reprints of my own, rather diffidently, to give you some idea of our work so far. I hope very much to develop this with controlled trials geared particularly

---

[88] John Bonica (1917–94), the widely acknowledged 'father of the pain field' and founder of the International Association for the Study of Pain.

to the needs of patients with intractable pain rather than to drug evaluation per se when we open a new unit for these patients in 1967.

Major General the Lord Thurlow

Reading, Berkshire

3 February 1966 I hope that this letter will be there to welcome you back and that it will not be too long before we know that you are safely back in this country and have had a good holiday. I gather from my own friends in Nigeria that things were not quite so dramatic as they sounded on the BBC but it must have been anxious and exciting and probably still is.

It will be very nice indeed to have you back and I am glad to be able to give you some good news to welcome you. Professor told me two or three weeks back that now was the time to make an application to the Sir Halley Stewart Trust towards the Outpatient Pain Clinic. This idea rather grew up just as you were going away and I am not at all sure we actually discussed it. As you know I have it in mind for the future but when we were talking about it on St Christopher's "Day" on the 4th December Professor Stewart said then that he felt very strongly that it would be important to start this from the very beginning. Mr Smith[89] immediately came up with the idea that the space in the hospice that would do very well for this was that planned for my own flat and so this was decided forthwith. I am sure I will have no difficulty in finding myself somewhere in the vicinity and perhaps it will be all to the good if I am not on the spot the whole time. Anyway, this was only going to be temporary accommodation and so I think it is important that we use it in this way.

I went ahead with the application to the Trust and I am enclosing a copy of that so that you have it for a reference if you want it and I also enclose a letter from Professor Stewart with the good news that the Trust were going to cover both the cost of the equipment and a doctor to deal with the research side of the work. I will start putting feelers out for the right person for this job as I have some good connections in this area. I am sure that the right person will be sent when the time comes.

The Annie W Goodrich Visiting Lectureship that he mentions in his letter is the appointment I have been offered at Yale for a month starting the 21st April. This brings me in a vast sum of dollars and I am going to be given a guest suite in one of the original buildings in the middle of the campus, for free. They are going to work me very hard indeed as I not only have to talk with students in the Graduate School of Nursing and all the members of their Faculty but also meet with members of the Medical School, taking Student Rounds on three days and discussing problems with doctors who deal with children of dying parents and also some other problems apart from terminal cancer. This is going to be extremely demanding and I know well who is going to learn most but it will be a good thing to be able to report to the Wolfson Foundation and others and also, incidentally, extremely enjoyable.

The other good news is a letter I had this morning from the City Parochial Foundation of which I also enclose a copy. This really is good news and I think that we will very happily have this in reserve if the Wolfson Foundation do not come up to scratch when their

---

[89] The St Christopher's architect, Justin Smith (usually known as Peter Smith) of Stewart, Hendry, and Smith, London.

Trustees meet, which I think is in April. As we are at the stage when we have to think of borrowing on our grants and/or the site of even the building it is very good indeed to have this suggestion from them and I do think we can be pretty optimistic about it. I think I told you that I took good care to get to know Mr Johnson personally and go and see him and show him pictures of the building and to write with full details as to what stage we had reached. When we did not get anything from the last Wolfson Foundation hand-out just before Christmas I wrote to all the Trusts who had given us grants to send our Christmas greetings and to bring them up to date with what was happening. I had an extremely nice set of letters from each one of them which I will show you when we have the next meeting. I hope you will come to the flat and have a lunch time meeting if you can face my stairs again[90] and do this soon after you get back.

The building looks splendid and seems to be growing at good speed. We have gone ahead to arrange the next St Christopher's "Day" because it is so difficult to get a Saturday from the Bishop and also to fit ourselves into Riddell House. We are meeting on the 26th March and this does seem to be the only possibility and I hope very much that it will be all right for you. I have suggested that we all meet on the site at about 11 am and I am sure there will be enough cars for those who have got there by public transport to get a lift back to the Hospital for a sandwich lunch and our afternoon meeting. Archbishop Anthony came on the 4th December and was really excellent and we had a marvellous discussion. I am not sure yet whether he can come on the 26th as he is in Moscow at the moment.

I think this is really all that has been happening while you have been away and I am look-ing forward very much to seeing you and filling in the picture a bit.

Dr Esther Lucile Brown

San Francisco, USA

17 February 1966 Thank you so very much for your very good long letter. I am enclosing a photograph of St Christopher's so you can see where we have got to. It was taken about six weeks ago.

Thank you for sending me Dr Sidney Cohen's article. I have written to him and had a note back and he was able to tell me that a book of his was just being published over here. I am on the waiting list for it at the Royal Society of Medicine Library and look forward to reading it. He pointed out in his letter that he is so often able to help patients without even using LSD because no-one has thought of using simple personal relationships to give them a feeling of security and understanding and one visit will make an astonishing amount of difference.

Someone else sent me a copy of *Awareness of Dying* and I was very interested in it indeed. Thank you so much for suggesting that you might send me your copy but now I am supplied. I will wait for your prospectus on which you were working when it is released for public distribution and will be very glad indeed to have it to pass it on to some of the nurs-ing leaders that I know here. I think that Miss Nuttall, the editor of The Nursing Times, would be particularly interested in it.

---

[90] This reference appears several times in the correspondence and concerns the seventy steps which had to be climbed in order to reach her flat in Connaught Square, London.

I was fascinated by your description of the two different Homes. I am afraid I will not have time to do any visits when I am over this time as after my very demanding month in Yale I lecture in the Department of Psychiatry in Cleveland and possibly pay two short visits to friends and then straight back home. I come over on the 19th April and really must be back by 1st June because I cannot stay away too long from either St Christopher's or other work at present.

I am not sure if I mentioned to you that I am speaking at the Pre-congress Colloquium at the International Congress of Gerontology in Vienna at the end of June. I was originally expecting to do only a very short part in a prepared discussion on training students in Gerontology, referring to, of course, training in the care of the dying. Now I find that I am reading the lead paper in the discussion on the role of social medicine under this general heading of Training in Gerontology.

This is one of these vague titles which you can use fairly freely I think and although I want to concentrate especially on my own subject as I do not think one has any right to do otherwise when speaking for the first time at some international meeting I would like to speak in wider terms as well. It does seem to me that this is a field in which one could expect to have the opportunity to talk to students about psycho-social aspects of patients in general, not only the elderly and that I could legitimately bring in some of the insights that you were giving us on cultural differences, the importance of real communication and so on. It seems to me that so often gerontology is concerned with helping the elderly person to live to the full and concentrates so much on this that it finds it extremely difficult to recognise the fact that some patients are no longer able to do this and that *all* are eventually going to die. It appears to be as difficult to recognise this fact in a very active geriatric unit as it is to recognise it in a general ward and once again the concept of a good death, of the immense importance of an active acceptance rather than a persistent and bitter denial are ignored. I would say that the first aspect of gerontology will be the one that is emphasised at the Congress and I do not think that I will be remaining unnecessarily in a rut if I concentrate on this side. I have to produce a paper by the 15th March but will be speaking to this and if you have any ideas and suggestions they would be most gratefully received. I do not think you will mind if I quote you as I think I may well want to.

I have a brother who is a business consultant and working in McKinsey's London branch. As you probably know they are a well known firm of American consultants and he is very fortunate indeed to be working with them. He was at Harvard Business School for two years after he did his degree at Oxford University. He is an extremely intelligent and alive person with a real social conscience and breadth of sympathy. He is not thinking of taking on responsibility in one of the usual charitable, volunteer organisations but he is interested in the possibilities of using his own specialised knowledge somehow for the common good beyond his actual work as a Management Consultant. We were having a fascinating discussion about this the other day. He is extremely useful to me, incidentally, producing excellent ideas on the organisation of St Christopher's from time to time and also has plenty of ideas about editing, planning and presenting the things that I write about my work. I mention him because as I think of you I realise how very much I would enjoy bringing you two together. Perhaps one day you will be in London and certainly this will be one of my top priorities when you are.

Dr Colin Murray Parkes

Harvard Medical School, Boston, USA

24 March 1966 Thank you very much for your letter of 28th February. I was very pleased indeed to hear from you again. I certainly look forward to meeting you when you get back to the Tavistock in September.

I am glad your work there is progressing well. I am certainly still interested in the possibility of your working with us at St Christopher's and I do hope that we will be able to plan something together. I have got more and more interested in trying to help the relations more than we have done in the past and now that we have just been given a grant to have an Out-Patient Pain Clinic from the beginning of our work I think this opens up other avenues also.

I was fascinated by what you told me about Dr Elisabeth Ross[91] and I am going to write to her because I am going to be at Yale for a month from the 20th April and I wonder whether there is any possibility of our managing to get together during that time. I am very lucky in having been given a visiting lectureship in the Graduate School of Nursing and this is certainly going to keep me extremely busy but I think I might have some time available. At the end of my month I have a few days to spare and am then going to lecture in Cleveland, to the Department of Psychiatry on my way over to Vancouver to see a Pain Clinic and have a bit of holiday with a friend. That bit of the schedule is rather tightly planned and I do not think I could fit Chicago in there now which is a pity for that would obviously seem the logical way to do it. However, we shall see.

Our building is going well and our fund raising also needs crossed fingers but so far has kept pace with demand. Perhaps there will be a chance of having a word with you while I am over for it is just possible that I might come to Boston for a day or two but I am trying not to fit in too many things from this side until I know what the demands will be once I get to Yale.

Dr Elisabeth Kübler-Ross

Billings Hospital, Chicago, USA

29 March 1966 I have recently had a letter from Dr Murray Parkes, currently working in Harvard University Medical School, in the Department of Psychiatry, who I understand recently visited you and saw something of your work with dying patients. I understand he mentioned that he had seen something of what we had been trying to do in this field. I am enclosing two reprints with this letter but am sending one or two others by surface mail and also a brochure about the new hospice that we are building at the moment which will concentrate on further work among these patients both in control of physical pain and in

---

[91] Colin Murray Parkes had become acquainted with Elisabeth Kübler-Ross whilst working in the USA and was clearly eager for her and Cicely Saunders to meet, which they did at an 'Institute' the following month, April 1966, at Yale University (see letter to Florence Wald of 10 June 1966, p. 105).

trying to learn more of how to help them in other ways also. We hope very much that we will have a link with Dr Murray Parkes and his work in due course.

I am shortly coming over to the States to spend about a month in the Graduate School of Nursing, and then a few days in New York, a lecture in the Department of Psychiatry in Western Reserve University on the 24th May before I have some holiday and return home. I do not know if there will be a chance of seeing you at all during this time. If there is I would so much like it because I am sure there is a great deal I could learn from you. Unfortunately, on leaving Cleveland I fly straight over to Vancouver to meet a friend and have really not got any time after the 24th but I suppose, on looking at the map, it would not be out of all reason to suggest that I might come to Chicago before Cleveland rather than after. I cannot possibly ask Professor Pearson to change the date of my lecture at this stage!

While I am at Yale the Dean of the Graduate School of Nursing who is arranging my trip with some connection with the Medical School also, is working on plans for an institute of people working in this area being planned for the 6th and 7th May. I have been writing to her today and have taken the liberty of mentioning your name to her. I hope you will not mind. She was optimistically talking about Dr Feifel and Drs Glaser and Strauss and Miss Quint, but, of course, they are all working in California and I doubt very much whether they will be able to come so far. Anyway, this is all very much in a tentative stage as far as I know.

If you have written on this subject I would be very grateful indeed for any reprints you may have. As I am leaving London on the 19th April perhaps it would be best if you wrote to me c/o The School of Nursing, 310 Cedar Street, New Haven, Connecticut. I do hope that there will be a chance of our exchanging views and information.

Dr Robert G. Twycross

The Radcliffe Infirmary, Oxford

14 April 1966 Thank you very much for your letter of 5th April. I am most interested in your thought that perhaps this will eventually be your own field.

My own preparation for this work was so unusual that I find it rather difficult to give you advice. It seems to me that there are several possible lines of approach and you will obviously know which is going to be the right one for you when the time comes. I am thinking of the possibility of doing some psychiatry particularly of the preventive kind, eg the work at the Tavistock Centre. Here I think it would be well worth your while talking with Dr Murray Parkes who has worked on problems of bereavement and who is at present over in Harvard for a year. We hope he will have a link with us at St Christopher's in due course. More and more it seems to me that one has to learn about the minds of men if one is going to have what Bettelheim calls "The Informed Heart".[92] We have to be able to teach students and I think possibly this is going to be a profitable line of approach to them.

Secondly, there is the possibility of concentrating on the problems of chronic pain and its relief. This is certainly a very open field. I am enclosing a copy of a paper I am presenting at

---

[92] Bruno Bettelheim (1903–90) studied psychoanalysis in Vienna and was a survivor of Dachau and Buchenwald concentration camps. He moved to the USA after World War II. The book referred to here appeared as B. Bettelheim, *The informed heart* (Harmondsworth: Penguin, 1960).

Copenhagen in the summer and also of another I am giving in Vienna. These, incidentally, are my two first visits to international congresses and I am very delighted but also somewhat apprehensive. Everyone who works in an Out-Patient Pain Clinic finds that these patients are jettisoned or abandoned by everyone else. To prepare for such work I think one has to concentrate either through neurosurgery or through anaesthetics on the problems of nerve blocks of various kinds. Another line, of course, is the problem of drugs which includes both chemistry and statistics. None of these are my own lines. I only know enough to manage somehow in this particular maze.

Finally, of course, there is just good general medicine or general practice both of which give the experience among all the other things that happen. Social medicine, on the whole, seems to concentrate on epidemiology and I do not think is yet a really good way in but knowledge of case work certainly would be.

Of course we hope there will be opportunities for you at St Christopher's! We will have a Research Fellowship for someone to concentrate on the clinical trials with drugs and we already have the money for this. I will probably have another older person as my co-doctor for the day-to-day work but I think we would certainly have more than one special project afoot and who knows how far the Out-Patient Pain Clinic and even a sort of family club or bereavement clinic may develop.

I am off to the States on the 19th April and back on the 1st June but please keep in touch and let me know what you think of these possibilities and what comes up for you.

Florence Wald

School of Nursing, Yale University, Connecticut, USA

10 June 1966 Safely back again, and I am finding that everything has gone on very well while I have been away. St Christopher's looks really splendid and the windows are in, the wiring being done and even some painting in the Grasshopper's Wing,[93] which is very well advanced. The builders are hurrying up and say they will be finished on time or even earlier! I am longing to show it to you and really feel very proud of its handsome appearance.

I managed to get both the record and the paper back of *The Fiddler on the Roof* before I left USA and so I now have them to remind me of an evening I enjoyed even more than I expected – and that was high enough. It was a perfect ending for such a lovely month with you.

This afternoon I spent three hours over at St Joseph's with the nuns. It was so good to see them – I really do miss working there, but could never have done all that has been fitted into this year if I had still been there.

I asked Dr Simmons if he could remember the horns of his dilemma because I liked that very much and I rather think that was one of the tapes that didn't come through – he thought he would easily remember what he said. I think that it was probably the statement which went best with what you said and would remind the rest of us of that last afternoon. It was so nice to see him and his wife again and we had a very pleasant evening together.

The tapes have probably given you all a great deal of trouble. It was very much your Institute – the success and all. Someone tells me that some of the sociologists and psychia-

---

93 The long-stay wing for older residents at St Christopher's.

trists interested in the dying have started a forum of communication and that Avery Weisman wrote something called "The birth of the death people".[94] Have you heard of it? I think that their title is worse than The Ghouls, and that our group must all the more keep together, even if they join in too. Colin Parkes will probably hear of it, I'm not even sure it wasn't he who mentioned it to me. He has just sent me a fascinating description of his picture of the possibilities of St Christopher's, particularly the thoughts concerning involving families. I am so glad he will be part of the team in some way. He has a most impressively clear grasp of essentials and the blend of objectivity and real caring which people will find so comforting and steadying. Once again St C's is going to be lucky in being sent someone.

I wonder if you have any news of someone else for the Graduate School? I hope very much to see you looking less tired when we meet here and that you will have news that satisfies you about it all. I also long to know something about the follow up meeting in the Pediatric Department, and lots of other things.

No news yet of any more money – but I cannot feel too depressed. I understand that the Wolfson Foundation meet towards the end of this month. I have to try and get the widespread interest in what St C's wants to do across to them without seeming to be perpetually bothering them but hope that it will just percolate through. I feel like getting you to write a reference for us and the idea!

This is a woolly letter, it is rather late and I am just wandering on on the typewriter thinking of you and how much I enjoyed it all.

Dr Olive Wyon

Cambridge

12 June 1966 I have been meaning to ring or write ever since Mrs Matthews came to see me last week and time has slipped by. However, first of all, I do hope that you have now quite recovered from the tiresome chest and that walking goes well also. I do hope that the move from the flat is progressing and that the new plans develop happily. Grasshoppers looks absolutely beautiful, with the dove cote being put into position and painting being done. It has sprinted ahead of the big building and they will even have the garden part tidied up for the AGM. They are pressing ahead generally and hope not only to finish in time (end of December) but even to be ahead! This does not mean that we will be hurrying everyone else, as I think we will use all the spare time for getting the equipment into place, but it does mean that this time next year sounds really well set for the big opening, and that people will move in gradually over the six months beginning March or so. I am all for doing all that in slow speed as then everyone can settle down without the pressure of all 70 beds filled. Finally, I have been told of a little cottage, newly built, within 3 minutes walking distance of the Hospice, but up a little side road with good trees etc. I like it and my brother's firm are investigating it and I am making an offer. That of course, is on me, but the rest of the building is needing either a Wolfson grant within this month – or – it has to raise a mortgage. I gather from Albertine Winner that both Sir Stanford Cade and Sir Charles Dodds are much on our side and they are the two medical trustees, but they have just given Professor

---

[94] She is referring to A. D. Weisman, Birth of the death people, *Omega: Newsletter of Time, Perspective, Death, Bereavement*, **1** (1967).

Hoyle all that money for Cambridge so the kitty may not be so rich as all that! I believe that we can go on praying quietly for this and do not have to agonize or storm the gates of heaven but I would be so glad and grateful if it would only come through.

I like Mrs Matthews immensely, and I was interested that she comes from Dohnavur. Some of Amy Carmichael's writings helped me a lot at one time. She seems to have a pull towards St C's and I would think that she would be a very likely helper generally and a very important person in the Chapel. She hopes that she may time her next trip over to our next Day probably early November – and will likely look for a house in our area! Your recommendation is enough of course, but I did like her very much and she would be good ballast I feel – we need to keep our balance between very convinced, very prayerful and the rest of their varying shades of thought and conviction. I'm still sure of being 'open' and have just had a good addition in a first class psychiatrist – Colin Murray Parkes, interested in the bereaved, Cruse Clubs and very intelligent thoughts on preventive psychiatry and work with our patients with and among their families.

Any hope of your coming to the AGM? I think that unless its *easy*, you should think twice … it won't be such a get together as sometimes. But it will be well attended and of course with a good chance of inspecting Grasshoppers. Anyway, bed reserved here if needed.

Dr Colin Murray Parkes
Harvard Medical School, Boston, USA

14 June 1966 Ever since I had your fascinating summary of your thoughts about St Christopher's I have been turning over in my mind what you said and planning out a proper answer. This is just an interim reply because I really want to sort out my thoughts about the use of the chapel and the religious and philosophical basis of the work a little more clearly as a definite answer. This is just to enclose two papers that I am not certain whether I ever sent you. They are in part an answer in themselves.

As it happens I have had two meetings in the last few days which are relevant both to the thought of a non-hierarchical staff structure and also the work of families both while the patient is ill and afterwards. In the first place I went over and spent a lovely afternoon with my special nuns at St Joseph's Hospice. The comment of one of them "The patients are never a problem, it is always the families" reminds me that the two senior sisters who are going to open up our first ward and who come from St Luke's Hospital in Bayswater are used to a routine in which there is not even a visiting time every day and in which this was not extended because "The relatives tire the patients out" and then to balance that I spent a very pleasant evening last night with Mr G and his mother-in-law. They were completely integrated into the life of the ward, never put a foot wrong in a very relaxed and informal relationship with sister and the many student nurses they knew over the years and remain two of my best friends. Mrs G's ward sister will be our senior sister at St Christopher's and Mr G our head porter. We are used to working together as a team but during all these years remain quite automatically 'Mrs G', 'Mr G', 'Miss Saunders'. Mr G and, incidentally, my excellent cleaner, Mrs Cherubim, fit entirely naturally into the St Christopher's group and, in fact, I do not think that anyone has to stop for a moment even to consider that this is in any way different from the relationship between any of the rest of us because, of course, it is not.

My thoughts are always in a more unkempt condition than yours but I will write you a full answer probably not before I leave for Vienna. I had an SOS telephone call from the editor of "Psychiatric Opinion", Framington, Mass, asking me if I would produce something to go in a number concerned with the care of the dying in August and this has had to be added on to everything else.[95]

St Christopher's building looks absolutely magnificent and the bills are coming in in equivalent proportion. We have a Council meeting tomorrow and have really got to seriously consider raising a mortgage because we are £10,000 in the red as far as cash is concerned at the moment. Do not get alarmed at this because we have £70,000 promised us in grants and the building and the land itself to be mortgaged. We have already paid out some £160,000 so far but this is a realm of high finance and you will probably be happy to hear that the ex-secretary to the City of London Parochial Charities joins our council at the meeting tomorrow.

Sir Kenneth Grubb

Downton, Wiltshire

23 June 1966 Please forgive me for not signing this letter myself but I am off to Vienna today to take part in an International Congress of Gerontologists.

I was sorry to hear from John Wilkins that you had not been well but I do hope that you are now better and are enjoying life.

St Christopher's is getting very large and splendid and the bills are matching it. At the moment we are patiently waiting to hear from the Wolfson Foundation whose Trustees, as far as I know, meet sometime in the next week or two. I know that the two medical Trustees are going to speak on our behalf as Dr Albertine Winner of the Ministry of Health has had a word with them as she fortunately meets them at various official occasions. One of our other Vice-Presidents, Lady Monckton, has also had a word with Sir Isaac Wolfson who is said to be interested as well but, obviously, I have not been trying to work my way down the list of Trustees and nobble everybody in turn. I did, however, have a chance to meet Sir Harold Redman who was very sympathetic but, of course, not at all forthcoming.

The present position is that we have paid out roughly £160,000 to the contractors, Fairweathers, who are making an excellent job of the work. It really does look very beautiful and very well finished. We also have paid £38,000 for the two sites and have approximately £70,000 in promised grants which are due to come over the next few years. We are now, however, at the end of our cash grants and therefore unless the Wolfson Foundation are kind to us or unless one of the others releases their money sooner than we expected we will have to borrow. Kleinwort Bensons, the Bank with which our Treasurer is connected have agreed to do a "long stop" operation but suggest that possibly the Midland Bank might do it at more favourable terms. Our Chairman, Treasurer and myself will probably go and see them when I come back from Vienna on the 2nd July if we have not had any good news before then. We still need a lot of money to complete the work but I also believe that it will come one way or another.

---

[95] The article appeared as C. Saunders, A medical director's view. *Psychiatric Opinion*, **3**(4), (1966): 28–34.

We have strengthened our Council very much recently by adding Sir Donald Allen who was, as you know, with the City Parochial Foundation for so many years. His knowledge of Trusts and Foundations is unrivalled and he has already had some very good suggestions to make. I have re-written our appeal and am about to send it off to be duplicated. We have never had it printed because the situation has always been changing and the brochure itself does do a considerable amount of the work for us. This is really designed for people who want to know something more about it and just because of the changing situation it has always seemed wrong to produce it in a more permanent form. I would be very glad indeed for any comments you might have about it and your usual helpful suggestions.

Lord Thurlow tells me that he has had a word with the Queen Mother's secretary and we are to put in our request for her to come and open the Hospice for us next spring or summer in August this year. I do hope so much that she will be able to come.

I think this brings you up to date. I do hope that there will be a chance of seeing you and talking about our plans sometime again soon.

Captain T. L. Lonsdale[96]

London

10 July 1966 After all their delay the Wolfson Foundation have at last said "No." I had a very nice and regretful letter from Sir Harold Redman yesterday with no chance of a come-back on their next meeting. This is rather hard, as although he wrote a discouraging letter originally, they have had two meetings since then and said nothing, and we had really encouraging remarks from Sir Isaac, and both the medical trustees. I guess that they managed to keep it in court for that time and then finally lost out. Albertine Winner, who happened to call me yesterday, was really surprised so I do not think I was being unduly hopeful.

Be that as it may, we now have a considerable wait before we are likely to hear from anyone else and so the position is rather acute. I think Alfred will have already spoken to you and sent off the cheque to Fairweathers, who had just written a restive letter. I feel rather guilty over them and very much so over Mr Smith, who is not having too easy a time with his own business at present and hangs back from sending us any bills. I suppose we should have written them the moment that last account came through, but I'm afraid I just said to Alfred that they would have to wait until we could meet with you and the Midland as I went off to Vienna. It is not likely to be any easier for them than anyone else at present is it?

So I hope that we may now hear from the Drapers. I am writing them by this post to plead again for that £30,000 they owe us and which would tide over this month. The next Fairweather bill is due before 20th I think. I will also write the Max Rayne Foundation but am less hopeful about their £20,000. But at least we haven't yet spent any money that we have no promise for!

I have a list of things to do about all this but with these two exceptions, no-one is likely to produce anything quickly. So the thought that you said that Kleinwort Benson had talked of acting as a long stop though at a high rate makes me hope that I won't land up in a debtor's prison or that the building will have to stop. But I will be calling you on Monday for reassurances!

---

[96] The St Christopher's treasurer.

I am writing now because it will probably be easier for you to have it in front of you. The things I have to do are as follows:

1   Meet the Ford Foundation person again on 5th August. We talked two hours and she will not only try to think of the best way to present our case to their trustees but also what other trusts might help and of which she knows people.

2   Write Sir Donald and hope that he may prod someone, including City Parochial.

3   Write City Parochial anyway as to position now we have heard from Wolfson.

4   Type up letter I have from Lady Monckton on Friday asking me to phone for a date and whether she could do any helping. She has just been having dealings with the Gulbenkian Foundation.

5   Make a bleat to Mr Peers of the King's Fund, Admiral Bingley of the Sembal Trust and perhaps Mr Young of the Nuffield Foundation.

6   Press on with publicity for the AGM but hope that all the builders won't be too worried themselves if they listen in!

7   The good prayers were mobilized some time ago. Perhaps they had best be directed to Kleinwort Bensons??

I think that it is no good just saying we are unlucky in that giving has been much more tight for the last 18 months and borrowing now very hard indeed and trust that it will be sorted out somehow. Albertine was most encouraging as always. She is truly committed to us and when she retires from the Ministry early next year will both be on our Council and also working with me as one of the doctors. She will be doing something else that fits in wonderfully well with our work. She said that there is little doubt about the Contractual arrangements. She spoke to the SAMO,[97] Dr Fairley, who said that their recommendation had gone through and that there was no reason to think that it would fail to be approved. She also said that there is nothing like a crisis to mobilise things and that in one way, we were a bit too successful earlier on to make the rest feel the urgency.

Meanwhile the building looks really marvellous. I was there on Saturday morning and things continue to sprint ahead. Excellent standard throughout too.

Sorry for a long letter – but it is probably better than a spate on the phone – and we have to do something rather smartly. I'm sorry I've been away so much but it does prove how many people believe that this idea is important. And it is the *idea*, not one individual, that will get us the means to go on.

Florence Wald

Yale University, Connecticut, USA

14 July 1966 Just a note to say how much I am looking forward to seeing you and hope perhaps you will call me from the Mitre Hotel when you get there if you feel strong enough. I notice however that you are not really in London until the 11th August for your ten day visit. On that particular day I will be in Copenhagen taking part in the Anaesthetists Congress and do not get back until Saturday 13th August. We must get in touch then and

---

[97]   Senior Area Medical Officer.

try and get you to Marian's atelier and so on. I know he is going to take a holiday sometime but I am not quite certain when.

I much look forward to taking Henry round the pipes and lighting of St Christopher's. At the moment our finances are in a rather shaky state because mortgaging on the land, premises and building is not too easy in this country at the moment and although we do confidently expect further grants at the moment we have a hiatus as the Wolfson Foundation has just turned us down.

Vienna was splendid and I was introduced to Miss Ollie Randall who I think you know and who sorts out some of the appeals to the Ford Foundation. I had a long talk with her in London afterwards and am meeting her again on the 5th August. I hope that possibly she may be able to present our case in a way that comes under their terms of reference but in any case she may be able to introduce us to someone else. Anyway I am plodding on in every direction and having a fairly hectic life as you may imagine.

Dr M. B. Bennett

Camps Bay, Cape Town, South Africa

14 July 1966 Thank you very much for your letter of the 4th July. Certainly you may quote from anything I write at any time and do not worry to ask.

I would be very interested indeed to see you when you are in London but I am afraid that I will only have an unfinished hospital to show you. I left St Joseph's at the end of September last year and am occupied at the moment in trying to get some writing done and trying to cope with all the problems of getting St Christopher's finished and open. Perhaps you would like to call me when you reach London and we will see what we can organise. If you are interested in seeing the unfinished building I would be delighted to take you down there and talk about the work.

I hope this will reach you before you leave Cape Town but I will get my secretary to make a note in the diary and drop you a line at the Barkston Gardens Hotel in case this misses you.

Sir Kenneth Grubb

Downton, Wiltshire

19 July 1966 Thank you so much for your long and helpful letter. I am very grateful to you for your suggestions and would most gladly take advantage of them.

I was sorry to hear from your secretary today that you are still getting trouble from this arthritis in your neck and I do hope that the pain will improve with treatment. I will look forward to seeing you in due course but quite realise that this is out of the question at the moment. I can only tell you how sorry I am that you have been having such a lot of trouble and send you my own personal good wishes and those of St Christopher's.

At the moment I feel rather like that small and diligent wader, the turnstone, who bustles up the beach turning over every single stone it meets to find what lies underneath. I have been in touch with everyone who has helped us and I know that they are getting together a bit and I believe that we will soon have some encouraging news. Tonight I go to dine with Dr Albertine Winner who will come to St Christopher's when she leaves the Ministry of

Health (where she is Deputy Chief Medical Officer) next spring. She telephoned me on Saturday to say that she had two members of the Wates Trust to lunch and that they were very interested in St Christopher's. This may possibly be the piece of good fortune for which we are looking but, of course, I am not flagging in the pursuit of all other possibilities.

It will be very good to have the Annual General Meeting in the unfinished building this Friday and I think we will have some 150 people there. I will be talking about it on Woman's Hour that afternoon and there should be an article in the Guardian that morning. I hope that none of this will give us the reputation of "A Home for the Dying" but that it will present the picture as it should be shown. Anyway, I am sure we will have a lot of interest and enquiry and perhaps something will come of that also.

The best thing about having any kind of trouble is the discovery of how much other people care and how nice they are. This, perhaps is one of the reasons why a hospital which specialises in our kind of care also specialises in goodness.

The Right Reverend the Lord Bishop of Stepney
London

27 July 1966 I am sorry that I didn't get this into the post last night but I am dropping it in by hand today so that there shall be no further delay.

Thank you so much for getting on with this, I hope that at least something of what we need may come to tide us over. But if it doesn't, well at least we've tried. The enclosed Appeal is a supplement to the Brochure and I sent it to the larger Trusts we approach. It keeps being altered of course as things change and as I slant it to the interests of those concerned. Not that we change our plans to suit them but with such a many faceted thing as St Christopher's there is always one aspect that can be brought forward while keeping all the rest still in the picture. The financial summary on the penultimate page is just to give a broad picture and as you see, leaves us with £212,000 odd to finish and equip. Mr Smith is occupied among other things in seeing what we could postpone, such as the laundry equipment, so that we can certainly bring this figure down somewhat, and I'm not worrying about equipment just at present anyway, what we want is to keep building so that it gets ahead and doesn't deteriorate. For this, we need some £150,000 during the next 6 months. This would be tight but I think would be all right.

The upshot of the long session with the contractors on Tuesday is that they will wait for their part of the money, with us paying it as it comes along, if the sub-contractors will do likewise. They will not carry the burden of all the money owing themselves, paying the sub-contractors as they finish their part of the work. Mr Smith is now speaking to each of them in turn, asking them if they will do this. So far, he has spoken to them (in preparation for Tuesday) and found that in principle they will all wait for some 3 months, knowing that this is a Charity with good sponsors and hoping that it will be settled by then. He is now doing the second round, saying that the contractors will hold their bit if they will in their turn. If they do not, then they make the building watertight, put in a watchman, and we begin again when the money has come in.

So far, we have been seeing a little light. The Drapers' £30,000 was what we already expected and does not come into the extra money we still need. Max Rayne will only release £5,000 of the remaining £20,000 already promised, but that is a help anyway. Since last week, we have had £5,000 from the Chairman of the Bank who couldn't give us the loan and another partner, who has already given us £5,000 has asked to see the Treasurer today about St Christopher's so perhaps he has ideas. Then I have had encouragement from the Ministry of Health to hope that they will give us some of their first ever capital allowance for a few research projects. I have applied for the capital cost of the Pain Clinic and ancillary rooms, if we get it it should I hope be soon and about £11,000. I hope to see them soon.

We are waiting to hear from any number of Trusts to whom I have applied. The Nuffield Foundation are prepared to be *asked* for a low interest loan in early October, but there is no guarantee that we will get it. It would likely be in the £30,000 – £40,000 range. Dr Winner and others are really trying hard for us. I think that I have done all that I can think of myself for the next few days – and then next week talk to the person who sorts out the appeals for the Ford Foundation who would truly like to get us under their terms of reference, but doesn't know whether she can. She will try for other American introductions and I am doing so by other routes also.

The Sembal Trust would have helped us but they have their Inland Revenue case to hold on for. That is in January. They will certainly help after that I think, and if they win would have a lot of money available then.

Somehow we will get it, and those who have helped us will not let it sink, but if the Church Commissioners would consider any kind of loan (giving is too much to ask I fear) then it would help immensely just to keep building.

Professor Gordon W. Allport

The Ella Lyman Cabot Trust, Harvard University, Cambridge, Massachusetts, USA

2 August 1966 You will be getting another newsletter about St Christopher's in the fairly near future which will give you a copy of the address I had to give at our Annual General Meeting in the unfinished building on the 22nd July. This was to say that unless we had some real financial help we had come up against the credit squeeze and the possibility of getting a bridging loan just at the moment when we were short of cash and had been turned down after a long wait by a big foundation. However, even since that time a great many things seem to have happened; a certain amount of money has already come in and the contractor and the sub-contractors have all agreed to go on building knowing that the money may come in rather more slowly than their bills will reach us. This is very good indeed of them and we are most grateful and all the more impelled to raise the rest of the money so that they do not have to wait. I believe it will come.

Since I wrote last the building has made tremendous strides and we have our work well ahead and could, indeed, have finished two or three months earlier than the finishing date we expected, towards the end of February. Now we will be going more slowly and probably, if all goes well, that will be the time of completion. We have also gone ahead with plans for involving the families and founding an Out-Patient clinic from the very beginning of our work and letting that develop if it seems right into both a certain amount of day care facilities and also domiciliary care for patients in their own homes by the staff who have known them in the wards. We are very fortunate in that Dr Colin Murray Parkes who has done some excellent work on the problems of the bereaved in this country and is currently finishing a year directing a project at Harvard in the Department of Psychiatry, is going to join us. Another great acquisition is the Deputy Chief Medical Officer of the Ministry of Health who retires next spring and who will come on to our staff and our Council. She is a first class clinician who has been in administration since the war but who I know from having watched come round St Joseph's on two occasions, has all the warmth and understanding that this work needs. She will also make certain that we keep ourselves well on the right administrative track!

There is one other reason for writing to you and that is to ask your advice. I have a Polish friend here, a Professor of Art (and also mathematics) whose son lives and works in Poland. He is some 30 years old now and has just got a doctorate in Pedagogical Psychology at Cracow University with first class honours. Incidentally, he had the opportunity to do this course after he had been removed from his teaching post because of a refusal to sign a general petition to stop religious teaching in schools. The end of his teaching appointment and the beginning of a grant to do this course at the University came together I understand from the Ministry of Education. Such can be things behind the Iron Curtain. But certainly his courageous stand was not done with any foreknowledge that this would be the result. Apparently, his professors have suggested to him that he should try for some form of scholarship or fellowship to enable him to do some further work abroad. As he is not a member of the Communist Party he is not likely to have any help from his own country but apparently would be allowed to travel should some place be found for him. I am afraid I do not know too much about the exact work he would like to do but have asked his father to get more particulars from him. He is a deeply religious person and from a letter his father read to me I would think that he is particularly interested in an existentialist approach to psychological problems and also in trying to see whether one can observe and learn something of what sounds to me a description of the contemplative state. If you could either tell me of any possibilities in your country or anybody else I might write to I would be very grateful. His father, who is unable to return to his own country, would, of course, dearly love to have him work in England but is far too generous not to try to find out whether it might be better for his son to work in your country should that be possible and I promised I would try and find out anything I could. You were the first person who came to mind. I am sorry to bother you but I know that you will understand. His father, incidentally, is the artist who is painting some really magnificent things for St Christopher's most of which he is giving us. As it is related to your own field I would be very grateful for any suggestions as to where he might work and possibilities of scholarships and so on.

There is no time in this letter to describe what a splendid time I had in Yale as a visiting lecturer for a month and also the fascinating afternoon I had with Dr Judah Folkman at the Boston City Hospital, to whom I was introduced by Dr Robert Shaw. I found myself lecturing again at Memorial and also in Mount Sinai Hospital and finished a very hectic five weeks by lecturing in the Department of Psychiatry at Western Reserve University. From this came an invitation to contribute to a symposium in Psychiatric Opinion in the August number which, perhaps, you may see. I got back to this country at the beginning of June and just had time to get things sorted out before I was off to Vienna to take part in the Congress of Gerontologists. Now I am about to set off again to talk about the use of intractable pain as a testing ground for analgesics at the Anaesthetics Congress at Copenhagen, this time to put in a strong plea that these patients should not just be *used* but that we should realise our responsibility to carry out the kind of trials that will teach us how to use these drugs for their benefit. All this is very exciting and very useful for St Christopher's because it means that we have first class contacts with people in many allied fields and should be able to make an impact in due course far beyond our own patients and their families although they will always be the centre of our concern.

I hope you had a good time in Honolulu. I was very sorry not to see you but greatly enjoyed a lovely evening with Father and Mrs Whitney Hale and heard of you from them.

Please give my greetings to Mrs Sprague. I was sorry I was not able even to speak to her during the short time I was in Boston but I did see Dr Friedrich and very much enjoyed meeting him once more.

The Reverend A. E. Barton

Brackley, Northamptonshire

15 September 1966 No money I am afraid. I am still waiting for news and, of course, may even have it before this letter goes off. I think I told you that I am due to ring Mr Johnston of the City Parochial on Monday, when he comes back from holiday and have had my opening remarks practically dictated to me by Sir Donald, bless him.

About the rail. I, myself, find it extremely difficult to get up and down for Communion without a rail as I am pretty stiff and I am sure that a lot of the Grasshoppers would find it even more so. I do not quite see how we would get round this by having to move benches and so forth but I suppose this is a possibility. Do you really have to have a chair? What is that for? If it is only for the Bishop, I am sure he would forgo it on behalf of the Grasshopper's bending or genuflecting, perhaps one should say.

I think we ought to get together about this sometime. I will try and get this organised with Mr Smith.

Florence Wald

Yale University, Connecticut, USA

20 September 1966 Just a note to send you these photographs which I do not think very outstanding but at any rate I have a picture of the Walds at St Christopher's which was an important occasion. Let us hope that next time the photography is rather better. It was a lovely day anyway.

I have just had a cheque for £5,000 this morning and this means that our total that we can pay out in October is £20,000 with September already covered. This is marvellous and added to a very unofficial talk with a Trust who are going to give us a very large grant in January has made me write a very much more enthusiastic letter to the contractor this morning. I think that we can go ahead with the finishing date of March DV and DG.

I have just finished an immense review article on the care of the dying.[98] If it gets printed in full, which I am beginning to doubt a little, it should be out in October and November and I will send you reprints. It means also that I can take a week's holiday in October which is a splendid thought.

I hope that you found that things were going on all right when you got back and that your own changes are beginning to sort themselves out.

---

[98] This appeared first as a series of three articles in the *British Journal of Hospital Medicine* and then as C. Saunders, *The management of terminal illness* (London: Hospital Medicine Publications, 1967).

Professor John Hinton

Department of Psychiatry, Middlesex Hospital Medical School, London

22 September 1966 This is just a note to send you my congratulations on your appointment to the Chair at the Middlesex Hospital Medical School.[99] I was very pleased indeed to see the announcement.

At the same time I feel that I ought to mention that I have quoted you several times in the review I have written for "Hospital Medicine" on the management of terminal illness. I understand that originally they asked you to deal with the psychological and social problems and as you were writing a paperback I was then given the whole assignment. I am sorry that you were not doing it but I look forward to your book and I hope you will not mind the number of times I have quoted you. In view of the scarcity of factual studies this was really inevitable.

You may be interested to know that St Christopher's Hospice is well on with its building, that Dr Murray Parkes has joined the team and that we are hoping to develop quite a lot of out-patient work and work among the families as well as just concentrating on the patients as we were doing more at St Joseph's. I look forward to welcoming you there one day.

Dr Henry K. Beecher[100]

Massachusetts General Hospital, Boston, USA

27 September 1966 I am afraid you must have been thinking that I had forgotten that I had promised that I would send you this reprint of Sir Theodore Fox's Harveian Oration. Anyway, here, at last, it is. The reason for the delay was that the finances of St Christopher's, which we are building, required every spare minute I had.

It was a great pleasure to meet you in Copenhagen and I was very grateful for an opportunity to talk with you about some of our problems in planning the work of St Christopher's. I am enclosing a note of the plan of work that we are contemplating. This, of course, does not go into any detail of the pain problems and analgesic trials that we want to consider but in this general context I hope we will be able to do some useful work. Certainly we will have a group of patients with comparable situations and the opportunity to learn about their needs and to do the sort of trials that I know are essential if we are going to have answers that are helpful to other people.

I was very delighted to meet Professor Lassner from Paris in Copenhagen and I am going to have the pleasure of taking him round St Christopher's unfinished building later this week. He, apparently, is planning a Pain Clinic rather on the lines of our own but had not had much thought about admitting patients. I hope we may persuade him into planning some sort of St Christopher's in Paris.

I hope possibly you will have seen Tony Brown in the States before he sets off home again to work in Vietnam.

---

[99] Recently appointed to a chair in psychiatry, John Hinton had already published some important research papers on the physical and mental distress of the dying and his book *Dying* (Harmondsworth: Penguin) appeared the following year, 1967.

[100] The noted pain researcher, who had first met Cicely Saunders in 1963.

I hope very much that we will be meeting again and particularly hope that we will have the chance of welcoming you to St Christopher's one day.

The Reverend Almon R. Pepper

Executive Council of the Episcopal Church, New York, USA

25 October 1966 There is no time now to write to you very fully but I do want to let you know of some very good fortune that has come St Christopher's way. Last week we had a grant of £12,000 from the Research Department of the Ministry of Health for the capital cost of the Pain Clinic to be followed by £5,000 a year for 5 years towards the running costs and then last Friday news of a grant of £25,000 from the Goldsmiths' Company of London, another of the City Companies like the Drapers'. This, with the *wonderful* number of smaller gifts which have come our way since July enables us to give the "Go ahead" to an accelerated building programme to the contractors and means that not only have we paid everything up to date as the certificates have come in but that everybody is tremendously impressed by the way it has all happened. I am so grateful to everybody for the gifts, large and small, and for everything they represent. We also have some news of some good fortune sometime towards the end of January and this means that we really can hope for a finishing date sometime in the spring.

There is no time for more now but I did want you to know this.

The Reverend A. E. Barton

Brackley, Northamptonshire

10 November 1966 We had a good session at St Christopher's yesterday. The more I think about it the more I think you are right in saying "No Altar rail," but the Bishop does feel, I believe, (and perhaps you might discuss it with him) that the older people will find it very hard not to take their Communion in the way they have always done. Perhaps we could come round this by having a moveable bench for those who feel like that about it but the rest of us will, perforce, be drawn back into the primitive way of receiving and not having room for a rail is a very good excuse to move that way. At the same time I don't think the Bishop thinks very firmly about the seat behind the altar so at best perhaps we can give you a tiny misericorde but I don't think anything else is really necessary, is it?

Could you send 1 dozen brochures to Albertine Winner please.

Sister Zita Marie

Providence Hospital, Kansas City, Kansas, USA

6 December 1966 You will be having our official newsletter coming by surface mail but I wanted to let you know that since our crisis in July we have now been given or promised well over £100,000! I feel we all ought to be going round with prayers of gratitude the entire time but, of course, this means that we are now pressing ahead fast and are organising practical things, choosing beds, fixing staff, and organising everything for a completion date from the builders of 31st March. I feel optimistic about getting equipment in during April and being able to take at least a few patients in May but perhaps this is really too optimistic and I will have to wait and see.

It does mean, however, that we can now give you some idea of when we will be more or less full and ready to welcome you to come and work with us. I suggest that you let us know what would suit you giving you as long as you feel you should have and some holiday before you have to get back by July 1968 as you told me in your letter of August 14th. I would suggest that perhaps October would be a good month but you let me know if you think it would be really valuable to come sooner and see us in our real throes of beginning, say, any time after June.

The story of all our money and the way things have dove-tailed literally from day to day is too long to put here but I will just repeat again the verse that came in my daily reading after I had come upstairs with a promise of £25,000 on the very morning I had to telephone the contractor to confirm that we could have a full speed ahead and a definite finishing date – "Of His fullness have we all received and grace for grace". Somehow "grace for grace" speaks to me of all the small sacrificial gifts (over £3,500 by October) which have come since July and which I am sure have called down the larger ones by their prayer and care.

With all good wishes to you and I hope that we really will be welcoming you for your time with us and that we can learn together.

Miss S. C. Cheng
Queen Elizabeth Hospital, Kowloon, Hong Kong

3 January 1967 Thank you so much for your very beautiful Christmas card. It was very nice indeed to hear of you again. I was delighted also to hear that you are having a block built for our kind of patient and I am sending you one or two papers by air mail and one or two other things by surface mail as you may find them useful or at least can pass them round.

We will put you on the list of Friends of St Christopher's so that you will get our regular newsletter and I am sending you the last two as they sum up what we are trying to do as well as anything.

I hope you will be back in England again and that we will welcome you to St Christopher's open and working.

Do let me know how your plans go and if you can send me any further information I would be very grateful for I think it is very important that we all know what is going on in different parts of the world in this field. I know there is just a chance that Time magazine may write something about this type of work when St Christopher's actually opens and it would be very nice if I could give your address and information from Hong Kong as well.

Dr Margaretta Bowers
New York, USA

19 January 1967 I must write by return to thank you so much for your good letter and for the various things you told. As you have written to Dr Sacerdote sending him on the literature I will not burden him with the whole lot once again but I will write him a note of thanks and enclose copies of the two recent reprints which I enclose now for you. As you see now the third one will have an immense number of references and I will send that on to you when I get them.

People are always after me about writing a book and I do intend to do this but truly raising the money, ordering the equipment, devising the structure, gathering in the staff and the patients and old people for St Christopher's is enough to keep me going for the moment!

Once I am there I will not be the only one by any manner of means and I do truly think that there will be more time free to do such things.

I hope you will not overdo it yourself and that perhaps you have some holiday coming up. Thank you so much for writing.

The Right Reverend the Lord Bishop of Stepney
London

23 January 1967 I wanted you to know that I had a very good discussion with Sister Helen Willans (our Church Army girl who is going to be in charge of our Old People's wing) this last Sunday about the daily prayers at St Christopher's. We are, of course, sure that whenever we find the right part- time chaplain we have got to start with our proper traditions from the first moment. We were both rather attracted to the idea of using the book of the Church of South India for daily prayers rather than Matins and Evensong, which to many people are rather routine. This, she would lead and those of us who wanted would join in and then we could develop, perhaps, led intercessions or silent prayer from there. I am sure we must have daily prayers when it is possible for most of the staff to attend if they want to. We both of us would have a daily communion in due course, again, normally at an early hour so that the chaplain can then go up to wards to patients who want communion, but at least once a week at a time when as many as possible of night and day staff can come if they wish.

The ward prayers, we feel, ought to go straight on from the St Thomas's tradition which, of course, you know are taken by Sister or the nurse in charge of the ward morning and evening. We think probably no services in the ward other than these but that she and eventually the chaplain and any of us perhaps could take it over sometimes. We could perhaps have a more informal type of evening prayers with music, reading and so on as people choose, going out over our own line on the earphone but taking place actually in the chapel. This, patients could tune into if they wanted but would not be broadcast on any loudspeakers which we are not going to have.

She is such a good person and I am very pleased indeed we have been given her. I think this makes me feel very much better about the present lack of chaplain than I otherwise would have done and perhaps the laity have got to pull their weight very much at the beginning and we may not even get a chaplain until we have our full complement of patients which after all will not probably be until the autumn.

Sir Kenneth Grubb
Downton, Wiltshire

13 February 1967 I know that you will rejoice with us to hear that the City Parochial Foundation has granted us another £50,000, available during the next two months. As you can imagine this makes our finances look somewhat different, although I must admit we still have some £90,000 to raise to pay off the grand total, but as a proportion of that total of approximately £480,000 it is not so serious at this stage I believe.

I do hope you have kept well since we were last in touch, and that your neck has not been giving you too much pain. I hope that the flat at the top of CMS House is a success.

I have been introduced to Dr John Taylor by the Bishop of Stepney and I am very glad to be going to meet him in the middle of March. We are changing our plans for a Chaplain,[101] and the administration is being split away from his duties so that we are at present in the throes of advertising for a Bursar (although we have a very good friend already in the Health Service). We will then need a part-time Chaplain, possibly somebody retired. It occurred to us that Dr Taylor might have some suggestions. I wonder if, by any chance, anyone comes into your mind?

Dr Elisabeth Kübler-Ross

Billings Hospital, Chicago, USA

20 February 1967 Thank you so much for sending me your reprint, which I was very glad to have.

In exchange I am sending one of my own, and I am glad to be able to tell you that our new Hospice is likely to take its first patients early in June, so I hope I will be welcoming you there one day.

I hope your work goes well and that you will send me anything else you write because I think it is most valuable.

Dr H. C. Ho

The Hong Kong Anti-Cancer Society, Hong Kong

8 March 1967 Thank you very much for your full letter describing your plans for the hospital. I was very interested in all of this but I am afraid I do not know anybody I could suggest might wish to spend a few years in Hong Kong. I will, however, mention this to a friend of mine in the Ministry of Health who has a much wider acquaintanceship than I have, and perhaps something might come of it.

I do hope you will keep us in touch with the development of your plans and of the work itself, and we will do the same.

Dr Robert Fulton[102]

University of Minnesota, Minneapolis, Minnesota, USA

20 April 1967 I was very glad to receive an invitation to your symposium on "Death, Grief and Bereavement" although I am afraid there is no possibility of my attending. I

---

101 There had been a parting of the ways between Cicely Saunders and the Revd Alfred Barton, who was to have been a combined chaplain and bursar at St Christopher's.

102 The sociologist and editor of *Death and identity* (New York: Wiley, 1965).

wonder if the proceedings are going to be published because if so I would very much like a copy and would be most grateful if you would put my name on any list you have of those interested.

May I take this opportunity of saying how much I appreciated your book "Death and Identity" and in particular your editorial comments on Weisman and Hackett's paper. I have on several occasions quoted the words in your last sentence there "A dignified death proclaims the significance of man".

You may possibly be interested in the enclosed memorandum about the work which we are planning for St Christopher's, which should receive its first patients during June of this year. If you are ever in London we would be delighted to welcome you there, and I would greatly appreciate an opportunity of discussing some aspects of the work with you.

Dr S. Krishnamurthi

The Cancer Institute, Madras, India

24 April 1967 Another Newsletter for you, and I am glad to say that St Christopher's is nearly finished and hopes to admit its first patients in June. I look forward to welcoming you there one day.

I am sorry you have such a struggle with your own Institute, and am also sorry that the Annual Report went astray and never reached me. I do hope you will find some way round your financial problems and difficulties in getting equipment. I feel we are extremely fortunate in all that we have, and have all the more reason to be grateful. Of course we do not have the problem of scientific equipment for St Christopher's in our particular branch of the work; our next project is going to be a Nurses Home and Teaching Wing so that we can expand the work beyond our own walls. Perhaps we will come into contact with you in this way one day.

Olive Randall

New York, USA

16 May 1967 Of course the builders have had delays and we are not going to get rid of them until June, but St Christopher's looks splendid and we are boldly going ahead arranging for some of our old people to come in at the beginning of June, and a few patients at the beginning of July! We can also announce a royal Opening, although cannot say who will perform the Ceremony yet, on July 24th. Is there any chance of your being in this part of the world and joining us on that day? You know how much I would love to show you the completed building and hear your comments. There is a chance I believe that Canon Almon Pepper and even Theodate Soule might be about. Theodate, as you know, is starting out in July for Australia and although she expects to go via the West Coast she might just change her plans.

If you are in England then I would so much like you to meet various members of the staff, a really splendid team is getting itself 'dug in' now and we actually have three people working in the building with commissioning, visiting our few residents and so on.

The Reverend Almon R. Pepper

Executive Council of the Episcopal Church, New York, USA

25 May 1967 I was delighted to have your letter. My reply has been rather a long time coming but I had a holiday during the first two weeks in May to prepare me for the summer and so my correspondence was delayed. I was very interested indeed in all your news and do hope that July 24th, might possibly fit in with your plans for this summer. We would love to welcome you there.

I was glad to have all your comments about St Christopher's responsibility of all the patients we will have; it would be frightening if we were not developing such a splendid team to try and help them. There is one gap about which we are concerned at the moment and that is the Chaplain. Mr Barton is leaving us to go back to parish work and we have been able to hand over the administration to a first class Bursar, Mr Leach, who was lately Deputy Treasurer of St Thomas's Hospital but we have not found someone to fit in with the part-time Chaplain's post so far although we shall have the help of local clergy and more than one person is prepared to help us out from time to time. As it is so important that we have the right person we are not hurrying over this because we believe he will come at the right moment and that either a temporary or permanent Chaplain will arrive by the time that we have our full quota of patients and will need him for supporting both them and the staff.

I was sorry to hear about your brother but am glad that he is being so well cared for. I hope you have been able to see something of him yourself.

The Right Reverend the Lord Bishop of Stepney

London

26 July 1967 You should not be writing to thank me – it is I who should be writing to thank you. I am sure no Hospice was ever dedicated with such love and sincerity and in better words.[103] You made me feel safe when I first went to see you in 1960 and now you have given this confidence to everyone here.

We love having your mother-in-law and we will do our best to keep her happy and it is nice to think that it means that Patricia will be coming to see us when you are home from Ireland, and will be in close touch.

Everyone was tired but so thankful for our lovely day on Monday, and today we are having our first Communion Service, with two patients down from the ward in their beds so we have really gone straight on with the important things.

Dr F. R. Gusterson[104]

Pulborough, Sussex

16 August 1967 I am sorry I was not able to write to you by August 15th, and have only just got round to replying to your letter. However, as I know how long everything takes and I have talked with you on the telephone I hope this will be alright.

----

[103] The hospice was dedicated by the Bishop of Stepney and opened officially by HRH Princess Alexandra, on 24 July 1967.

[104] Dr Francis ('Gus') Gusterson, founder of St Barnabas Hospice, Worthing, which subsequently opened in 1973.

Thoughts have come into my mind as I look at your memorandum as follows:-

1 I think you should certainly have at least one nurse on your Council and, if possible, find your Matron at this stage and have her in on your discussions with the architect.

2 I am glad you already have contact with the statutory body concerned because I am quite certain that it is impossible to run a Home of this kind without contractual arrangements for at least some of the beds. I think all these contacts need to be rather personal and the Regional Hospital Board certainly likes to be kept in touch throughout developments.

3 I heartily concur with your idea of avoiding fund raising professionals and would recommend that you concentrate on personal application where you have an introduction to some member of a Trust.

4 At this stage I do not think it is wise to print but rather to duplicate any memoranda you produce. Each one needs to be slanted to the Trust to which you are applying and, in any case, one's thinking alters and develops as the plans continue. You do, however, I think need some kind of visual aid and I would recommend that your Architect produces something in the way of sketch plans and the Quantity Surveyor is asked to give you the cost of these so that you really know for what you are asking.

5 I would also recommend that you consider having some mixture in the type of patients you take. It is not helpful to your future waiting list to become know as a Home for the Dying, or a Home for cancer patients exclusively. Long-stay patients, temporary in/out visits and convalescence for those difficult to place elsewhere are possible ideas.

6 There is no doubt that there is a great need in your area and I think you would find this confirmed by the Marie Curie Homes Committee. I do wish you the very best of luck and hope that we may see you, and your Architect also, at St Christopher's sometime.

Dr Donald P. Conwell

Department of Public Health Education and Welfare, Arlington, USA

13 November 1967 I feel very guilty that I did not reply more quickly to your letter of September 19th. Some of the delay was caused because of my change of address and the rest because of the pressures of opening St Christopher's. We have had a splendid but most demanding time. We have just added to our staff a Catholic Nun from Kansas City,[105] who having done 25 years in religion as a nurse, tutor and administrator, has come for 6 months post-graduate experience. She is an immense asset and I hope that she will learn as much from us as we from her.

I am enclosing a copy of our plans but must emphasis that all the out-patient work at the moment is still a dream and that getting the first two wards really working is as demanding as it is exciting. I shall be delighted to keep in touch and let you know how we are going on.

---

[105] Sister Zita Marie Cotter; see letter to her of 13 August 1964, p. 74.

I know you will be pleased to hear what a tremendous success the "Grasshoppers" are – to all our efforts I would add their contribution – they pray, they sew, one of them is really an assistant chaplain, friend and shopper for the patients, another looks after the plants – but the stability of their living in their wing so happily gives most of all.

With greetings to you both from Verena Weist and myself – do come and see us in the midst of it all some day!

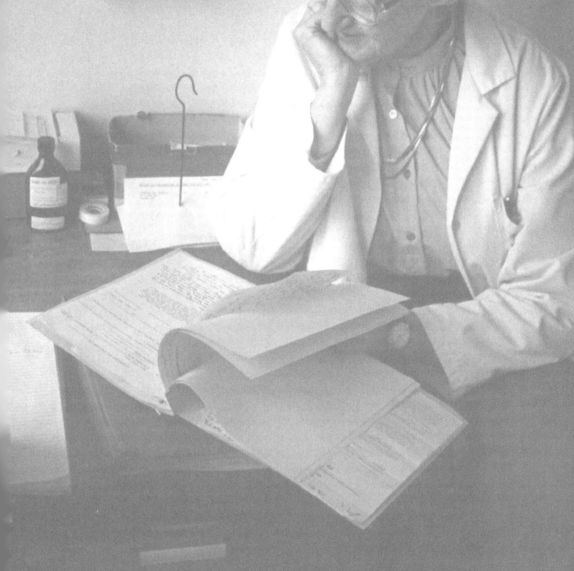

Part 2

The expansive years (1968–1985)

The opening of St Christopher's Hospice marked the culmination of one aspect of Cicely Saunders' vocation, but also the mere beginning of its true purpose. For now the work of the hospice had to be developed in earnest, and its ideas and principles would require testing in practice. Above all it should begin to serve as a source of inspiration to so many others, elsewhere in Britain and around the world. From the opening of the hospice in the summer of 1967 to the autumn of 1985, a period of seventeen years, Cicely Saunders was its Medical Director. The job involved a huge quantum of daily clinical work and numerous organizational responsibilities. Concerns about finance were never far away. There was also the constant round of travelling, lecturing, and writing. With all this came a growing recognition for the movement which she had founded and the global contribution she was making to improvement in the care of the dying. It brought a measure of fame which Cicely Saunders might hardly have contemplated in 1959. There were awards and honours, plaudits and frequent publicity. At the same time her personal life became more rewarding and eventually led to marriage. So we might characterize these as *expansive* years, professionally and personally rich, lived at full throttle.

Establishing St Christopher's

After the excitement of the official opening, it was necessary to begin to establish the daily routine of the hospice; new staff continued to be appointed, procedures and policies were developed and refined, and the credibility of the service in the local area had to be earned. At a symposium in October 1970 an overview of the work of the hospice emphasized several points (Saunders 1971). Despite a continuing reliance on charitable grants and gifts, the National Health Service now contributed two-thirds of the running costs; indeed the research programme together with the experimental outpatient and domiciliary service were at that time wholly supported by NHS funding. The hospice included fifty-four inpatient beds and the Drapers' Wing, of sixteen bed-sitting rooms for elderly people. Its teaching unit was now under construction, and over time a whole cohort of junior doctors would come to St Christopher's for their training, working closely not only with Cicely Saunders, but also with Tom West, her deputy. By 1970 some 400 patients died at the hospice each year and between 40 and 60 were discharged home, at least for a short time. Soon a majority of patients had their first encounter with the hospice's services in their own homes.

At the same time plans for other hospices, modelled substantially upon St Christopher's, were beginning to emerge in Sheffield, Manchester, Worthing, and elsewhere in the United Kingdom. There was a constant flow of communication between the staff of St Christopher's and others across the United Kingdom who shared similar aspirations. As a critical mass of enthusiasm developed, policy makers began to take a closer interest in the subject and the first national symposium on the care of the dying was held in London in November 1972, with the proceedings published in the *British Medical Journal* (Saunders 1973).

A paper by Cicely Saunders which appeared in 1968 in a Catholic quarterly elegantly captures St Christopher's orientation to care in the last stages of life (Saunders 1968). It calls for a positive approach which sees this as a time not of defeat, but of life's fulfilment, recognizing that there will be many different paths to life's ending. Here comfort and care become the prominent aims in a 'middle way' between too much and too little treatment, where understanding and compassion are vital. In subsequent years we see growing attention to notions of personhood, particularly in the family context. This greater focus on families was regarded as an important distinction between care at St Christopher's and earlier work at St Joseph's. The emphasis on *person* speaks in turn of a growing influence from psychology and theology on Cicely Saunders' developing thinking; here *person* is seen in interrelationship, and it is a matter of how the person is *being* in the face of physical deterioration. At such moments 'full-time concern for the patient' becomes essential. Elsewhere this is neatly captured in the statement that professional work in this area has two key dimensions: 'we are concerned *with persons* and we are concerned *as persons*' (Saunders 1972: 275).

But such caring, it is acknowledged, can be costly to those who give it. At St Christopher's the emphasis from the outset was upon the development of a multidisciplinary team, which could work together to explore the needs of individual patients at the deepest level, but which could also support and enrich itself, not only through the inclusion of a range of professional perspectives, but also by the involvement of volunteers, as well as the children of staff and also the elderly residents living in the Drapers' Wing. By these means a sense of community was fostered and enriched which might also serve to ameliorate the consequences of work involving constant exposure to loss, sorrow, and bereavement. In this context some attention is needed to the support of staff, and this was fostered at St Christopher's through small-group discussion and the regular involvement of the psychiatrist, Colin Murray Parkes.

Between 1970 and 1974 a working party of the Church of England Board of Social Responsibility sought to develop an Anglican contribution to the debate on euthanasia and two of the chapters in the group's report were drafted by Cicely Saunders (Saunders 1975). All members endorsed the recommendations, including the undesirability of extending the term euthanasia to incorporate the withdrawal of artificial means of preserving life or to include the use of pain-relieving drugs which may marginally shorten life; the recognition that if all care of the dying was at the standard of the best then there would be no prima facie case for euthanasia; and finally the belief that such standards are more hindered by ignorance than by money and staff shortages. A few years later Cicely Saunders was active in commenting on and expressing opposition to Baroness Wootton's Incurable Patients Bill of 1976, wherein she feared the *right* to die might be interpreted by some as a *duty*. Likewise, in 1977 and 1978, she took part in debates at the Royal Society of Health and the Union Society, Cambridge, where in each case motions in support of the legalization of euthanasia were defeated. Her position was clear: euthanasia is not a matter of desisting from active treatment, it is a killing act and the person who requests it has been failed in some way by others. She did acknowledge, however, that both sides in the euthanasia debate have a vendetta against pointless pain and impersonal indignity, though their solutions are of course radically different.

From the outset there was an emphasis on the science and the art of caring at St Christopher's.

The early research programme had three predominant themes: psychosocial studies of grief and bereavement; attempts to evaluate the St Christopher's approach in relation to other forms of care organization; and pharmacological work on the relative merits of different narcotics and their management. These endeavours marked a consolidation of the work of the early founders of terminal care in the late 1950s and early 1960s (Clark 1999).

Nevertheless, in a 1973 volume on health services research, it could be stated quite starkly: 'The position of terminal care in this country is at present unsatisfactory' (Saunders and Winner 1973: 19). Although interest in research into terminal care was growing, much of it remained descriptive and anecdotal and high-quality work was desperately needed to promote a rational approach to the care of the dying. Small achievements could therefore be significant, as when Cicely Saunders was asked to contribute a chapter on terminal care to a volume on the scientific foundations of oncology (Saunders 1976) and the editors thought it necessary to explain their reasons for including a contribution from such an under-developed medical field whose scientific foundations were only just being laid.

By 1978 some important evidence was emerging from research studies conducted at St Christopher's. Work by Colin Murray Parkes showed that unrelieved pain, as reported later by families, was found among 8 per cent of patients at St Christopher's Hospice, compared to 20 per cent of those in local hospitals and 29 per cent of those being cared for at home. Building on the work of Robert Twycross, it was also possible to state beyond reasonable doubt that morphine had become the preferred analgesic to diamorphine, and that the previously much heralded mixtures containing alcohol and cocaine should be discontinued (Saunders 1978). A constant stream of enquiries about drug regimens flowed into the hospice from all around the world, and these frequently required careful and detailed responses, not only in the giving of clinical advice, but also in offering support for strategic and policy changes oriented to improving opioid availability elsewhere.

Despite the concern for research, Cicely Saunders could also observe that whereas 'science tries to look at things in their generality in order to *use* them; art tries to observe things – and people – in their individuality in order to *know* them' (1971: 37). So in the photographs which she used in her lectures and publications, many of them taken by her American friend Grace Goldin, there could be seen the daily character of care at St Christopher's and the rich and stimulating environment it offered. Patients were encouraged to write about their experiences in prose and poetry; others made drawings and paintings which served as a window on suffering. Such an approach was also fostered through the sense of St Christopher's as a community in which many who served felt supported by some form of religious commitment.

By 1976 *Nursing Times* was publishing a revised set of the articles which had originally appeared and had caused so much interest in 1959. There was a sense that the field of terminal and palliative care was beginning to consolidate. There were opportunities to review changes which had occurred over the previous seventeen years and to address new debates and issues, such as 'living wills', 'furore therapeutics', and 'meddlesome medicine'. By now the increasing use of the term *palliative care* was coming to denote the transferability of ideas developed in the hospice into other settings, including hospital and home. In 1978 Cicely Saunders' first book, which it is clear from her correspondence so many had awaited for so long, finally appeared. It was an edited volume with many contributors who had been involved directly with the work of St Christopher's. Her first chapter was important in opening up a debate about the relationship of terminal care to the 'cure' and 'care' systems, arguing that no patient should be inappropriately locked into one or other system (Saunders 1978). By the early 1980s she was at even greater pains to suggest that the 'terminal' condition of a patient may not be an irreversible state (Saunders 1981) and 'active', 'palliative', and 'terminal' care could each be seen as overlapping categories.

The professional and clinical achievements of these years cannot be allowed, however, to mask the organizational issues and difficulties which also had to be overcome. There were losses which affected the whole of St Christopher's. In 1970 Dr Ron Welldon, the hospice's first research fellow, died suddenly, the news reaching Cicely Saunders just as she was about to give a lecture in the United States. The following year the death of Lord Thurlow after a period of illness marked the loss of a chairman in whom she had great confidence. Other blows could rain down. There was unwelcome publicity following the screening on German television of a film about the hospice. There were periodic financial crises, including a major one in 1974. And sometimes visitors to the hospice, on writing up their experiences, could say critical things about staff morale and the management culture, which was said to be authoritarian and inflexible, concerned only for the patients and not for the staff. By 1979 a Foundation Group was looking again at the early statement of aim and basis, which had been drafted by Olive Wyon, but could find little reason for any significant reorientation.

In 1980 St Christopher's held its first international conference, characterized as the hospice's 'bar mitzvah' and involving participants from seventeen different countries, the proceedings of which were subsequently published (Saunders, Summers, and Teller 1981). The contributions contain a growing conviction that the work of the hospice should be integrated with general medical practice, forming a complementary resource and service. Indeed, there was now a growing confidence that ideas and influences developed in the world of charitable hospices were beginning to affect the mainstream healthcare system.

Wider influence

Another way in which the reputation of St Christopher's was established in these years was through continued writing and publication. Between 1967 and 1985 Cicely Saunders produced, individually and with others, around eighty-five publications; they appeared in several languages and numerous countries. She wrote for clinical journals and prestigious textbooks; for religious publications; and for the wider public. During these years three clinical and organizationally oriented books on hospice and palliative care appeared, and one of them was soon produced in a second edition. There was also a collection of poems and prose pieces produced for patients, families, and professionals encountering suffering and disease – an early example of a contribution to the *medical humanities*. Her work appeared in the proceedings of symposia and conferences, it was described in magazines and newspapers and became the subject of documentary films. Links with overseas colleagues produced a growing cross-fertilization of ideas. It was contact with the Montreal surgeon Balfour Mount, for example, which led to the increasing adoption after 1974 of the term 'palliative care' to describe the work which was being undertaken.

Over this period there was also a growing reflection on the state of the 'movement' which was developing around hospices and similar centres. As her work matured, we see Cicely Saunders reflecting more on the origins of homes and hospices for the dying. We also see an increasing recognition that palliative care is something which can be developed in many modes and settings. It can be extended beyond its initial successes with cancer patients to include those with non-malignant conditions, initially motor neurone disease, and in due course the challenge of caring for people with AIDS. Above all, its major purpose comes to be seen as the improvement of care within the mainstream setting; not through the continuing proliferation of hospice units, many of them independent charitable organizations, but rather through education and training and the broader diffusion of appropriate knowledge, skills, and attitudes. Accordingly, we see at this time the first discussions taking place about the creation of national representative bodies which will promote the interests of hospice and palliative care more widely. Two key examples are *Help the Hospices* and the *Association of Hospice Doctors* (later the Association of Palliative Medicine).

Of course St Christopher's Hospice had a vital role to play in these processes. Initially it was the only centre for specialized education and training in the new field of terminal care. We therefore see in the correspondence in this section of the book evidence of the tidal wave of requests from around the world to visit, to work, and to spend time at the hospice. Initially these were encouraged, even fostered. By 1975 there were 2000 visitors per annum; special times were set aside for visitors each week, and in due course some visits were conducted in French. They had to be contained within special slots within the week; sometimes too, as the letters show, there could be irritation at those who wished to make extravagant journeys to St Christopher's at the expense of overlooking growing expertise nearer to home.

There were also many who wished Cicely Saunders, increasingly acknowledged as the founder of the modern hospice movement, to come to them. From the late 1950s, she had developed a special relationship with colleagues in the United States (Clark 2001) and made three important visits there before the opening of St Christopher's. In her years as Medical Director she visited North America around a dozen times and developed close professional links as well as an enduring friendship with Balfour Mount and the palliative care service at the Royal Victoria Hospital, Montreal, regularly attending the international conferences which he hosted every two years from 1976. First visits were made over several years to many countries, including Yugoslavia, Belgium, Australia, Israel, and South Africa.

Her network of collaborators expanded, her influence and reputation grew. In time formal honours began to appear, first in 1969 in the award of an Honorary D.Sc. from Yale University, but soon from many other parts of academe, in the United States, Britain, and elsewhere. She was made a Fellow of the Royal College of Physicians in 1974 and was awarded the Lambeth Doctorate of Medicine by the Archbishop of Canterbury in 1977. There were honorary doctorates from the Open University in 1978 and from Columbia University and Iona College (both New York) in 1979. In that same year she became the first woman to receive the Worshipful Society of Apothecaries' (London) Gold Medal in Therapeutics. In 1980 she became a Dame of the British Empire, adding to the Order of the British Empire which she had already received in 1965. In 1981 she became a Fellow of the Royal College of Nursing and also received the prestigious Templeton Prize, awarded for outstanding contributions in the field of religion. In 1983 she was awarded the Cabrini Gold Medal. The early 1980s in particular saw a long string of honorary doctorates and one fellowship from universities and colleges in Britain, America, and Canada: Creighton University, Omaha, together with Marymount Manhattan College, New York, and the University of Western Ontario (1981); Jewish Theological Seminary, New York (1982); the universities of Essex, Leicester, London, and Sheffield (1983); as well as Queen's University, Belfast, and the University of Kent (1984). A further mark of recognition came in 1982, when Shirley du Boulay embarked on a biography of Cicely Saunders, which was duly published two years later (du Boulay 1984).

Health and happiness

A schedule such as this would inevitably make huge demands on personal resources. A life devoted to giving needed also to receive support and nourishment, both through the realm of faith and also in relationships with others. Cicely Saunders was capable of prodigious quantities of work at this time, but she could also be vulnerable to illness. A life lived out in the public domain also needed to foster some private areas for reflection, recuperation, and intimacy.

In 1968 Cicely Saunders' mother died in St Christopher's; she had remained active up to the end and her loss seemed capable of acceptance. Then, just over two years after the hospice opened, there was a long period of sick leave, from the autumn of 1969 to March 1970. Complications after a hysterectomy, followed by the side effects of influenza and then a recurrence of long-running back problems all conspired to keep the St Christopher's Medical Director away from her work. Even so the hospice's programme continued and after that good health seemed to return.

From 1963 her relationship with the artist Marian Bohusz-Szyszko had been developing, slowly and intermittently. He was born in Poland in 1901 and had studied fine art and painting at the universities of Wilno and Cracow and the Warsaw Academy of Fine Arts. He spent most of World War II as a prisoner of war before making his way to Italy in 1945. Subsequently he settled in London where, in the autumn of 1963, he held a major retrospective at the Drian Galleries in Porchester Place. Here his work had come to the attention of Cicely Saunders. She fell in love with the paintings and then with him. She became his patron, and his work was prominently displayed in the hospice from the outset. He had professed his love for her, but was not free to marry. His long-estranged wife in Poland was still alive, he continued to support her financially, and his Catholic faith precluded any divorce. It seemed an arrangement that suited him, but over time an appropriate solution evolved. In 1969 Cicely Saunders moved from Lambeth to Sydenham to live closer to the hospice. There, with Polish friends of Marian, she purchased a house where two couples could share accommodation. They thought of it as their 'kibbutz' and it was to prove a lasting domestic arrangement. In 1975 Marian's wife died, but it was not until 31 January 1980, seventeen years after they had first met, that Cicely Saunders and Marian Bohusz-Szyszko were married. She was sixty-one and he seventy-nine. At first their news was kept secret to all but a tiny group of close friends, but gradually it became public and delighted many. Her last five years as the hospice Medical Director were spent as a married woman, secure in her status, and content as never before with her personal life.

References

Clark, D. (1999) Cradled to the grave? Terminal care in the United Kingdom, 1948–67. *Mortality*, **4**(3): 225–47.

Clark, D. (2001) A special relationship: Cicely Saunders, the United States and the early foundations of the hospice movement. *Illness, Crisis and Loss*, **9**(1): 15–30.

du Boulay, S. (1984) *Cicely Saunders: The founder of the modern hospice movement.* London: Hodder and Stoughton.

Saunders, C. (1968) The last stages of life. *Recover*, Summer: 26–9.

Saunders, C. (1971) The patient's response to treatment. A photographic presentation showing patients and their families. In *Catastrophic illness in the seventies: critical issues and complex decisions*. Proceedings of the Fourth National Symposium, 15–16 October 1970. New York: Cancer Care Inc., pp. 33–46.

Saunders, C. (1972) A therapeutic community: St Christopher's Hospice. In *Psychosocial aspects of terminal care* (ed. B. Schoenberg, A. C. Carr, D. Peretz, and A. H. Kutschereds). New York and London: Columbia University Press, pp. 275–89.

Saunders, C. (1973) A death in the family: a professional view. *British Medical Journal*, **1**(844): 30–1.

Saunders, C. (Member of Church of England Board of Social Responsibility Working Party) (1975) *On dying well: an Anglican contribution to the debate on euthanasia*. London: Church Information Office.

Saunders, C. (1976) The challenge of terminal care. In *The scientific foundations of oncology*. London: Heinemann, pp. 673–9.

Saunders, C. (1978) Appropriate treatment, appropriate death. In *The management of terminal malignant disease* (ed. C. Saunders). London, Edward Arnold.

Saunders, C. (1981) Current views on pain relief and terminal care. In *The therapy of pain* (ed. M. Swerdlow). Lancaster: MTP Press, pp. 215–41.

Saunders, C. and Winner, A. (1973) Research into terminal care of cancer patients. In *Portfolio for Health 2. The developing programme of the DHSS in health services research*. Published for the Nuffield Provincial Hospitals Trust by the Oxford University Press, pp. 19–25.

Saunders, C., Summers, D., and Teller, N. (1981) *Hospice: the living idea*. London: Edward Arnold.

Letters, 1968–1985

Dr Robert Twycross

Lancaster

26 March 1968 It is now some months since you called in and unfortunately missed me, and I am wondering how things are going with you. I think you were tackling your Membership, and I hope it went well.

I know you are very interested in this field and it occurred to me the other day when I was thinking around the problems of starting our Pain Clinic and launching our analgesic research that you might possibly be interested in doing this for a year or two. We have a grant of registrar level salary waiting for the right person. We have a Research Committee which is in the process of planning the work and a possible Nurse Observer interested in doing the day-to-day chores concerned.

I do not want to 'bounce' you into anything but it occurred to me that as you are interested in this field you might like to do this and get some slightly unusual experience at this stage, and that it might fit into your programme – and to ours also![1]

Let me know what you think about this and do come and see us again – but not during the first three weeks of May when I shall be away on holiday.

Mother Leo Frances

Mother House, Sister of Charity of Leavenworth, Xavier, Kansas, USA

13 May 1968 I think Sister Zita Marie will reach you just about the same time as this letter. I saw her safely off on Saturday last with great regret that the end of her time at St Christopher's had come.

I cannot begin to tell you what a blessing it has been for us to have her for these six months and she goes with grateful love from everybody here. Surely our Lord knew how much we were needing her faith and enthusiasm at this early stage of our work and she has made a contribution to our daily life and our thought and prayer which will always remain as one of our very precious foundation stones. Her faith is the kind that lights up that of others and her willingness to expose her own thoughts makes it easier for others to understand and contribute their own. So she has not only helped very many of our patients with the physical and spiritual burdens of their illness, and helped them to a happy death, but also enriched our own possibilities of continuing to do the same. She has given all this with such gaiety and cheerfulness that we feel at the moment rather as if a light has gone out.

I hope that perhaps in the future her experience here will also bear fruit in the work of your own Community. I am sure that this is one of the unmet needs of our day and a place where the positive values of Christianity stand out in great contrast to modern thought, or refusal of thought about death. The number of visitors we have here impresses us daily of the need for such Christian contribution, not only to the care of the patients we have and of their families, but also in teaching many students and graduates in the medical and nursing fields. It would

---

[1] In the event Robert Twycross did not join the hospice until 1971, and the medical research post went to Ron Welldon, who died in 1970.

be a great joy to have links in such work in the future with your Order should this develop. But whatever happens in the future we have some wonderful memories here and once again send our grateful thanks to you for sparing Sister Zita Marie for so long.

With our prayers and best wishes for your future work and for your Chapter this summer.

Florence Wald

Connecticut, USA

18 June 1968 Thank you for your letter. Splendid! We are so much looking forward to having you. Do telephone me when you arrive in London (778-9252) and then we will get everything organised.

There is no need for you to bring anything with you except your shoes and things. We can supply you with some of our own uniforms but do just what you like. How I am looking forward to it but I hope you have a good holiday first because we are quite hard work!

Mrs W. Pearce

Seal Beach, California, USA

3 September 1968 Thank you so much for your letter. We were really fortunate in that my mother[2] died here and she was really on "the crest of the wave" and happier than she had been for many years or, indeed, at any time in her life I think. She was driving her car until she had the first minor cerebral haemorrhage and was convalescing from that when she had a very severe one. So until a month before she died she was in full activity and we can only be thankful.

I knew Ida was thinking of moving but did not get her new address so I am wondering if you would share your Newsletter with her as there has been a hold-up because of this in sending one direct to her.

I am coming to the US to give a lecture in Philadelphia and am just collecting up one or two engagements in California to earn enough to get over to see you and also to see Sister Zita Marie in New Mexico on the return journey. She was a tremendous asset here and I shall enjoy seeing a new part of the country.

I am delighted to hear all your news and that you seem so well and energetic!

Reuben A. Holden

Secretary, Yale University, USA

15 November 1968 Your letter has just reached me and I am most deeply honoured by it. Nothing would give me more pleasure than to accept the honorary degree of Doctor of Science from the President and Fellows of Yale University, and I shall be grateful if you will convey my thanks to them.

I could arrange to take some holiday around the time of the Commencement Exercises of the University and will be very glad to attend.

---

2 Christian Saunders (née Knight) b. 1889, d. 16 May 1968.

I know that this honour expresses your concern for the care of the patients I attempt to represent and St Christopher's as a whole will feel that it is linked with Yale University.

I am sure you know we had Mrs Florence Wald with us for three weeks this summer and we hope perhaps there may be other exchanges. We found her visit of very great value as well as enjoyment.

I will look forward very much to meeting you next summer. My thanks are really those of St Christopher's as a whole.

Florence Wald

Connecticut, USA

14 January 1969 Bless you for your letter. I have copied out one paragraph for both my brothers as they have both at various times had business trips to the USA and might be able to manage something! It would be lovely to have someone there.

We loved your other letter, which is still on the board, and we are very thrilled at the thought of St Christopher's in the field.[3]

I would certainly enjoy discussing Protocol but I do not think I must let the whole trip be more than a week or ten days at the most; but I must admit that I would wait years for a pilliated woodpecker!

Sue Ryder

Sue Ryder Foundation, Suffolk

4 February 1969 We much enjoyed Dr Hessek's visit and I think you have certainly found someone who will work for all the right things as hard as he can. He impressed us very much, patients as well as staff, and we were glad to give him a gay week-end at Professor Bohusz's Name Day party, and a spate of classical music to finish up with. If he has extra time and another day or two spare in London we would love to have him back again.

When we were talking about the quality of our nursing staff here we offered to have a nurse from Poland to work here for some three months. We have had several people from abroad as well as from different parts of the British Isles and believe that three months is really needed for a proper learning visit. He is going to try and arrange this from his end and will I expect already have talked to you about this. We would be able to provide accommodation and pay Nursing Auxiliary rate of salary (I am almost certain we do not have reciprocal registration and would not be able to give her full registration salary). We would love to do this and if possible in time for the opening of your new pavilion at Olztyn.

More than any other visitor I think he has made us realise how blessed we are in the amount of space, equipment and so on we have here; one should not be ashamed of one's blessings I suppose but only continue to give thanks and try to use them with proper responsibility.

I do not need to tell you how important it is that the place should be a community of some kind if the individual people are going to be able to go on with the very demanding

---

[3] A reference to the plans which Florence Wald and others were making to establish America's first modern hospice, in Connecticut, USA.

work, and there are two things above all that I would love to feel he could aim for at Olztyn. I would suggest that if possible you should add two good sized rooms to your next pavilion, one for the use of families to sit, either with the patients or on their own if they are waiting around, and the other for a playroom for children of married staff and/or volunteers. Dr Hessek was obviously impressed by the way we have found both these things help in the life of the Hospice and with the morale of patients, families and staff. He is quite aware that these two ideas of volunteers and people coming to work with children to be parked in a play group, as so many of ours do, would be new and might be difficult to carry out.

It would be quite impossible to experiment with either of these ideas without space but no space would ever be wasted should this not come off. I think myself he really needs somehow to have a corner for someone to organise volunteers and perhaps you might think of this when you are planning the office accommodation, which I know is in short supply anyway!

I think volunteers must be a very strange idea to Poles, so many of whom have to do two jobs in order to survive, but we are very impressed by what they contribute here. But it is important that if they are going to be used adequately there must be someone to organise them.

I would love to come and see you when I visit Cavendish on April 17th, and perhaps I could slip in about tea-time.

Margaret G Arnstein

Yale School of Nursing, Connecticut, USA

17 April 1969 I wonder whether my visit in June is now allowed to be known officially? I am building plans for a holiday around the visit and must apply for some money above our rather meagre travel allowance. It would be a help if I could say officially why I am going!

Also I would love to know what sort of clothes I shall need to wear, that is, what colour is the gown and do you wear as we do at Oxford, a "sub-fusc", which consists of a black coat and skirt or equivalent with a white blouse, and black shoes and stockings? I guess you probably do not do anything like that but I probably need something discreet and the equivalent of the male dark suit. Also what am I likely to have to wear for the Principal's Dinner the evening before?

I am so much looking forward to this. I am going to have about a week's holiday with a friend in Montana and then fly to you at the week-end preceding June 9th. After leaving Yale I hope to spend a couple of nights with Marty Hermann before coming back here.

Dr Claire F. Ryder

Department of Health, Education and Welfare, Virginia, USA

27 June 1969 It was an absolutely wonderful experience to be at Yale and to realise that the care of the dying was of sufficient concern with the University for me to be honoured with a degree. I have the very strong feeling that every single patient I had ever looked after, including the group you visited with me so long ago at St Joseph's, were on the platform or around somewhere on that occasion. Anyway, someone managed to burst a balloon which bobbed in front of my brother's camera at the crucial moment; it exploded quite inexplicably so that the proper photograph was duly taken!

I am now writing to let you know that I am going to have to be really fierce with myself in my autumn trip. I have just had a couple of days' investigation in hospital and, *although there is nothing whatever to worry about*, I do have to be a bit more sensible than I usually am on such trips. I am very fit indeed at the moment but there is a chance that I have an elective, unworrying operation hanging over my head. I am sticking to my initial programme of Boston, a short stay in New York and then Philadelphia, going on to Duke University and then to New Mexico for a few days holiday before returning home. I feel that I just must leave Washington out. This is very disappointing as I would absolutely love to see you again, but I have to be sensible for once in my life.

In any case, I do find that I hate being away from St Christopher's too long and this very viable and happy institution does have its teething problems and I should not really be away and let them accumulate for too long.

Dr Esther Lucile Brown

San Francisco, USA

27 June 1969 I have just returned from the very memorable visit to Yale and after a brief two days in hospital, I am managing to catch up with everything. One of my first letters is to you because I have to write with great regret that, after all your efforts on my behalf, to say that it just looks impossible to extend my time on your side of the Atlantic this coming autumn as long as I had hoped. I do not think I ought to come to San Francisco at all, after all.

Whilst you are drawing breath and saying what you think of me for this, let me hasten to explain. In the first place I find that I have got an entirely unworrying and elective operation rather hanging over my head and, although I am not at all worried about this and am extremely fit at the moment, it is obviously not going to be very sensible for me to give myself such a testing programme as I had originally hoped to fulfil. Secondly, I have come back to the Hospice to find that, although it has managed well enough in my time away, it is not yet really established sufficiently to be too happy with my absence for more than two or three weeks at a time. This probably sounds as if I have not managed to establish a viable institution, but you must remember that we are not quite two years old. I know that other people can do pretty well everything but a child of two years old does rather need its mother to feel sufficiently secure. Dr Winner is more than able to take my place but is only part-time and has got her pretty heavy commitments for the next year or two.

I will write direct to Anselm Strauss and to Dr Weinstein and Professor Kaldman. I do not want to emphasise my potential need of medical care but I think I have to in order to make my apology adequate and it is the reason that has tipped the balance. I would have managed everything else but this, I feel has to have proper consideration.

I am going to suggest to Anselm Strauss that, as he is probably already in touch with Dr Melvin Krant, of the Lemuel Shattuck Hospital of Boston, he may be interested to know that Dr Krant has visited here and is setting up a Conference in Boston at the end of September when I shall first be over in the States. I feel in many ways that, if they could get together, if they haven't already done so, it would be an extremely valuable thing.

I spoke to Sister Zita Marie while I was over and, whatever happens, I am going to finish up with her in New Mexico. I think I shall make my way there from Duke University, which I shall be visiting after Philadelphia, and then come straight back home from there.

Messrs Cottrell and Leonard

Albany, USA

8 July 1969 I was very happy to receive an honorary Doctorate of Science at Yale University this June. I have your address from the Hood which was presented to me on that occasion but I was only loaned the cap and gown to go with it and now wish to acquire these.

I wonder if you can give me some idea of the cost of the cap and gown and also whether the blue gown which I saw various people wearing (although not those on the platform with me) is acceptable. If this is so I would much prefer it. If the cost is very great it is obviously not going to be easy for me to produce the dollars although I have a small quantity from an honorarium received at the conference on that occasion. If I find that the cost is prohibitive I wonder if there is any possibility of you sending a specification so that I can have the gown made over here.

The Reverend W. Benjamin Holmes

Church of St Martin-in-the-Fields, Philadelphia, USA

6 August 1969 Cancel everything! I have to go in for surgery – only an hysterectomy for fibroids but to battle on with pills seems to be no longer possible and my staff have put down their collective feet. I go in about ten days' time and dare not think that I shall be fit for an American trip by October. I do not feel so badly about you because you are so relaxed and understanding about it all, but when I think of what must be being said about me in the Pennsylvania Hospital, my spirit fails me.

However, one does not plan these things and there appears to be no choice in the matter. Perhaps it will be only a postponement as there are so many people in Philadelphia and, if they are prepared to see me after all this, I hope it may be possible to make plans for another time.

Major General the Lord Thurlow

Etchingham, Sussex

8 August 1969 I was delighted to hear your voice at home the other day and hope all is going well. May I send you the official greetings of the Council with their hope that you will speedily be quite better, but insistence that you do not try to do too much too soon.

I have to retire to hospital in a week or so. It is nothing serious but I shall probably be off for about two months. We are fortunate in having a young locum and I am sure all will be well. I will come back here to convalesce as I shall be far better looked after here than in a flat on my own!

Henry and Florence Wald

Connecticut, USA

24 November 1969 Don't worry too much about our deficit. I am on an all-out drive to raise funds and I am sure it will come. I think I shall get beds endowed through the

Teaching Hospitals and some of the big givers but probably in the meantime we shall have to live by faith, as usual, and the money will come just as it is needed.

John Brown

College of Aeronautics, Cranfield

2 December 1969 I do not know whether you will recall that right back in 1964 I wrote to you after reading your talk "The Shrinking Consciousness" which was reprinted in The Listener. You wrote me a note at the time and I have often quoted from this from time to time in lectures.

It seemed unlikely then that our fields should overlap but I am now writing about an idea that has occurred to me. You will see from the enclosed Annual Report and newsletter that we have a certain financial problem for the maintenance of St Christopher's. I am not too depressed about this because since writing it I have already been promised support for the extension of the Out-Patients side and also two hospitals have agreed to support a patient for six months or the equivalent thereof and others are interested. This means, I hope, that our contractual arrangements will rise again to a reasonable figure at our increased costs.

It is on the question of increased costs that I feel we must make continual efforts. It is very difficult indeed, of course, to measure value and particularly value of such intangible things as listening and doing things slowly and treating people as individuals. It would be nice, however, if we had some outside and objective assessment of the difference between the care we give and that of other places whose charges are nearly half. I am extremely loath to have an ordinary management consultant here, not only because we could not afford it but also because the staff find it a very threatening procedure and as we are such a new institution I think this would be very difficult for them to bear. However, it occurred to my brother, a member of our council and an ex-member of McKinseys, that some place such as your college might have a good student who needed a project for the summer and who might come here and look at something quite different from the usual management enquiry. Obviously there is a great deal of thought needed about such projects but before I discuss it with our committee here my deputy and I feel that we would very much like to have your views on the subject.

I am sorry to write at such length and give you rather a lot to read as well but I hope you will forgive me and if there is any chance of such an idea being a possibility could we have your ideas on the subject.

Dr Avery D. Weisman[4]

Massachusetts General Hospital, Boston, USA

23 March 1970 I am sorry to have been so long in answering your letter of 14th January 1970, but I am afraid I only got back today from a rather prolonged sick leave. Due to an oversight your letter was not acknowledged in my absence.

---

4   Dr Weisman later became a Professor of Psychiatry at Harvard Medical School; Cicely Saunders was particularly interested in his notion of 'an appropriate death': see A. D. Weisman, *On dying and denying. A psychiatric study of terminality* (New York: Behavioral Publications, 1972).

The invitation to St Christopher's was, I hope, taken for granted by you and you would be welcome to come for as long as you like. I think probably the best plan would be for you to stay for two days, if you can, and for this to include a Tuesday when we have staff meetings which you could attend: I would be grateful if you would perhaps be prepared to discuss your own work with us.

I expect you will be visiting with Colin Murray Parkes – I am not sure which particular field you want to follow up, or quite what to suggest, especially as you have probably discussed it with him recently. Presumably you know all about our "Samaritans" and will be seeing the Reverend Chad Varah.

You may be interested to see our brochure we have just produced for prospective patients and their families. We are, I think, justifiably anxious that we should not have an "abandon hope" atmosphere. It seems essential to do this as it is often only when patients really feel safe with us that they begin to face up to what is happening at all.

Dr Robert Twycross
Romiley, Cheshire

30 April 1970 I hope that you have had our Newsletter at your new address.

I assume that you are now working in the Manchester Royal Infirmary itself. I wonder how things are going with you and whether you are still interested in terminal care? We filled the post that I wrote to you about with a Senior Registrar in Psychiatry, and the Department is flourishing although beset with illness, like all the doctors in the Hospice at the moment.

I am writing now because I am really interested in what you are thinking and doing and also to know whether you have heard of the project for St Anne's in Manchester. If you are still interested in this type of work I think you would like to meet the people concerned with it.

I know there is little time for anything when you are a Registrar but it would be nice to hear from you.

Mrs Y. Dale
Woking, Surrey

14 May 1970 I promised that I would write you a letter about some of the problems on starting new Homes for terminal care.

I think in the first place you must realise that it is going to involve much more work and much more expense than one can possible envisage at the moment.[5] I feel strongly myself that a project like this should not be embarked upon unless one literally cannot help it because the compulsion that it is the right thing is so strong.

If you are going to have such heavy nursing cases you will need either a purpose built place or somewhere that has excellent reconstruction. It is not ideal to nurse these patients in single, or even in double rooms; they are lonely and it is much heavier on the nurses both emotionally and physically. We find that we are really like an acute intensive care unit and

---

[5] In fact a hospice appeal was not launched in Woking until the early 1990s and the Woking Hospice received its first patients on 5 December 1996.

need a nursing ratio of one-to-one (this means one nurse to one patient over a whole year, including night duty, holidays and such "unproductive" persons as Matron and her deputy). If we had single rooms I think it would be more difficult still to give the kind of care these patients really need. It is very important that they live until they die, and this is more than just keeping them safely in bed and free from pain.

You will need above all a doctor who is really interested in this work. It will not do to have the patients just looked after by their general practitioners; they will find it hard to come in regularly and some of them may not be interested. Those who do come in will often order different things and different routines and make it extremely difficult for the Ward Sister to keep her drug rounds and the rest on a rational basis. They should certainly be encouraged to make social and semi-clinical visits if they wish but I think your ideal would be a married woman doctor who would act as a clinical assistant and co-ordinate everything on a daily visit. I know some Homes only have a doctor once or twice a week but I do not believe that this is enough.

You will get staffing problems whether you anticipate them or not but this is rewarding nursing and once you begin to tap married part-timers and the cadet nurses and have a proper supply of volunteers you will be alright – apart from the devastating crises such as when all the children have measles etc.!

I think in one way or another you must get round the problem of identification solely with cancer or death. In our case we have a mixed group of patients and also an out-patient clinic with a visiting Sister. I think the latter would be difficult to incorporate into a small unit but if you had the good fortune to be linked with a group practice which had a Health Visitor or nurse closely associated with it then perhaps you could have such a liaison to fill this need. We find increasingly that the fact that we can visit quite a large number of patients in their own homes before they come to us means not only that they come at the right moment – right psychologically as well as physically – but also that their families feel much happier about the whole thing. We have had tremendous help from nearly all the local family doctors as we develop this work. Another possible mixture is to have people in while relatives go on holiday or to have some patients with longer term illness.

You will have to think not only of raising money for capital but for maintenance. I think that you need to talk to your local Medical Officer of Health and then gradually consider informal discussions with relevant people in the Regional Hospital Board. You can by no means take it for granted that you will get contractual arrangements with the Regional Board, and it is very important to involve everyone like this at an early stage.

I think all this has to be thought through before you reach the stage of setting up as a charity with its own Council of really dedicated people. As I suggested, I think you should consider first of all talking with people who are doing something on the same sort of scale, such as Mrs Saunders-Brown (Cromer, Norfolk) and Coppercliff Nursing Home, whose leaflet you had, and who, incidentally, manage very well with single rooms.

There is no doubt at all that there is a tremendous need for Homes of this type, for the smaller ones as well as the larger ones like St Christopher's. You will have to find out how great the need is in your own area and go on from there.

Very good luck to you. Do let us know how you get on.

(If it is right, it will happen.)

PS I am sure you would like to know that Miss H slipped away very quickly after your visit – she was not at all afraid.

Marty Herrmann

New York, USA

3 June 1970 Bless you for your letter – I could feel nice loving wishes coming over the Atlantic and did not feel at all neglected. I am not exactly blooming as I am, at the moment, supported by a most uncomfortable surgical corset!

I shall be on holiday in July – from the 10th to the 24th. I would not miss a chance of seeing you and would love to see you at the Hospice again. Jane has planted us a wonderful mound now and it is going to be beautiful.

I am looking forward to the Symposium and also to staying with you. I hope to get over two or three days ahead of time, if that is all right. Please give Rene my greetings and say how much I look forward to coming to what I think of as my home in New York.

So glad you have had your kids with you and that you have a spell with Amy; very glad to hear that there is a job at a specially good place coming up.

Dr Esther Lucile Brown

San Francisco, USA

17 August 1970 Very many thanks indeed for "Nursing Reconsidered"[6] which arrived on my desk at the weekend. I have only had time to glance at it but I am looking forward to reading it myself before passing it on to our senior nurses.

You will be having another Newsletter from St Christopher's in the not too distant future but one piece of news will interest you which will probably not appear in the letter. We are at present having a visit from two members of the faculty of a School of Business Management. This plan was initiated some months back when I was very concerned about our finances and wished to have some objective assessment of our work in comparison with units caring for similar patients. At the same time I felt that after three years working we had probably reached the stage where we needed someone else to look at our organisation, formally and informally. We have been most fortunate in that two very able people have offered to do this for us in their vacation time for travelling expenses only. They are still in the early stages of their work but I am already finding it most helpful. The girl is working as one of our volunteers and visiting the different departments of the hospice. As she works she has time for informal discussions with the staff and she is obviously a very sensitive person so that although her time with us is comparatively short she has great awareness of what is going on and I feel optimistic that the final discussion and report will be very helpful.

Professor F. J. J. Buytendijk

Amsterdam, Holland

19 August 1970 I was very glad indeed to hear of you from Dr Zuyderduyn when he visited this hospice last June and now he has found your address for me.

---

6   E. L. Brown, *Nursing reconsidered. A study of change* (Philadelphia: J. B. Lippincott, 1970).

You may remember that I wrote to you after reading your book on "Pain" and we had some discussion one evening when I was staying in Amsterdam with my mother. Since then we have opened St Christopher's and have had a number of visitors from the Netherlands. I remember your concern that it would be very difficult to have such an institution in a small country but we have found that by having an out-patient clinic and domiciliary visiting service, some mixture of patients, but above all by coming to know the community around us, we do not seem to have the depressing and forbidding image some people fear. However, one is never able to control all one's public relations and I was sorry to have a letter from the Netherlands with the inclusion of "for the dying" in our title. It seems that this is being passed around and it is one of the reasons why I accepted the invitation to participate in the Conference on Cancer Chemotherapy in Leiden on September 5th.

Your work is of great interest to us here and I am glad to say that we have two psychiatrists,[7] one in charge of our research into the control of pain (both in the way of controlled clinical trial of drugs and in extra pharmacological effects) and the other concerned with problems of families during and after terminal illness.

I do not suppose there will ever be a chance of you visiting us but if you were in London we would welcome you most warmly.

Marty Herrmann
New York, USA

27 November 1970 I tried to call you but missed you in Washington but no doubt you had my message. I wanted just to say Good-bye and that I was tied up with my usual little bout of engine trouble. We were two hours late in leaving Dulles airport and an hour and a half arriving in London. However, dear Marian was safely there waiting for me and I had had some sleep in the plane as we were rather empty.

What I wanted to tell you was that while I was in Lexington I had a cable with the terribly sad news that Dr Ron Welldon, heading our research here, had died suddenly in his sleep. I am afraid that dreadfully careless thing of having sleeping pills beside you and taking extra by mistake. No doubt at all that it was by mistake, but devastating and an irreplaceable loss. He was a dear person and I have tried to express his originality in the obituary that I wrote for the Lancet. It was far better done by Chaplain Dobihal speaking at his memorial service here yesterday. That was a wonderful occasion in that the whole family managed to pile itself into the chapel and his small son of 9 months chatted away to himself all through. But oh dear, how very much we miss him.

It is good to be back though there is a lot to be done. I would never, never survive these trips if I did not have you to lean on. If anything good comes out of it you take a lot of the credit but I did enjoy it and I loved meeting everybody again and feeling that I have a real link.

The Reverend W. Benjamin Holmes
Church of St Martin-in-the-Fields, Philadelphia, USA

1 December 1970 Many thanks again to you both for giving me such a good visit. I thoroughly enjoyed it all.

---

[7] Colin Murray Parkes and John Hinton.

I know you have the newsletter but you have missed out on some reprints and I am sending some over by surface mail. They are a bit heavy to go with this. I am enclosing though some literature concerned with one of our doctors. I had the sad news of his sudden death by cable when I was in Lexington. It is not easy yet to believe fully that he has gone. I think you will see from the service and the other things the kind of person he was and what a very sad gap he is leaving. He was a most enabling person and certainly I used to go down to his department for solace. I now go down to the two girls there just as often and we have found ourselves forming a St Christopher's Weight-watchers with a considerable amount of hilarity. We must do something to keep us going over this initial phase. God knows where we will find the replacement and I do hope he will let us know soon.

I had the news just as I was going in to take a ward round and really Ron did that and certainly the big lecture that evening. I had an exceptionally nice thank-you letter after that saying that a candle had been lit. It was certainly lit by Ron about whom I did have to speak because I had to put together those two thoughts – 'Death is an outrage' and 'Death is all right', and Ron's fascinating way of turning things upside down. One does turn medicine upside down when you care for the dying and strange things happen when you do this. By that time I had met up with Sister Zita Marie and as when I called at the Hospice they were determined I should have my three days holiday with her we went on into Kentucky, near Gethsemane, Thomas Merton's Trappist monastery. We stayed in a Conference Centre run by the Sisters of Charity of Nazareth, Martin Luther King's Center and in that chapel there and in Gethsemane we really had a retreat and somehow it all got gathered up. The chapel is fascinating. It is the only cruciform building that I have been in that is so plain with so little decoration and an almost invisible crucifix that one was suddenly made to realise that the whole thing was the Cross and you had come inside. That, and the Gethsemane statues away up in the woods to which we plodded our way on a very rough path made up the retreat. If you ever have a chance to go there may I recommend it most heartily.

I refrained for so long because I found it impossible to go into retreat because my Father died while I was on one and suddenly I was given one without my volition and all was well.

Dr Elisabeth Kübler-Ross
Flossmoor, Illinois, USA

24 December 1970 Thank you very much for your card. I am afraid we were the same over addresses because you have my old one! It is always best to write to me here at St Christopher's.

I have wanted to have news of you and have been wondering about your mother. Just my thoughts and sympathy to you whatever has happened.

I have been meaning to write to you ever since I got back but life has been more than hectic as our young doctor in charge of research died suddenly just before I returned. He is a great personal loss. I had the cable just as I was going to lecture to the Medical School at Lexington. I found myself talking about death as an outrage and yet somehow that it was alright at one and the same time. Ron Welldon very much gave the lecture for me. Now we are very happy in that his wife and baby son seem to be establishing themselves once more and that a young doctor who has been interested in our work for five years is just at the stage at which he can give two years to our drug study and get this done. So life goes on.

I hear from Bob Neale that you spoke exceedingly well at the Euthanasia Educational Fund Conference. I understand that you focused on the distinction between a "good death" and killing people. As I am on the Church of England Commission which is trying to write a pamphlet on this subject I was delighted to hear this too. It is not a distinction which is very easy to get across to philosophers and lawyers.

Admiral J. M. Holford

Department of Health, London

29 December 1970 You will remember that when you came down to see us the other day I mentioned I was in touch with a young doctor who might be suitable to take Dr Welldon's position. His name is Dr Robert Twycross and he came to see us on December 22nd, and spent the whole day here seeing Dr Winner, Dr Parkes, Dr Robbie, the two girls in the Research Department and, finally, Dr Duncan Vere at the London Hospital. Everyone liked him and Dr Vere was very impressed by the grasp he already had of the particular research problem we are tackling.

I spoke to Professor Stewart on the telephone and Dr Winner and I made the decision to offer him the post subject to a satisfactory reference from Professor Vincent Marks the next day whose comment was that Dr Twycross was the most able and likeable person he had had in his department and that although he had no formal research training he was very keen and given encouragement he was sure he would do extremely good work.

I have also spoken to Professor Hinton and I hope you will agree with us all that we should offer the post to Dr Twycross. Professor Stewart has said that he will take the decision on behalf of the Halley Stewart Trustees but I have already spoken to one of the other Trustees and she feels certain that they will confirm the grant at their next meeting on January 6th.

Professor Marks commented that we would be extremely lucky to get Dr Twycross and as I have been in touch with him for the past five years and know something of his real concern about terminal care and of his very courteous and considerate personality I agree with him.

With all good wishes for the New Year.

Professor G. R. Dunstan[8]

King's College, London

29 December 1970 Thank you very much for sending me a copy of the Minutes. I have only had time to go through them once but I can see something of what a very fascinating afternoon it was. In a way I think it may be comparable to our discussion about prolongation of life and the distinction between "letting things take their course" and taking active steps to end life. When we have other medical members I would like to come back to this discussion and I think I would like to try and write a paragraph or two on the control of pain and dis-

---

[8] The Reverend Canon Gordon Dunstan, Professor of Moral Theology and founder of the journal *Crucible*, and from 1974 a member of the Council of St Christopher's Hospice. The letter refers to an informal discussion on ethical issues which Cicely Saunders had been unable to attend.

tress and on the difference between relevant and irrelevant treatment, or perhaps in the older phraseology, ordinary and extraordinary measures.

A discussion with some of our theological and pre-medical students and with two or three patients yesterday was extremely pertinent to this whole problem.

With all good wishes for the New Year.

Sister Raphaella
Our Lady's Convent, London

1 January 1971 Thank you so much for your Christmas greetings, and now for the delightful little vase for a rose and the special remembrances. It is lovely to have these from you and I look forward to a holiday in Italy again one day. Assisi and Perugia are two of my favourite spots, especially Assisi, where I spent a wonderful week in one of the Convent Guest Houses.

The Editor
"The Times", London

1 June 1971 You will see from the heading of our writing paper that Major General the Lord Thurlow, whose obituary appears in the "Times" today,[9] was the Chairman of our Council of Management. I understand from the Mission to Seamen, with which he has been intimately connected for many years, that they are writing to you to ask if something more might be added to the obituary which appeared today. I enclose a brief statement but it is not easy to sum up how much Lord Thurlow gave to the Hospice.

St Christopher's was once referred to in your columns as "St Christopher's Hospice for the Dying". The last three words are not part of our title and I would be very grateful if you could be sure that this mistake, which can be very disturbing to our future patients, does not occur again.

The Matron
St Ann's Hospice, Cheadle, Staffordshire

14 June 1971 I must congratulate you on a most successful Opening Day. I am sorry it was so cold for you but what a blessing there was no rain.

I was very pleased to have the chance of going round before most of the guests arrived and appreciate you taking that time when I know you had so much to do.

I think you have a good nursing staff and potentially excellent. We found we had so much to learn together when we first opened here because this work is so different from other ventures. We hope to be having days of discussion for staff working in Homes similar to our own in the future and I do hope we shall be welcoming you and some of your staff then.

With my grateful thanks, and every good wish.

---

[9] Lord Thurlow had died on 29 May 1971.

Lt General Sir Derek Lang

Perthshire, Scotland

15 June 1971 It was very nice to have an opportunity of speaking to you about St Christopher's last night although I am afraid it was rather costly for you. I appreciate that you will have only a sentence or two to say about the Hospice but Lord Thurlow was a great friend to us all and I think he would like it to be mentioned.

As I told you on the phone, we became a charity in 1961 and Lord Thurlow joined us through a personal connexion of our treasurer, Captain T L Lonsdale, who was also treasurer of the Mission to Seamen. He therefore joined us at an early stage when we were very small and struggling and before we had most of the money for building. He was a great support at that stage and signed the contract when we still had only about half the money given or promised.

After we were opened in 1967 and gradually became financially respectable, Lord Thurlow continued to come down whenever he could so he not only became a friend of the Council but of the residents in the Drapers' Wing and of many of the staff and patients. We looked after his old dog, Tammy, when he was in the Bahamas over Christmas. I was glad I visited him at home and that Dr Winner was one of his last visitors in Millbank.

As you appreciate, it is difficult to describe our work in a way that will be both honest and unalarming to our future waiting list. I think, on the whole, a phrase such as, "St Christopher's is unique in that it offers care, research and teaching into the problems of patients with chronic and terminal pain, and the needs of their families both at home and in the Hospice." It is a religious as well as a medical foundation and Lord Thurlow had both sides very much at heart.

The brochure I enclose is out of date as we are reprinting at the moment. The patient's brochure shows the kind of image that we try to present before they come to us, and the duplicated sheet sums up a few facts about the Hospice. I hope I have not inundated you with material.

Dr Margaret Thompson

Mount Zion Hospital and Medical Center, San Francisco, USA

30 June 1971 Thank you for your letter. I am enclosing a copy of the "Care of the Dying" and another reprint which may be of use to you.

We have a number of doctors coming here for study periods and a great many more students. We are just starting to build a residential and teaching block and I am afraid until then I am unlikely to have a space free for you.

I would suggest that if your interest continues you might like to write to me more fully in about a year's time so that we can think about making plans. For example, I shall not have any money available for a Fellowship for you and although our living expenses are not high (£1–£1.50 per day), you would need a certain amount of money if you were going to live comfortably on the outskirts of London.

I am sorry not to be able to say "yes" immediately but I am sure you will understand we are very pressed by visitors and at the moment I am trying to keep open for doctors in this country who want to come to us, of whom there seem to be an increasing number.

Herr H. Michalsky

Hamburg, Germany

13 August 1971 I was very interested to read your letter. In due course there will be a publication from the Television Centre which will, I think, answer all your questions.[10] I understand that there has been a certain amount of discussion in your country so you may find other writings later.

1   The total cost of the Hospice was about £500,000. This included £27,000 for the site and approximately £30,000 for furnishing. As you will see, we will eventually be using our top floor (at present full of students) as a ward. This will bring the cost per bed to £5,900. There are other Homes which have been built more cheaply where they have been in areas where land was less expensive. They have also been able to have buildings with less expensive foundations.

2   As a Charity we do not pay tax. Under our system we are able to reclaim tax paid by donors of covenant gifts.

3   It costs us £7.45 per day per bed. I am afraid I have not converted these figures into Dm, but I am sure you can do this through your local bank.

The real founders of St Christopher's are the patients and I think that the people planning any similar institution should be in touch with patients and must include professionals so that the vision can be translated into reality.

I am sure that one could be carried away by a need such as this without really counting the cost, not only in money but in care and work and professional skill. There are several groups in this country who are opening or planning this type of work and in each case they have had to work very hard in the early stages. There are no short cuts.

Dr Elisabeth Kübler-Ross

Flossmoor, Illinois, USA

15 September 1971 I am absolutely delighted to hear that you are going to the special Conference at the Katholische Akademie in Bayern on October 23rd/24th. I much look forward to seeing the second film taken at the Hospice – still more to the chance of meeting you again.

I shall be coming almost direct from Africa as I am having three weeks holiday with a friend in Nigeria and fly back on October 22nd. I will come on to Munich on October 23rd with our Deputy Matron/Director of Studies, who will stand in as my deputy should I by any chance get delayed by a sand storm in Kano or for any other reason cannot get back to London in time.

I expect you will be taking this chance to visit your mother and family in Switzerland and I do hope that you have good news of them. It is very hard to be so far away and deal constructively with the problems which one has in one's own family.

---

10   A film about St Christopher's had recently appeared on German television, leading to some unfavourable comments in the press both there and in the UK.

I wonder if you will have a chance of visiting St Christopher's. If you can come back with us on October 25th and come down and meet some of the staff on October 26th, staying with us if you wish or in London if you prefer it, that would be a great delight to us all.

Dr Colin Murray-Parkes asks me to give you his greetings and to say how much he hopes we shall see you here. We normally have a big staff meeting on the afternoon of Tuesday and if you are not too tired, and if it were not an imposition, we would love you to join us and talk a little. I know that a large number of our staff have read your book[11] and have found it extremely helpful. I know also how many demands there are upon you and how everyone tends to think that they are the only one – but I hope you know us well enough to say "No" if you really only want to be a visitor and observer.

Dr Daniel H. Schwartz

Montefiore Hospital and Medical Center, Bronx, New York, USA

1 December 1971 Thank you for your letter of November 15th. Correspondence should be addressed to me at St Christopher's as I now only visit occasionally at St Joseph's as a consultant.

I am very interested in your request and would suggest that probably the best way for you to approach it would be to have a consultation with Mr and Mrs Wald, of Connecticut. Mr Wald has recently completed a year's course at Columbia University and written a dissertation on "A new English Hospice". This was based on his visits to St Christopher's and many discussions we have had with him and his wife. They are currently very concerned in setting up something similar in the New Haven area and I think discussion of your different problems would be enlightening. His thesis includes plans of St Christopher's and I think it would be helpful for you to discuss them with someone who has seen them from outside as it were.

We, ourselves, find the hospice is very well suited to our work and that much of its life and enthusiasm, which is so noticeable to patients and their families, stems from the fact that we are a separate institution. There are problems in carrying out similar work on a separate floor of a larger establishment. If it is at all possible for you to plan for a separate pavilion I would strongly recommend this for the following reasons.

i   Your staff must work as some kind of community if they are going to do it adequately.

ii "Terminal Care" is really a specialty and should have its own physician(s) with their own skills and enthusiasm. In my experience I have found that where a separate ward has been established there has been the difficulty consultants find in handing over their patients to others. The tendency is for them to fail to do so and yet not to attend to their patients on the new ward either.

My comment on our plans is that I would alter very little except to enlarge the day room area on each floor. It might be ideal to have a second bed lift but the problems involved in our present set up are not great enough to wish we had incurred the very considerable extra expense.

I shall be very interested to know how your plans develop.

[11]   E. Kübler-Ross, *On death and dying* (New York: Macmillan, 1969).

PS   We will have more single rooms for those who are admitted for their last few days only when we open the 4th floor.

Dr Austin H. Kutscher

The American Institute of Life-Threatening Illness and Loss, New York, USA

1 December 1971 A friend sent me a copy of the "New York Times" magazine with the article "Learning How to Die" by David Dempsey. On the whole I felt it was a good summary of the work I know in your country but I wonder whether each report has the hint which I detect in that about our work. Thank you for your kind comment but I hope that you do not really think we use drugs in order to produce "a terminal euphoria, or 'high'". What I try to get across when I talk is that [I try] to help patients' mood of depression and sadness with drugs only as part of the whole approach. I am quite sure that our patients are not "high" but are enabled just to go on living as ordinary people at a normal level with the burden in manageable proportions. I would like to point out, too, that we never use narcotics merely to change the mood but they are used specifically to control pain and breathlessness. I am sure that it is the relief itself which helps most. I do hope you will not suggest that we encourage the use of LSD. I think this is a most dangerous drug and I have never used it and do not intend to do so.

I can see I must try and find time to write more but it is very difficult to do so with all the demands that are going on at the moment.

The reprints from you will be a help and I look forward to having them. In the meantime I would be most grateful to have copies of the books in which the various articles which you have been asked to reprint have been included.

The Reverend W. Benjamin Holmes

Church of St Martin-in-the-Fields, Philadelphia, USA

9 December 1971 Thank you so much for the reprint and copy of the article you sent in September. I think they are both excellent and contain some very "quotable quotes".

You do not mention Dr Howell and I wonder if you have seen her. I still continue to worry about her from time to time.

You will see from the enclosed Newsletter that life has been a bit heavy here recently. I am afraid there is no way of avoiding this sort of misunderstanding and at the same time try to respond to what one considers to be responsible and important demands. I believe it is part of our teaching function to try to help people who wish to spread this kind of work in other places. Even if one does nothing but continue with ordinary lectures and teaching rounds there may happen something like the reference in the "New York Times" and "Newsweek" last week of which we had no knowledge before it happened. Fortunately, few people read these papers in this country but to link our work with drugs with someone else's work with LSD in the States is not a juxtaposition I would ever have chosen. I suppose this must be an accepted risk in responding to requests for talks etc.

All this has been an anxiety but we had a big discussion group with the staff this week on how to get through times like this which was immensely cheering. The staff really have cohered as a community, and a very mixed one at that, which is the strength of the whole place.

Professor Dr A. Sikkel

Academisch Ziekenhuis, Leiden, Netherlands

31 May 1972 Thank you for your most interesting paper. I was particularly interested in your comments on loneliness. I am afraid I do not agree with you at the end where you suggest that we may have to come to the place of active euthanasia. This really needs more detailed discussion than just a comment in a letter but perhaps I could summarise a conversation I had with a patient this last week-end.

She had been talking with one of the Sisters and had said "I would like to ask for something to end it". They had talked round the problem and she appeared quite determined on such a course had it been possible. However, when I went to see her our conversation went briefly as follows.

"Sister has told me about your conversation. You know I cannot give you an overdose but suppose for the sake of argument I could. Would you like me to do it now?" The instant response was "No, not now". "When would you want me to?" I asked. "If the pain got too much or if I got desperately fed up with it all." I replied to the effect that we would certainly be able to control pain, although we might have to make her rather sleepy. She had been refusing doses because of fear of sleepiness. I said we could certainly help feelings of anxiety and desperation and maybe she would need to sleep and I told her she could certainly send for me if she wanted to do so. She went on to say that this was really what she wanted but added how hard she found it for her husband to see her like this. We discussed that and how she would feel had things been the other way round. She then asked me not to tell her husband what she had said. I said, "Well, we have only been talking about pain, haven't we?" I think that was the truth of the matter.

As it happened she saw her two lots at grandchildren that evening, had a small increased dose both before and after and went to sleep but was awake to speak to the night nurse.

Incidentally, I only increased the dose by one quarter and that certainly was not lethal. I think too this sort of request is so often near the end and comes from the utter weariness which we can help. Never when I have asked "Do you want it now" have I been given the answer "Yes".

The main argument against euthanasia, legalisation, signing of forms, medical requests, etc, is I think one of relationships – above all, relationships among the family. I do not think they can withstand the pressures. I think one should remember the trauma of suicide and multiply this.

Dr Morris A. Wessel[12]

New Haven Hospice Inc., New Haven, USA

31 July 1972 I was very pleased to see "To comfort always" in the Yale Magazine. I think you have got a lot across in a comparatively short space. I am always glad to see anything from the New Haven Hospice Inc, and am much looking forward to seeing you when I come in March 1973. I hope you will have gone a long way by then.

---

[12] Morris Wessel studied medicine at Yale and later became a professor of paediatrics; he was also actively involved in the work of the New Haven Hospice.

It seems rather churlish to say it but you have made a slight mistake about our routine giving of drugs. We have a 4-hourly schedule and I think where you have picked up $3\frac{1}{2}$ hours was when I said it was rather an "Irish 4 hours" and could be plus or minus $\frac{1}{2}$-hour – a $3\frac{1}{2}$ hourly routine would be rather difficult for the nurses! I mention this because you might be printing it and I think you would need to say "Why not every four hours routinely?"

Incidentally, like many others, you have spelt my name wrongly but that does not worry me.

Dr Elisabeth Kübler-Ross

Flossmoor, Illinois, USA

22 August 1972 I am delighted to know that we are going to be on a platform together again. I am looking forward to meeting you at the Congress of the Association of Operating Room Nurses in Chicago in March 1973. This is a long way ahead but of course it is inevitable that we should be planning like this.

We have recently had two students from Illinois, both from the University of Illinois Medical Centre. I think they came because of a recommendation from you and I am very grateful for the things that you say of St Christopher's. There is one slight problem, however, in that USA programmes and ours are so different that whatever you say I am afraid people who have heard you talk about us tend to have expectations somewhat at variance to what they actually find. We write letters such as the one of which I enclose a copy but in spite of this they come over expecting to work as medical students and not as members of the team of St Christopher's nurses and orderlies. This is obviously difficult for some of the more senior students. I have had exactly the same problem from a student who heard me talk in Lexington so please do not think that I believe you are misrepresenting us. I am sure this is to do with the emotive area of death and the need of so many to isolate their patients behind some kind of academic barrier.

Of course our teaching programme is very much in the developmental stage. Miss Nevell, our Director of Studies, whom I know you heard in Munich, has an unusual gift for meeting with students of different disciplines and we are all working on the programme together but inevitably it is part of the total care of St Christopher's. Incidentally, our Teaching Unit building itself will not be open until next Spring when Miss Nevell will then have more help, and so will I.

My second problem may also be due to people's difficulty in listening. I had a visit a few days ago from an Episcopal priest from Los Angeles. He had heard you speak and say some good things about us but he was convinced that you had called us "St Christopher's Hospice for the Dying". Please, those last three words are not part of our title. We are trying very hard not to have the image of caring only for patients in the last few days and weeks of their lives. We have the other groups such as the elderly residents and those who are discharged again with their pain controlled. If they are left out of the picture the Hospice could seem mysterious and rather dreadful and frightening to its future waiting list. It is not that we do not want to be frank with them in due course – it is just that we do not want some kind of "abandon hope" invisibly over the door.

I was very interested in the report of your evidence to Congress in our "Sunday Times". I know one or two other people who will be appearing there and I shall be glad to know whether anything comes of this. One of the initial reactions has been a request from the ABC News London who want to make some film. I am not going to let them come into the wards here but it is possible that we might find ourselves able to make a documentary of our own that we could let people use. I am constantly trying to fight off publicity while at the same time we want to get across a different attitude to all these problems. I know you have the same difficulty.

The reports I have read on the Congressional Hearing reveal the usual difficulty people have in defining euthanasia. In our country it has come to mean the taking of active steps to kill a patient at their request. We are trying to emphasise that the with-holding of antibiotics in the case of terminal pneumonia or a patient with a severe stroke or terminal malignant disease, is relevant medical care and not euthanasia. The difficulty people have of distinguishing between these two seems to bedevil everybody on the subject and I think it is very important to keep them separate. The reports from the States make me think that the word "euthanasia" is used for the second and I am afraid this may add further misunderstanding between our two countries – yet another case where we think we are speaking the same language and are in fact not doing so at all.

Grace Goldin[13]

Hamden, Connecticut, USA

5 September 1972 I hope all goes well and both you and Judah are recovering from all the vicissitudes.

I am just embarking upon our Annual Report and as it is five years since we opened as well as the Annual Report before we open our Teaching Unit I want to do a little bit of survey as background. This led me to looking up the description of hospice in the Encyclopaedia Britannica, which as you probably know is given as follows:-

"The name frequently given to the guest houses established for the reception of pilgrims and travellers within the precincts or upon the property of religious houses."

I am now asking you as a hospice and hospital historian whether you can throw any more light on the development of the word to cover our kind of work. I know Mother Mary Aikenhead used it for the Sisters of Charity's first hospice about the middle of the last century in Ireland but I think it must have been used before then.

I have not got chapter and verse but I have always thought that medieval hospitals must have welcomed many people who were at the end of their lives due to the rigours of pilgrimages. After all, it was certainly a way of paradise to die upon a pilgrimage. It was also

....

13 Grace Goldin (d. 1995) the photographer, poet, and medical historian first encountered Cicely Saunders when her husband heard a lecture given at Yale University in 1966. A voluminous correspondence ensued between the two women over the next thirty years. Grace Goldin wrote on the early history of St Luke's House, London; on hospital architecture; and in particular produced a major photographic essay on the history of hospitals which contained two chapters on hospices: G. Goldin, *Work of mercy. A picture history of hospitals* (Ontario, Canada: The Boston Mills Press, 1994). She visited the UK and undertook photography in several hospices and palliative care units, but especially at St Christopher's, supplying Cicely Saunders with many images for use in publications and teaching. Her husband, Judah Goldin (d. 1998), was Professor of Classical Judaica at Yale University.

true as you say at the end of the two reprints which I have ("A Walk through a Ward of the Eighteenth Century" and "A Painting in Gheel") that a hospital was a place in which to die, where the chapel took over from the secular side.

Do you have any further details about this which you can send me briefly on an airletter? I do not want to make too much of this in the Annual Report but I would like to have a couple of sentences which I wish to be accurate.

Sister Raphaella Alberti

Perugia, Italy

17 November 1972 You sent Freda and Mary back so happy and uplifted that they have spread their gratefulness all around the Hospice. Thank you so much for all you did to make their visit such a memorable one. It will be a long time before we hear everything there is so much to tell.

Thank you for the lovely card, the kakies and the cards for everybody, which have been distributed and received with much pleasure.

We had a lovely AGM yesterday and are busy making plans for the next developments. Life is very busy so we greatly need your prayers and are very glad to know that we have them.

I nearly always take prayers in our chapel on Monday morning at 9.30 a.m. and I wonder if this would be a good moment for us to keep remembering you and for you to remember us in turn. We have many links with people like this and it would be nice to set aside a special time as you suggest.

Dr Brian L. Mishara

Northville State Hospital, Northville, Michigan, USA

6 December 1972 Thank you for your letter of November 29th. Perhaps you do not have so many Bank Holidays in your country over Christmas as we do here but I assure you nothing in London will be normal from December 23rd until December 27th. I think only a psychologist without clinical responsibility could ask a Medical Director to take him round a hospital over Christmas. I am sorry to sound so unwelcoming but have you any idea how many things one has to do at this time and how many staff have to sort out their own Christmas with their families and the work with patients?

Having I hope made you feel badly about asking I will now say perhaps we may be able to find a mutually convenient time but I am afraid you will not find the Hospice working quite in its usual fashion. The best day of those you give in your letter to me is Friday, 22nd December. May I suggest that you come down that afternoon? I am afraid Dr Murray Parkes, our psychiatrist, will not be here as he is only here on Tuesdays and of course Tuesday, December 26th, is a Bank Holiday, but there will be other members of staff available as well as myself.

You do not say where you are staying in London and I would suggest that you telephone us in the morning of December 22nd and we can then give you some suggestions about travelling. The easiest way is for us to send a car for you. This will only cost about £1.50p from Central London.

If you cannot manage December 22nd, my only other hope is December 27th, as I shall be taking a couple of days off on December 28th/29th. I work through Christmas and enjoy it.

Dr Colin Murray Parkes
Chorley Wood, Hertfordshire

22 December 1972 This is a bit out of "The Foolishness of God"[14] which I said I would send to you. It is really an extension of your summary on the religious attitude. I think it is important that we think not of ourselves going on into after life but about being safe in the thought and love of God. I remember hearing Sydney Evans talking about us living in the memories of those who love us and saying God is the great Rememberer.

Incidentally, if you ever feel like reading theology "The Foolishness of God" is a superb book. We are studying it at the Foundation Group.

Dr Elisabeth Kübler-Ross
Flossmoor, Illinois, USA

26 March 1973 Many thanks for a most lovely evening. It was the greatest delight to see you in your own home and to meet your family. I do hope your 'flu is better. I must say that I think you are even worse than I am in running yourself into the ground in trying to answer all requests. I do not have so many as you but I am also beset by this missionary type of reaction about responding. But please preserve yourself – you are very much needed. I am delighted, however, to hear of those July and August pages being torn out of your diary.

This is just a brief letter to get these off straight away. I think possibly I could add one thing to these and that is the regime which has been developed by the doctor in charge of the Pain Clinic at Yale.

This is obviously a good regime and I would be very interested to try it out. It is really much the same as our methods and it might produce less reaction in the States than trying to get someone to make up our mixture with morphine or another opiate available to you.

I do hope that your lady goes safely and peacefully.

Sister Mary Etienne McDonald
Mount Carmel Infirmary, Dubuque, Iowa, USA

23 May 1973 Thank you so much for your letter of April 30th. I have delayed answering this until we had the enclosed check list of reprints duplicated. I thought you would like to

---

14 J. Austin Baker, *The foolishness of God* (London: Darton, Longman, and Todd, 1970).

know about this and also I am enclosing some reprints written by patients with motor neurone disease.

Now to try and answer your questions. I think the enclosed list of drugs we most commonly use for our patients with terminal malignant disease will probably answer your first question. For patients who have arthritic conditions there are, of course, a whole set of drugs which you could consider and I do not think I need emphasise them.

We have used various medications for our patients with motor neurone disease (which you refer to as "ALS"). Most of them have needed some form of tranquilliser but they very much dislike being made to feel dopey and some of them have been resistant saying that each drug we tried made them feel awful. However, I think I would first of all try a small dose of diazepam (Valium), and this of course has often helped where they have had fasciculation. The other drugs we have tried successfully are promazine (Sparine), chlorpromazine (Largactil). You have of course a range which you might try. I do think that they get extremely frustrated and that a small dose of drug in this group can take some of the edge off of this kind of anguish.

Many of them have done well with a small dose of diamorphine elixir. You do not have diamorphine and I would suggest that you use a small dose of whatever opiate is easily available given by mouth and not until later suggest by injection.[15] This medication is certainly of real value when they start to feel breathless because it does control this very unpleasant sensation. It is also valuable in controlling feelings of thirst and hunger.

We do not insert nasal-gastric tubes. Although we ask these patients with two exceptions they have all refused. They often have a great deal of saliva and sometimes a lot of mucous in their chest. We find that tapping and slapping only exacerbates the situation. We use Atropine or other belladonna mixtures by mouth and by injection towards the end if necessary, when our choice is hyoscine (Scopolamine).

I am fascinated that your sister blinks the Morse code. Valerie Morton did this and we had a long correspondence by this means. We also had buzzers fixed to the last thenar muscle that worked and at the last stage she could manage something with her big toe calling people at night.

I shall be very interested to hear if any of these suggestions are of any help.

---

[15] At this time a diamorphine 'elixir' was still in common use at St Christopher's. Known elsewhere by various names, most commonly 'The Brompton Cocktail', it also could contain morphine (instead of diamorphine) as well as cocaine, alcohol, syrup, chloroform water, and a phenothiazine. By 1977 the research of Robert Twycross had concluded that morphine or diamorphine could be used just as effectively in a solution of chloroform water, and that the other elements of the 'cocktail' could be abandoned. This letter also highlights the fact that, unlike in Britain, diamorphine was unavailable for clinical use in the USA. See also the letter to Robert Twycross of 17 May 1977, p. 173.

Dr J. Menges

Hulshorst, Holland

20 June 1973 I was interested in your long letter but I am very sorry that we are not able to help this time. As you may imagine a number of people ask us to co-operate with them in this way and we can only do this for a limited number of them. We have reached the limit of people we can possibly have here this year.

We have recently been working with a radio programme for your country and I took part in a Television programme made a few years ago. I gave then my own views on Euthanasia and do not think I can usefully contribute any more.

I am enclosing a paper transcribed for a talk given in this Hospice. It is for private circulation only but it would perhaps clarify some of the issues. We feel as Professor Dunstan does that proper medical care which includes desisting from irrelevant treatments and the prolongation of life in the irreversibly dying should not be termed Euthanasia or "negative Euthanasia" as I think the Dutch church has defined it. It is good clinical judgement to decide the time is past for such activities.

I emphasize this because I think that one of the most important issues at the moment in this debate is that we should be clear in our definitions. If we are, there need be much less polarization if we all keep clear our desire to relieve suffering.

I entirely agree with you that any request for active Euthanasia is made because someone has failed the patient, and the answer is better care not the negative solution which would bring such harm to society.

Professor A. N. Exton Smith

London

2 August 1973 I was delighted to see in the Medical News of the British Medical Journal that you are now a Professor. Congratulations on a most well deserved recognition.

This is also a warning ahead that Princess Alexandra is coming to open our new Study Centre on October 11th sometime in the afternoon. If there is a chance of you getting down that day we would be delighted. You will have our more official invitation in due course, this is just a hope that you will be able to book it.

For my sins I am a member of the Church of England's Board of Social Responsibility Commission on Euthanasia.[16] Have you ever had any further thoughts in this field since you did your original article in which Dr Leonard Colebrook was so interested? Do not worry if you have not, but if you have I would dearly love to know if you have committed them to paper.

---

[16] Its report was subsequently published as *On dying well: an Anglican contribution to the debate on euthanasia* (London: Church Information Office, 1975).

Jósef Trzeciak

Warszawa, Poland

14 January 1974 Thank you so much for sending me the Polish paper with the book review. Marian translated it for me. I owe so much of what I know to Antoni Michniewicz that it is good that now something is translated into Polish.

I have just been telling my secretary about our amazing meeting. I wish I could tell you in Polish how much he still means to me and how our meeting has influenced St Christopher's. One thing I can say is that I know he was happy and that the nuns at St Joseph's Hospice where he was a patient those last 7 months thought that he really was a saint. I still go to his grave and I have often remembered you there, one of his greatest friends.

I hope all is well with you and that someone has translated this letter for you.

Dr Ivan Illich

Centor Intercultural De Documentacion, Morelos, Mexico

29 July 1974 I much enjoyed our meeting earlier in the year and I hope that you were not too disappointed to think that St Christopher's Hospice set out to relieve pain and perhaps did not have the emphasis you expected. I am only sorry that I had not read Medical Nemesis[17] at that time because I would have been a little better prepared for the onslaught.

I assure you that you fulfilled your usual purpose of challenging assumptions, although I hope that perhaps we have some concern that people should die their own deaths and that our efforts are directed that way rather than towards introducing new techniques for their own sake. I hope you will still come and see us one day.

I am writing now also because the London Medical Group have asked me to take the Chair at their 12th Annual Conference on February 7th and 8th 1975. I understand they wrote to you a second time with the programme of this conference. I know they are most anxious for you to come.

I have been associated with that group since it began and I have discussed this present programme with their President, who worked here as a student for a month earlier this summer. There will be an excellent audience of some hundreds of students. The conference is one of the highlights of my own year because this is a self selected group of people who are interested in the human side of medicine and who really have the possibility of changing attitudes. I do not think you could speak to a better group in this country.

If you come it would be my great pleasure to introduce you. Knowing your interest in students I hope very much that you will.

---

[17] Ivan Illich's famous critique of modern medicine, *Medical nemesis*, was published in New York by Pantheon Books in 1975, so this early reference is curious and is likely to refer to a manuscript version. Born in Vienna in 1926, Illich had been working in Latin America since 1956 and was a co-founder of the controversial Center for Intercultural Documentation.

Dr Ann Cartwright

Institute of Social Studies in Medical Care, London

14 August 1974 I am enclosing the section on general medical considerations which I have written for our report "To Die Well" for the Church of England Board of Social Responsibility. You remember when I telephoned you I asked you whether your interviewers had heard of any requests for euthanasia and that as this was not a question you could really give no definite answer. I have not reported you as personal communication but as I have quoted extensively from "Life Before Death"[18] I want you to see this. I hope I have given you sufficient acknowledgement and if there is anything else you would like me to say the paper is just having its final typing.

The more I read "Life Before Death" the more impressed I am by all your work and that splendid last chapter. I only hope it is sufficiently noted by all concerned.

The bulk of my medical discussion appears in the form of discussion of a series of cases and I have not bothered you with those. The rest of the pamphlet is written by philosophers and theologians, the other medical member was Lord Amulree; though we took evidence from various other people.

Thelma Ingles

Blue Hill Falls, Maine, USA

25 September 1974 Thank you so much for your letter and gift in memory of KS. Her death was a real shock and we still miss her, she was a lovely person.

I wanted to write to you straight away, and if I find out any more about salbutamol I will write again but I would like to check this up properly.

I made no comments about your report at the time because I did not know what to say. You were here at a particularly difficult time when Marian Nevell, Sister Spears and Nurse Cosser were all going to leave for various reasons, and I know that you had problems of home sickness and were very worried about Fran Reiter. I am very unhappy about the idealistic image of St Christopher's which some people produce and perhaps what you say will be a good corrective. I do not have your copy any longer but both Jenny and I remember the words "much hostility" standing out. I am really unhappy about these two words, if you could just use the word "anger" I think it would give a different feeling and one more correct. Perhaps it is that we use hostility in a different way.

I am sorry that you still do have severe asthmatic attacks, but I hope that in general your health is improving.

Mr E. A. M. Lee

Williams and Glyn's Bank Limited, London

22 October 1974 Your letter to the Association of Nursing Religious has been passed to me by Reverend Mother of St Joseph's Hospice, with which I have been associated in various

---

[18] A. Cartwright, L. Hockley, and J. L. Anderson, *Life before death* (London: Routledge and Kegan Paul, 1973), a highly influential social survey of bereaved relatives.

capacities since 1958. I discussed it before with Sister Superior at the Hostel [of God] by telephone some 10 days ago and have now had opportunity to speak with our Council which met last week.

You probably did not think of St Christopher's Hospice as a nursing community but Reverend Mother knowing that the Catholic nursing orders are fully committed with their present work has strongly urged me to write to you. We all, of course, feel that it would be a tragedy if the Hostel of God should be lost to terminal care after all it has given over these many years.[19] May I ask to come and see you and your Chairman at some time in the near future? Or if you would prefer it we would be delighted to welcome any, or all, of you at St Christopher's.

I have had opportunity to discuss the situation before with the Mother Provincial of the Little Company of Mary, as several of that Order have worked with us on visits and we have two of their Sisters coming on one of our month teaching courses in November.

David Frost[20]

London

1 November 1974 I know that you have been kept fairly well up to date with news of the people here through Jenny and Helen. The latest news is that K's father became very ill, was admitted to hospital and she was able to visit him several times before he died. She then went home and was a marvellous support to her mother. She is back with us now, but the special pain controlling injection for which she was admitted some 3 weeks ago is doing well so far and we hope to be able to send her out again.

Mr V continues to lose more and more use of his hands and I am afraid the idea of his finger painting came to nothing. It was not possible even for him to start. He keeps up his courage but it is hard work sometimes and he is the one who would most appreciate seeing you again if you ever had a moment to spare.

Libby may have told you that we are being asked if we would make a tape together for the Journal of Medical Ethics second issue which should appear in the Spring. I am a member of a fairly august editorial board and the whole question of care of the dying is one of the first topics they want to tackle. When they asked me for an unusual way of doing this I suggested a "Shoot of Sacred Cows" of terminal care. I am now of course asked to provide suggestions of cows and marksmen. The Editor, who had seen our interview, and is a young Philosopher wrote to me saying –

> "I have been wondering about doing a kind of 'David Frost talks to Cicely Saunders' …
> This would be along the lines of the television programme but perhaps more fixed on particular questions. I have the impression that he might be willing to do this for us more read-

---

19 The Hostel of God had been founded in Clapham, London, as a result of an appeal in *The Times* in 1891 and was run successively by two separate orders of Anglican sisters. At the time of this letter discussions were taking place about its future, and in particular transfer to a lay system of governance and management, which duly occurred in 1977. It was re-named Trinity Hospice in 1980.

20 The well-known television interviewer and broadcaster, who had conducted a 'Frost Interview' with Cicely Saunders, broadcast in September 1974.

ily than writing a full article. If this idea appeals to you would you be willing to approach him in the first instance? I can then follow up with a letter."

Do you think we could do this? I think it would take a bit of preparation, or rather good editing afterwards – but at least we could leave the second to somebody else.

David Frost

London

13 January 1975 I am sure you will be sad that dear R died a few days ago. Completely unafraid to the last she slipped away very peacefully after only a few days of increasing weakness. The ward is most desolate but very proud that she never lost her courage or her faith, and went in most happy expectation. I certainly find it very strange without her but glad she never reached the stage of losing her voice and was able to be in charge to the end.

The family left us the picture you sent her and at the moment it is hanging over her bed. KW and her other friends were very sad but proud. K is now the only one left of your 4.

I wonder if you have had time to think about our doing a tape together for the Society for the Study of Medical Ethics. The debate on euthanasia is hotting up again and I think it would be helpful contribution. When I think of the debates on TV which are looming up I am so glad that you made your programme with us in the way you did.

Dr Elisabeth Kübler-Ross

Flossmoor, Illinois, USA

6 March 1975 I was delighted to see that you are chairing the Council for Hospice Inc. I hope you are now doing less racing around the country with lectures and you and the rest of the family, specially your husband, are well. It was nice seeing you in Columbia City.

We have had our usual 3 or 4 letters this week asking for massive amounts of information about St Christopher's. Many of them refer either to your book Questions and Answers[21] or to a conversation with you. Postage has become so prohibitive that as we are battling inflationary salaries we have reluctantly had to decide that we have to send literature by surface mail unless people send us international postage vouchers. Surprisingly few people do this. I am truly sorry if I sound churlish and unco-operative but the amount of publicity we get one way and another is a real problem to us. If you could suggest to people that they either find what is written in American literature for themselves or make a realistic contribution to what could be sent by air mail I should be so grateful.

Miss O. Burrage

'Copper Cliff' Nursing Home, Brighton

17 April 1975 It may have reached your ears that St Christopher's Hospice Choir is giving a concert in Brighton on April 26th, at 6.30 pm. I enclose our programme. Richard Baker, who you will probably know from his television appearances, is playing the piano for us and

---

[21] E. Kübler-Ross, *Questions and answers on death and dying* (New York: Collier Macmillan, 1974).

has offered to make a short announcement about the work of St Christopher's. We would like to couple this with the work of Copper Cliff, the Tarner Home, and St Barnabas in Worthing. This is not an appeal for money, although I think we may have a collection which we will split between us though I do not anticipate much from that. We were thinking of having some copies of our own Annual Report available for anyone who was interested but would not feel happy about this unless there was something from you as well. I hope you might come and bring some literature with you.

Cyril Clemens
Mark Twain Journal, Kirkwood, Missouri, USA

9 July 1975 I found your letter on my return from holiday. Thank you so much for electing me as a Daughter of the Mark Twain Society. I am afraid I did not know of the Society before but am delighted to do this now. St Christopher's as a whole thinks it is a great honour.

The Right Reverend the Lord Bishop of Southwark
Streatham, London

28 October 1975 I am indeed glad to have the opportunity to write to you about the Hostel of God. We have been concerned for a number of years about the references to it from patients and from doctors. There is no doubt that it has gained a somewhat alarming image as the "end of the road", and indeed the last comment by a family doctor from the area to one of us was, "We can only send our patients there when they are becoming unconscious and we can reassure the families that they will not really realise where they are going." This is a problem to most Hospices that have been open for some time unless a real effort is made both to have a mixed group of patients with some going home and to meet the local community with Open Days and so on. Added to this however I feel I must say that we feel that this is terminal care as was being carried out 20 years ago but not terminal care as can be developed today. Sister Superior seems to me to have vision but I fear there seems to be very little openness to the real possibility of this work among those of the senior staff with whom we talked. The Sisters have not had the support of either imaginative doctors or Trustees and although they have done a marvellous job in many ways it is terribly sad to see the present standards of care.

No one today should be trying to care for very ill patients in that beautiful old building but it has a wonderful potential for opening it out as I suggested in the memorandum. At the same time it is very sad to see the lack of involvement with the staff in thinking of any kind of future planning. They are very insecure at present.

It seems to me so important that a Christian foundation of this kind should be able to move into the present day. It need not in any way detract from the Christian side but it must be more professional than it is at present. To see it close rather than see it take a leap into the future would be a major tragedy. I think they will have sent you a copy of our Annual Report but I enclose another because it gives some idea I hope of the potential of a Hospice today.

I can assure you that St Christopher's Committee speaks out of deep concern for the work, true appreciation of what has been done and real excitement about the possibility for the future of a Phoenix Hostel but no thoughts of taking it over.

Grace Goldin

Swarthmore, Pennsylvania, USA

6 November 1975 Bless you for sending the pictures for my Christmas presents for which I enclose a cheque for what is I am told just over $24. I think you will have no more trouble in converting it over there than we have the other way round. I am also returning most of your precious slides. I am using those I have not sent and if you will spare me the ones I have kept I will be very grateful. I think I am sending you back the ones you really want, but I have one of a very ill Mr S and the very rubicund Mr F. These are really much better than the duplicates and I will be using them a lot. Do not worry about the Resurrection picture. We have a post card, even though I think it is not as good as yours.

I have now lectured several times with them and I am really delighted, they have got this year's message across.

I am not quite sure what you meant about our former chaplain. He left because his wife wanted to move. We were sad to see him go and I do not think there was a fuss about that. There was a fuss about a temporary or "trial for 3 months" chaplain perhaps that is what you were thinking of.

Bless you for this, it is a most enormous help to me.

Dr J. Beatson-Hird

Birmingham

23 December 1975 Thank you for your letter. It is a little difficult for me to give you constructive suggestions about general practitioners' coverage as on the whole I do not think it is adequate for proper Hospice care. I know that it is unlikely that many family doctors will ever find time available to come in and care for their own patients, although it is very good to be able to have case conferences with them. I know also that Dr Ronnie Fisher, The Macmillan Unit, Christchurch Hospital, Christchurch, Dorset finds that he needs to be a very whole time medical Director and to have several general practitioner sessions as well. I suggest that you would do well to write to him and perhaps with Dr Gusterson, St Barnabas' Home, Columbia Drive, Worthing, who runs units of a similar size to your own.

Our own situation as a teaching and research Hospice is obviously very different, but to give real care to families as well as patients, support and teach your own staff, be available as patients are admitted and do adequate ward rounds and keep a consistent way of prescribing which the nurses can use with confidence and a proper degree of flexibility means a whole time person.

Grace Goldin

Swarthmore, Pennsylvania, USA

4 February 1976 Much pleasure from all the family who received the photos for Christmas! Now much pleasure from me for that splendid book.[22] I would have read more of it already

---

22 A reference to J. D. Thompson and G. Goldin, *The hospital: A social and architectural history* (New Haven and London: Yale University Press, 1975).

because I find it truly fascinating but we have a euthanasia Bill coming up in our House of Lords and this has involved me in a great deal of work. It has also meant that I now have to write a second edition of my original booklet. I am well on with it and then I will be able to write a bit about yours. So far I know I will be most enthusiastic.

You bore with me on Faith – here is a mini contribution on Hope.

Dr Balfour Mount[23]

Royal Victoria Hospital, Montreal, Canada

5 February 1976 One of our troubles is that contrary to general belief we do not speak the same language and you should have heard Jenny and I exclaiming over "opportunity for exposure to Dr Cicely Saunders" etc! Seriously I will do my best because although when you read through the letter it seems like a merry-go-round I think basically it should work. I will certainly be prepared to talk at the public meeting bringing in perhaps St Joseph's as well as St Christopher's on the first evening and do a presentation in the morning of a more technical nature. I have an excellent set of slides now which are a ward round, ie all the patients in each of the 3 wards during one week. It is too many really to get round the whole Hospice but very possible to do one ward plus illustrations from the others. This gets across that we are not using our best patients but the sort of thing you would find at any time when you walk into the Hospice. If I do those two sessions it would probably not be a good idea for me to do the one on Management of Intractable Pain, though I might get up and add something. In any case I will have talked about pain as part of the philosophy of total care.

I am very prepared to be a discussant now and again and also to present a fairly brief session on Colin's work on bereavement; and incidentally the informal sort of work that goes on here anyway which in some ways is more important.

My plans for this trip include quite a lot of holiday. I am hoping to arrive in Vancouver to stay with a friend in Powell River from about Friday 22 October to 1 November when I come back to you. This would give me time to get my astral body along side me! And I think that would be the time for socialising. Then I really would like to leave on Saturday, 6th because I might well find myself performing in New York the following week, either with Thanatology or almost certainly with Carleton Sweetser in St Luke's before I get back to St Christopher's the week of the 12th. The rest of your session seems to me the fruit of plenty of thought. I look forward to hearing Melzack and of course to meeting you all and seeing how it is getting on.

---

23 Balfour Mount, the Montreal surgeon, had first visited St Christopher's in 1973 and went on to open the Royal Victoria Hospital Palliative Care Service in 1975. It is he who is credited with first use of the term 'palliative care' to refer to a wider concept of hospice and related activity and in particular their transfer into acute hospital settings. The letter is referring to the first of what became his important international conferences, held in Montreal in the autumn of 1976, in the form of a seminar.

Dr Hendrik P. Ventner

Welgemoed, Bellville, Republic of South Africa

29 June 1976 I am delighted to hear from you and know at last where those gorgeous grapes came from. They were accompanied by deliciously ripe pineapples and all of the patients and most of the staff had a few each. They were deeply appreciated.

Keep struggling and if you can find a respected, probably older, physician who would be interested in finding ways of setting up a symptom control team that might be a way of beginning.

Sandol Stoddard[24]

Tiburon, California, USA

26 July 1976 Many thanks for your letter. Interestingly enough the quotes you sent me from Henri Nouwen were picked out from those two books by Tom West when he was at Gethsemane in Kentucky recently and I bought "The Wounded Healer"[25] when I was browsing round the Yale Co-op some time ago. When we write our next Annual Report I am putting in a prayer about creating space as well as time for the people who need the hospitality of St Christopher's. I wrote this just a few days before your letter came so obviously the idea is in the air somewhere.

I suggest that you might see quite a lot of St Christopher's if you came to us for the day of Sunday 19 December arriving in time for chapel at 11.15 am, coming round with me in the wards and finishing the day with some discussion. I will send you one or two up to date reprints by surface mail and also put you on our mailing list if you wish.

Professor Bob Fulton

Minneapolis, Minnesota, USA

2 August 1976 Ever since I was at the New Haven conference I have been thinking of you because I was told that your wife was very ill. I am sending general thoughts of support and hope that when you feel like it you will write and let us know how things are. I was just reading again Death and Identity and being impressed by it and as I may want to quote a sentence or two in our own little text book due to go off to the printers next year I wonder if you will give me permission to do so. The dignity of all men is one which I have often used lecturing and it seems to ring a bell. Since you wrote that we have had too many people using the word dignity and we are going to have to begin to search for another I fear.

---

24 Sandol Stoddard was at this time engaged on a book about hospice care, by way of preparation for which she later worked for a time as a volunteer at St Christopher's. See: S. Stoddard, *The hospice movement. A better way of caring for the dying* (New York: Vintage Books, 1978).

25 Henri Nouwen (1932–96) was born in The Netherlands and ordained as a priest in 1957, moving to the United States in the early 1970s, where he was later professor of pastoral theology in the Divinity School of Yale University. The letter refers to H. J. M. Nouwen, *The wounded healer* (New York: Doubleday, 1972).

We much enjoyed Mel Krant's film Dying and want to try and buy a copy. I think the best way to do this will be for us to ask you to hold our royalties on our tapes to that end and I wonder if you could some time let me know how they are going.

Dr W. P. L. Myers

Memorial Sloan-Kettering Cancer Center, New York, USA

16 August 1976 I was fascinated to have your letter and to know that the working group had been formed at Memorial.[26] I do hope that this will be fruitful and gradually become an accepted resource in the hospital as a whole.

I am delighted to tell you that we seem to be making progress towards introducing this idea in my own teaching hospital and last week I was discussing it with Professor Symington of the Chester Beatty Institute. I think it is very interesting that the St Luke's team which grew out of their inability to acquire a few beds of their own should have turned up such a constructive new approach.

I think you have a great strength in that Dr Houde is already involved but I think the team will need to expand to take in several other disciplines.

Please keep in touch, and if you can spare a copy of your protocol when it develops I would be most grateful. In the meantime here is our latest drug sheet.

Professor A. N. Exton Smith

St Pancras Hospital, London

16 August 1976 Thank you again for a very pleasant visit with your group. I wish we saw more of you and I wonder if you would ever think of bringing some of your team out for a round here?

We have recently been discussing with our nursing staff the confusion which many patients experience and we agreed that, all too often, this is and remains somewhat of a mystery. I wonder if you have done any research in this area at all and whether you have any papers on the subject or articles by others which you could recommend. There are obvious organic and biochemical problems which can be sorted out. It seems to me, however, that there are other factors which we ought to be defining and dealing with and that there are probably too many patients who are accepted as being "confused".

I would be interested also in knowing what you commonly find most satisfactory as a tranquillizer or whether you use any at all. The Lennard Hospital use chlormethiazole a great deal but other people I know think little of it. We seem to make it work sometimes. The same goes for thioridazine. The last geriatrician I asked about this felt that promazine was considerably better than chlorpromazine. Have you any views as to where we really are in this somewhat confused field?

---

[26] In June 1976 Cicely Saunders made one of many visits over the years to the Memorial Sloan Kettering Cancer Center in New York. Here the Chairman of the Department of Medicine at the Center has written to inform her that, following the visit, a working group has been formed to deal with how the care of terminally ill patients there can be improved.

Dr Sylvia Lack[27]

New Haven, Connecticut, USA

19 August 1976 All sorts of things are happening and I cannot wait to see you. I hope your coming to the 'Think Tank'[28] on October 12th still stands. It is quite a short programme with people limited to around fifteen – one or two presenting specific things, eg Ken Calman on "Why we are doing this" and Robert [Twycross] on his prednisolone study. A short seminar at the end on "Anorexia, nausea and vomiting" will be led by Professor Laurence. This was originally billed as by St Christopher's but as he is a member of our Research Committee and is an excellent teacher, I thought it better than getting one of us to do it.

As you know, Robert got the Oxford job and Southampton did not make an appointment. I think this is no bad thing because it will underline to the NSCR [National Society for Cancer Relief] that it is really useless to set up units and have no thought as to who are going to be the staff. I believe that they have had rather a disaster at Northampton so this is an excellent moment to get this across. I am, incidentally, having a meeting with one or two 'high-ups' from Marie Curie (not Ronnie Raven), NSCR, Gill [Ford] (as from the Department) and a couple of us. This is ostensibly to sort out "Where are we now?" geographically. From my point of view the message I want to get across is the need for proper medical backing and nursing experience. The latest draft of "Components of Hospice Care" is enclosed.

I am more than happy to wait until you arrive to discuss possibilities concerning Robert's job which, of course if you do want to do, would give a chance of a further degree. We will need more clinical involvement in St Christopher's, I think, especially with our extra beds. We start altering the fourth floor in September and, as we finish it, will decant into its twelve single rooms the patients from Alexandra and City in turn in order to put a bathroom in each six-bedder with the loss of two beds and do a thorough spring-clean at the same time. This means that we will not have full 'beddage', ie 62, in the Hospice until next summer I would guess. Our finances are so much better now we have a better contract with the Region that I believe we can pay for this.

St Joseph's has Mother Paula back again and she is really blowing through the place like a good fresh breeze. She has acquired a maintenance team, has had long talks with Dr Winner and Richard Carter and me and has asked Dr Winner to chair a medical committee which would include everybody. She is also setting up some kind of a council which

---

27 Sylvia Lack was a Senior House Officer at St Joseph's Hospice, Hackney, London, from 1971 to 1973, from where she moved to work as a physician with the newly created Connecticut Hospice. Throughout this time she worked closely with Robert Twycross and they later jointly published a number of important textbooks and pamphlets, including R. Twycross and S. Lack, *Symptom control in far advanced cancer: pain relief* (London: Pitman, 1983) and *Oral morphine in advanced cancer* (Beaconsfield: Beaconsfield Publishers, 1989).

28 The terminal care 'think tank' was first established at St Christopher's in May 1975. It brought together leading medical figures and other professionals in the field and its agenda concentrated on clinical and particularly research issues.

would have representation from the doctors as well as from the Sisters and VIPs from out-side. This would really give continuity beyond the reign of an individual reverend mother. As they already do this at St Vincent's I do not think it would be disbanded by the next holder of the title. They have a good SHO [Senior House Officer] at the moment – a nun from the Medical Missionaries of Mary – she (Reverend Mother) will wait for an active medical director and they are prepared to wait for the right person. Mother Paula likes Richard Lamerton and, although he has been very quiet as far as I am concerned, I think he likes her. The RHA [Regional Health Authority] suddenly stopped his grant and Mother Paula asked what kind of contract we have so that we could use the same for him. As you know, we only have a letter of appointment so they are, no doubt, still sorting this out.

The Hostel [of God] is advertising for a matron and an administrator. I think they just did not feel they could be bold enough to implement change. I happened to run into Dr Brown in the shops the other day and he says he knows nothing more of what is hap-pening and continues to be treated as a child.

There are, in fact, a row of 'Macedonians' asking for help but none of them, except pos-sibly Southampton, needs any kind of answer until you come over and have a chance of taking bearings. I just hope it will be UK somewhere!

I have had a fascinating discussion with Professor Symington, of The Chester Beatty, and I think that some kind of interchange of registrars to and from the Sutton Marsden and/or up-grading of our SHO post to registrar anyway is on the cards. In fact, the whole thing is rather like a good stock-pot with some interesting ingredients bubbling away and, like most good stock, will be better for not being hastened.

I wonder what your reactions are to the enclosed? I think I remember Claus from both Working parties. I am writing back to ask him to let me know who else is involved: you really do have to tell people who else you are asking when you send these sort of letters!

Dr Balfour Mount

Royal Victoria Hospital, Montreal, Canada

23 August 1976 Thank you for the programme. You really have gone to town over this conference and I only hope we will stick to our brief or we will all be saying the same thing over and over again. The list of references is not very long because I am really not certain what is in print in your country. I think you know what I would suggest anyway. My own Care of the Dying should be in print by then and I think I could arrange for some to be sent over for the conference if you would like that. I was surprised how easily it updated from 1960.

I hope there will be time to fit in the Standards Group meeting as suggested and I look forward to it all.

Please could you tell me what the temperature range is likely to be so that I can consider my wardrobe?

Angela Tilby

BBC, London

25 August 1976 After talking to you and relaxing about the idea of doing something for "The Light of Experience"[29] my sub-conscious quietly got to work and this enclosed script emerged over the weekend. I am not sure about length but it does give the idea of what I would like to do and I thought it best just to send it off as it is.

Should you feel it fits in with a television programme I think illustrations would be a bit difficult but I have made a few suggestions and also of music in pencil around the script.

Thank you for being most helpful. I think I have needed to get this off my chest for quite a long time and even if it does not get used for yet a while I am glad to have done it. This is the first time I feel I have told the story of how St Christopher's began truthfully.

Dr Robert Twycross

Sir Michael Sobell House, Oxford

17 November 1976 This is a follow up from Jenny's letter in which she sent you the protocol. They have been visited by NCI and are hoping for a grant for them this time. It still seems to be doing alright. Bal's unit got its approval from the hospital to become a permanent part of the scene. I expect you saw the reprints from the Canadian Medical Association Journal of 17 July 1967. I much enjoyed meeting Melzack who is very enthusiastic about the Brompton cocktail and it seems that this is the name we are going to have to accept from the North American scene. He hopes to be visiting here when he comes to England in July. Incidentally he feels there is no need for anybody to do any further comparative trial of regular giving of such a mixture and prn analgesia.

Sylvia is going to be in England for December on holiday. Once she had written to Southampton she knew that it was not what she wanted to do. She is taking her licensure exams in November but has not made up her mind about the future. I hope very much she will meet Thelma Bates while she is here.

You still have not sent us the copy of your paper from Pain.[30] If you remember you showed me your only copy and took it with you. I would like to have a copy so that we could make the cheaper reprints here rather than wait for its publication. If you agree would you write on it how you would like it to be described.

---

29 A religious affairs programme on BBC television, featuring accounts of the life and work of particular individuals. It was in this broadcast that Cicely Saunders was to recount in public for the first time the story of Antoni Michniewicz and the part he played in her subsequent thoughts, feelings, and actions. See her letters to Dr T. J. Deeley of 15 March 1960, p. 26, and to Sister Françoise of 9 August 1960, p. 34.

30 R. G. Twycross, Choice of strong analgesics in terminal cancer: diamorphine or morphine? *Pain*, **3** (1977): 93–104.

Professor Patrick Wall[31]

University College Hospital, London

14 April 1977 On coming back from holiday I was delighted to find that you were coming to talk to St Christopher's on 1 June. I wonder whether you would have time to see a little of the Hospice at the same time and perhaps discuss our work on pain control?

You may not have seen the enclosed reprint which sums up much of the work Dr Twycross did here as our Clinical Research Fellow. We have not replaced him for the moment as we want to think with our Research Committee (which includes Professor Desmond Laurence[32]) and with others around the subject till we are certain what would be the most important area for us to look at. Our Annual Report will give you an idea of our work in general.

I have twice met Ron Melzack in Montreal and had very stimulating discussions with him and it seems very wrong that I have not met you yet to discuss our work. Would you like to come for lunch or stay after your talk? I will gladly fit in with whatever is more convenient for you but hope you will be able to give us some extra time.

Dr H. A. Copeman

Royal Perth Hospital, Perth, Western Australia

15 April 1977 Thank you for your letter of 9 March. I look forward to the visit and am glad it is beginning to fall into shape. My present plan is that I arrive in Perth some time over the week end of 2/3 September and will be ready to go by Monday 5 September. I would like to spend that week visiting the centres which are concerned with terminal malignant diseases and for this I refer to my letter to Miss Sellick of 14 April 1976 of which I enclose a photocopy. In my original letter from here it was agreed that the first week should be visits and include a few wild flowers, birds etc.

I am happy with the suggestions for the main seminar and obviously will have more understanding of your local scene after the previous week of visits. My lunch time talk would I think be best titled "Philosophy of Total Care of the Terminally Ill". This is the title I took at a big conference in Montreal last autumn and it does enable one to cover the ground fairly thoroughly. It is essential that I should be able to speak with slides, colour transparencies of the usual size which require a good blackout and a strong projector if it is a big hall.

I will enjoy the public meeting and am prepared to be involved in the programme as the Programme Committee asks adding that I think The Nature and Management of Terminal Pain, Home, Hospital or Hospice or A Death in the Family would cover the topics I would cope with generally in the presentation mentioned above, in more specific detail.

---

[31] Patrick Wall (1925–2001), leading researcher in the pain field and responsible, with the Canadian psychologist Ronald Melzack, for the gate control theory of pain: R. Melzack and P. D. Wall, Pain mechanisms: a new theory, *Science*, **150** (1965): 971–9. He later joined the research committee of St Christopher's Hospice.

[32] Professor of Pharmacology at University College, London.

I recently had two trips to the States. One on a Visiting Professorship to Galveston, the programme of which I sent to Miss Sellick for her interest, and the other for a holiday. The former was travelling first class and the second tourist. The Galveston trip was the first time I had travelled first and I hope you will be able to be equally generous. I am six feet tall and getting arthritis in my knees and last winter had a crush fracture of my spine so I think I am not fussing when I say that a trip of those dimensions has got to be done in this way. The first class return fare to Perth is 2,800 Australian dollars.

My present plan is to work in the University of California San Francisco the week before flying from there to Australia and I have a holiday in Jerusalem after that. I will obviously have to pay my flight from here. St Christopher's will pay the fare. All money ever paid to a St Christopher's staff member is, under the terms of their employment, paid to the Hospice so any help you can give towards my flight whether in my name or that of the Hospice goes straight to them and does not go through any tax procedure.

Can you tell me what the temperature range is likely to be?

I much look forward to coming.

Dr John Fryer[33]

Temple University, Philadelphia, Pennsylvania, USA

28 April 1977 Your letter of 14 March has just arrived. It was nice to hear from you and I shall be interested to know what happens to your friends.

So far I am impressed by what I have heard about Bill Lamers'[34] work and have enjoyed meeting with him and a few of the group. It is good that they have got accepted for Medicare and I understand that he and Hospice Inc are working hard with the insurance companies. I am going to San Francisco in August to meet with them and do one or two things and hopefully seminars and a lecture at the University Hospital. This is being co-ordinated by Sandol Stoddard whose book on Hospices seems to be going rather well and whose husband is Professor of Medicine there. We much enjoyed having them here at Christmas time.

I am most interested to see that the IWG [International Work Group on Death Dying and Bereavement] is meeting in conjunction with the Euthanasia Education Council. It seems to me that much of what they say is good and I know Sam Klagsbrun[35] has been involved with them. He, as you probably know, has been here twice and is a good friend. I am concerned however when their work on pressing for the withdrawal of inappropriate care shades into suggestions of active "mercy killing". If you can concentrate on definitions and keep the issues clear I think it would be a great help to the movement as a whole. This

---

[33] One of the founders of the Ars Moriendi group, from 1974 the International Work Group on Death, Dying and Bereavement (IWG).

[34] Bill Lamers, the American psychiatrist who founded the Hospice of Marin in California. Later he was Assistant Clinical Director at the Tom Baker Cancer Center, Calgary, Canada (see letter to William Lamers, 7 February 1984, p. 246).

[35] Sam Klagsbrun trained in psychiatry at Yale and heard Cicely Saunders speak there in 1963, finally meeting her in the early 1970s, after which he began a series of annual visits to St Christopher's and from 1985 became the hospice's official Visitor.

may be difficult but I think better clinical judgement, if necessary backed by the California Law because of malpractice problems is what we should all be 'working for'. If we keep talking together with our definitions clear there would be, I think, less need to polarise and have the Euthanasia Education Council on a totally different side of the fence from the ordinary Hospice workers.

It seems really impossible to me for there to be a law making possible an active killing however apparently justified in an individual situation without pressuring everyone else. No one would feel they had a right to longer term care once the short way out was available and society would very quickly endorse that impression.

I am really looking forward to seeing you at St Christopher's. Not as a worker but as a short term visitor!

Mr V. Brandon Melton

Methodist Hospital of Indiana Inc., Indianapolis, Indiana, USA

29 April 1977 I can hardly add up the number of people who write letters similar to yours. I know we have many years of experience but I think it is more important that you learn from the people who have already spent several years adapting our basic principles in the American scene. Our staff and our staff patterns are very different from yours. The whole financial scene is totally different, the kind of ways in which we support each other are not the same either.

However I am enclosing our last annual Report and a Personal Communication on Components of Hospice Care and I think you will find most of what you think you want in these. If you can afford something towards the postage we would be most grateful.

Dr Robert Twycross

Sir Michael Sobell House, Oxford

17 May 1977 I thought you would be interested to know that St Christopher's moves over to morphine by mouth as from next week, but maintains diamorphine by injection.[36] We will let you know how it goes and hope to be well established before producing our usual drug control of common symptoms later this summer. This will be printed as before in World Medicine who I hope will give us a good supply of reprints.

Mary Baines and I were discussing patients with high dosages yesterday. She had just had an Out Patient Clinic for two patients, one on 90 mgms and one on 80 mgms orally. Both were keeping to a 4 hourly schedule but were needing an occasional booster of Dextramoramide. Mary had found that this rather short acting booster was right rather than shortening the interval. As you say so firmly in your chapter that the larger the dose the shorter the interval may be, she asked me to mention this to you and have your comments. As you know we only shorten the interval very occasionally and have found that on

---

[36] This was an important moment in which the results of extensive research by Robert Twycross were acted upon. The 'Brompton Cocktail' was abandoned and morphine (a drug more readily available than diamorphine in many countries) became the analgesic of choice.

the whole this is right and we pass it on in this way when we are teaching. Would you consider making a foot note or some comment to this effect in your chapter?

Helen J. Nowoswiat

Roswell Park Memorial Institute, Buffalo, New York, USA

24 May 1977 I was interested to receive your letter, having spoken for a meeting organised by the Buffalo Hospice group last autumn.

Today St Christopher's is changing from the use of heroin or diamorphine to morphine. We did extensive trials of these two drugs which are summed up in the enclosed reprint and have felt that for teaching purposes we should no longer use a drug which is unavailable in most of the world. I do not think there is any need for your physician to conduct a further study in this area.

I am interested that you mention only one strength of morphine in your mixture. We use many different doses as enclosed. We are however still using diamorphine by injection because of its solubility and the equivalent doses to which we are changing are as enclosed. As you see we have tended to round up in order to simplify the change so that it is not exactly on the 1.5 to 1 ratio which we found correct in our pilot studies. You may be interested in our drug sheet. We will be producing a new one later this summer when we have settled down to the use of morphine. I believe we will find, as in our studies, that there is no clinically observable difference.

Dr Richard Lamerton[37]

St Joseph's Hospice, London

28 June 1977 Thank you for sending me your review with which I agreed on most points.

We have a real problem with the Brompton Cocktail. As you no doubt know it is becoming an acceptable form of treatment in the US under that title and with a flexible dosage and usually without cocaine. It may be that we have to accept it putting it in quotes and pointing out that it is by no means the same dose every time, nor was it when it was first concocted at the Brompton as far as I know. Now we have diamorphine elixir in the BP I suppose we are some way to standardising it but as we are stopping diamorphine anyway that does not really help.

Perhaps this would be a good topic for the Therapeutics Conference in November.

Thank you for the figures. I think they are slightly offset by the much smaller amount St Christopher's spends on capital and replacements. All our money goes to nurses. All the same it is amazing what St Joseph's does for the money it spends and as you know I never criticise St Joseph's in public.

---

[37] Richard Lamerton trained as a junior doctor at St Joseph's and St Christopher's before becoming the physician at St Joseph's Hospice, Hackney, where with Sister Mary Antonia he developed the home care service. For his recollections of that period see R. Lamerton, *East end doc* (Cambridge: Lutterworth, 1986).

John Whitman

Cornwells Heights, Pennsylvania, USA

18 October 1977 The enclosed literature will answer those of your questions for which we have the needed information. We are not required to keep details of the exact number of visits made to patients at home but I should point out that there is some information in the Annual Report and that only a small proportion of our patients die at home, most are admitted to St Christopher's. You will see that our discharge rate goes up slowly but is still in the region of 10%. We do not have a detailed breakdown of our staffing available but it may help you to know that we have through our 10 years had a bed cost per week of 70% or less of that in a teaching hospital in our area and 80% or less of a non teaching general hospital.

Hospice care is neither a cheap nor an easy option although it is both cheaper and more effective for the patients who need this care than a general hospital. It is more expensive than the ordinary nursing home.

Sister Mary Greaney

Ruttonjee Sanatorium, Wanchai, Hong Kong

19 October 1977 Here is our last Annual Report and some reprints which I think will answer most of your questions.

Our patients' relatives have almost invariably been informed of the seriousness of our patients' illness. It is more unlikely that the patients will be fully in the picture although there is a tendency in general hospitals to be somewhat more honest than say 10 years ago. We try to find out what the patient's insight is when he comes, both from the family and from him. We encourage the family to share if they can, but some maintain an attitude of denial and we do not try to force truth into that situation. It is usual to get their consent to talk if the patient wants and needs to know more, but somebody may go peacefully through an illness without discussing it directly and we would not be unhappy about that. Certainly more people know than do not at St Christopher's but there is no real general rule.

All good wishes in your own work

Henya Elkinud

Beth Hakerem, Jerusalem, Israel

25 October 1977 I know Tom [West] has written to both of you but I wanted to wait until I had the enclosed Annual Report to send you. Thank you again for the most wonderful evening and the best food and company we had in Israel. We hope very much we will have a chance of entertaining you here one day. Meantime we look forward to coming back and to hearing that there are some developments in Hadassah. It will not be a Hospice like us, but I am sure there is a unique Hadassah way of helping dying patients and their families.

Dr Walter Baechi

Zurich, Switzerland

28 October 1977 The Voluntary Euthanasia Society have sent your letter on to us. They are not involved with any clinics but passed it on with a friendly note knowing well that we consider that a Hospice is an alternative to mercy killing.

I enclose a memorandum on Hospice care which I hope your friend will find helpful. It is based on our experience and development and a great deal of correspondence and interchange of views with people planning this type of work in various parts of the world. May I add that we believe very strongly that a Hospice is not only for dying and that this should never be part of its title.

Dr Esther Lucile Brown

San Francisco, California, USA

9 November 1977 I thought you would like to know that early last week I had a brief, but I think very profitable, meeting at the National Institutes of Health with Mr Burke and his team and the head of the Division, Dr Fink. I was able to go over on Concorde and so able to lecture to the Division as a whole in the first afternoon and then spend the whole of the next day discussing standards and staffing, which of course means costs and evaluation.

Mr Hackley was at the first meeting and also two people from one of the other contractors. I think we have really got across that our own proportion of volunteer hours to salaried staff hours is very small. I gave them a copy of the enclosed and you will be interested to know that we have about 700 hours of volunteer help in a week.

Dr Fink was satisfied that this is a medical programme and I am sure that includes an understanding of levels of staffing needed.

They were aware of the problems of research in an evolving situation but I was able to give them a report of his work by our social psychiatrist which was carried out during our first 3 years. I hope this will solve some of the problems.

Dr John J. Bonica

University of Washington, Seattle, Washington, USA

11 November 1977 Many thanks for your letter. As you know I have booked the time in Venice[38] and would be happy to take part.

In your letter you mention both a lecture and participation in the general discussion "as well as your participation in the Special Problems on Saturday". I cannot find my name earlier in the programme so I am not sure what you mean by "your lecture". I would gladly tackle something to do with the family or the components of a Hospice programme, though I do not quite see where you would put it in. You may have other ideas and I would fit in with what you ask of me, if I can.

---

[38] This refers to the first International Congress on Cancer Pain, organized by Professor Vittorio Ventafridda in Venice, May 1978.

It was very good to meet you at last and to have a chance of taking part in this important symposium.[39]

Professor Kenneth Calman[40]

Department of Clinical Oncology, Glasgow

6 December 1977 Since the beginning of October next year's diary has got worse and worse and I am now looking at it in considerable despair.

Since you got on to me I have had an SOS from Aberdeen where they have a Continuing Care Unit opening with little public relations done with the doctors beforehand and a great need of an open meeting. I enclose a copy of my letter to them and I wonder if there is a possibility of my combining the 2 sessions. That is flying from Aberdeen to you or vice versa and doing it all in 2 days. You will have to have the same lecture. Perhaps the best thing would be for you to get on to Dr Brunt.

I am sorry about this but there has been a rush of important things.

Ava Tagore

Oakland University, Rochester, Michigan, USA

8 December 1977 Thank you for your letter. Your name makes me think that a very good way of approaching this problem would be for you to study Gitanjali by Rabindranath Tagore published by Macmillan and Company Limited, St Martin's Street, London. Embedded in this beautiful poetry are some extremely helpful thoughts on the nature of death coming from a totally different culture than our own.

I am enclosing our latest Annual Report and a copy of a memorandum on the components of Hospice care. From this you should be able to discover that St Christopher's has carried out research in clinical pharmacology and some psychosocial studies. I think that it is basic research in practical care that is needed in your country.

You might get further information from the Public Relations Officer, Hospice Inc, New Haven, Connecticut.

Dr Balfour Mount

Royal Victoria Hospital, Montreal, Canada

11 January 1978 Lovely to have your card and to know that you have had such a good time. I am very glad you were in Marseille, it was really important that you should be there. I look forward to some more feed back about that.

I did not know Faye had actually got her BTh. Many congratulations from us all.

We are much looking forward to your contribution to our conference but really would like to know what day you hope to arrive.

---

[39] They had recently met in Bethesda, USA.

[40] An important supporter of palliative care developments and later Chief Medical Officer for England.

You must have been getting requests from one or two people that we have passed on to you but I feel this is a fair exchange. Now I have a more personal request.

I have a niece who will be taking exams next July and November and will hopefully be going to University to read medicine. She will have a gap from Christmas to September (78/79) for travelling/working. Is there any chance of someone needing an au pair in Montreal? If you think there is any possibility of you knowing someone who would like an English teenager who would also like to learn French I would be most grateful. I would also arrange for her to come up and see you while you were here in February. My brother lives in Cambridge and she is the middle of the family and a bright girl who has done extremely well with riding in Pony Club trials and so on and is gaining in confidence all the time. She needs something extra to give her a boost as her older brother and younger sister are bouncing cheerful extroverts who find life considerably easier than she does. This may be impossible for you but I would be very grateful for help.

Dr R. J. Evans

University of Toronto, Toronto, Ontario, Canada

11 January 1978 Many thanks for your letter and for the kind effort in looking for the Joan of Arc reference and for answering my own letter in detail.

I think the point of our study among the community and from the memories of bereaved families is that this was the "pain" that they remembered a year later. As the groups who died at home or in general hospitals had no access to a clinic such as yours I am afraid a great deal of this was "physical pain". However I am equally glad to have your figures for discussion with such people as the Voluntary Euthanasia Society because it does point out that properly treated intractable pain is rare.

I do take you up however in saying that "retrospective assessments from relatives are of no use at all". The difference in the figures at St Christopher's from those in the other two settings are I hope an illustration of this.

I think the pain field is fascinating at the moment and will let you know how things progress.

Dr Robert Twycross

Sir Michael Sobell House, Oxford

6 March 1978 I enclose my precious and only copy of *Peace at the Last*.[41] It appeared on the desk of the Secretary to the City Parochial Foundation the day I first arrived in 1960 and Hughie of course was on our Council for a long time after that so it has been very important to St Christopher's. He took it from the collect.

I agree with you about the BMJ [British Medical Journal] title. In fact this was written by Daphne Gloag whom I met at the LMG [London Medical Group] conference.

You did not enclose your draft so I cannot make any comments at the moment. I will keep the original one under wraps.

....

[41] H. L. Glyn Hughes, *Peace at the last. A survey of terminal care in the United Kingdom* (London, Galouste Gulbenkian Foundation, 1960).

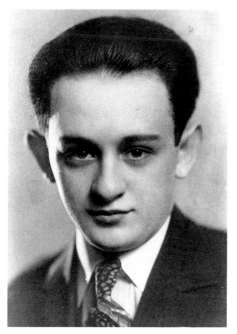

Plate 1 David Tasma (d. 1948): the inspiration for Cicely Saunders' subsequent work with the dying.

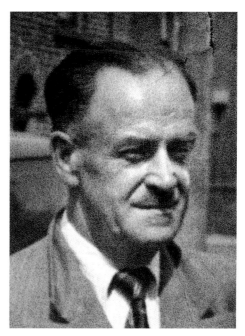

Plate 2 Antoni Michniewicz (d. 1960): cared for by Cicely Saunders in St Joseph's Hospice, and with whom she developed a deep and intense relationship in the final months of his life.

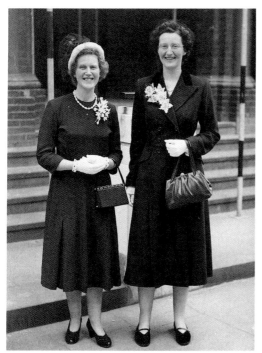

Plate 3 With Rosetta Burch (left) at a wedding in the early 1950s.

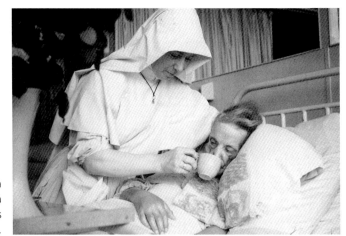

Plate 4 Sister Mary Antonia gives a cup of tea to a dying patient at St Joseph's Hospice, Hackney, c.1963.

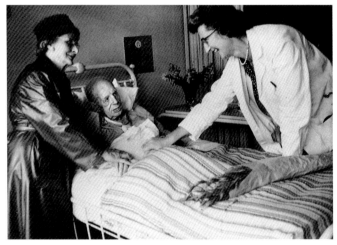

Plate 5 With two patients at St Joseph's on their golden wedding anniversary; he is in the bed where Antoni Michniewicz was cared for.

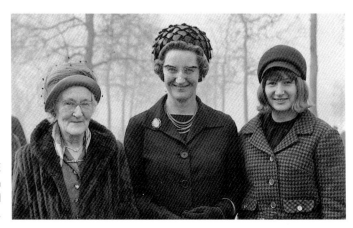

Plate 6 Receiving the OBE on 9 March 1965, with her mother (left) and niece, Penelope (right).

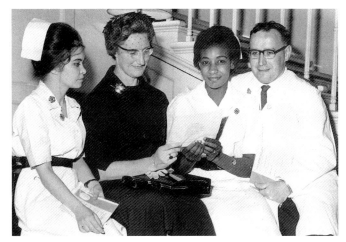

Plate 7 Awarding nursing prizes at London's Royal Marsden Hospital, probably 1965.

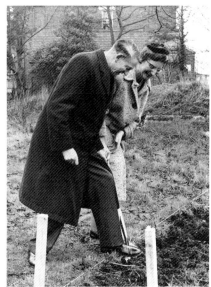

Plate 8 Lord Thurlow and Cicely Saunders dig the first spit to mark the start of building at St Christopher's Hospice, Sydenham, on 22 March 1965.

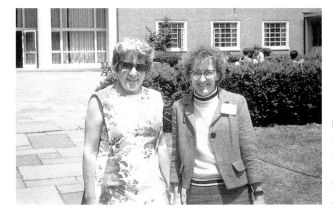

Plate 9 Florence Wald (left) and Elisabeth Kübler-Ross (right), pictured at the Yale University meeting of April 1966, at which they met with Cicely Saunders and Colin Murray Parkes.

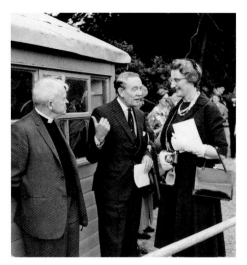

Plate 10 With Lord Thurlow (centre) and Almon Pepper (left) at the dedication and laying of the hospice foundation stone, 22 July 1966.

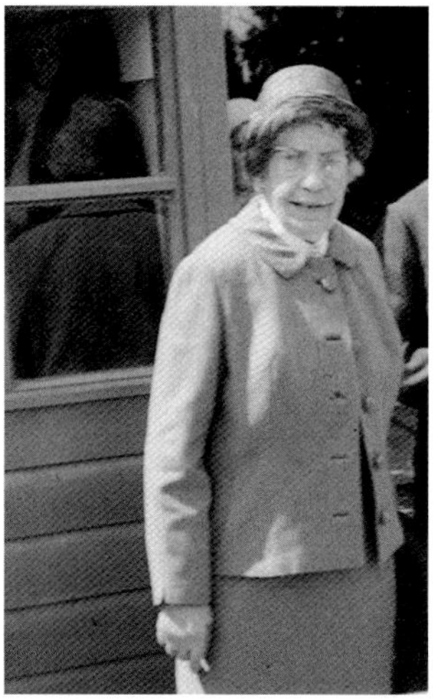

Plate 11 Olive Wyon, theologian and adviser to Cicely Saunders, on 22 July 1966 at the dedication of the hospice.

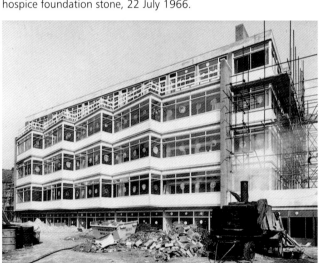

Plate 12 St Christopher's under construction, spring 1967.

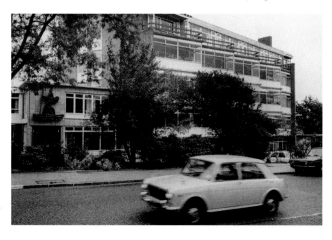

Plate 13 St Christopher's soon after opening.

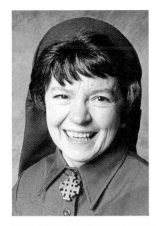

Plate 14 Sister Zita Marie Cotter, who came from the USA to work at St Christopher's soon after its opening.

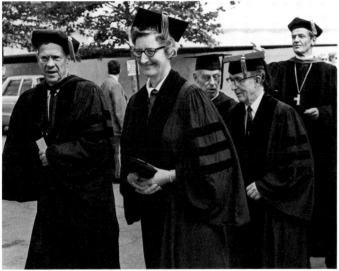

Plate 15 Receiving her first honorary degree, at Yale University, on 9 June 1969.

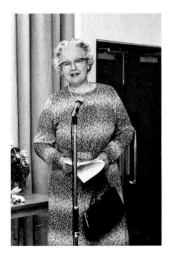

Plate 16 Dame Albertine Winner at the official opening of St Christopher's Study Centre in 1973.

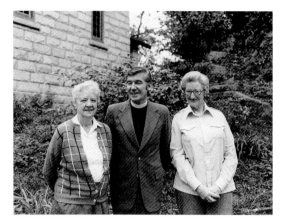

Plate 17 With Miss Betty Lestor and Carlton Sweetser in front of St Christopher's Chapel, Hyden, Kentucky, USA, 1978.

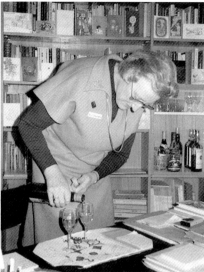

Plate 18 Drinks in the office, mid-1970s.

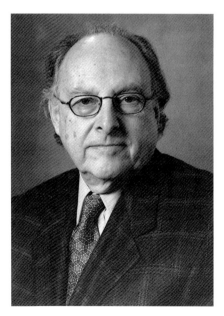

Plate 19 Dr Sam Klagsbrun visited the hospice annually to give organizational advice and was appointed Visitor in 1975.

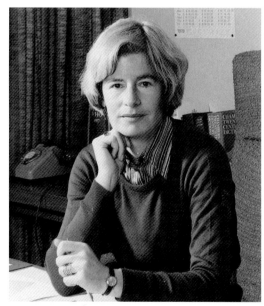

Plate 20 Dr Gillian Ford, long-term friend of Cicely Saunders and supporter of St Christopher's, in 1979.

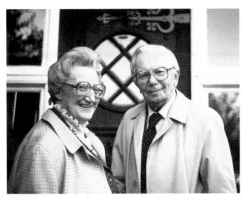

Plate 21 With her husband Marian Bohusz-Szyszko, outside their home in Sydenham.

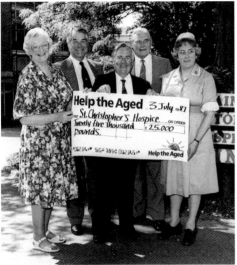

Plate 22 Over the years, fundraising was always a feature of life at St Christopher's. With (left to right) Tom West, Tom Breen, George Moore (of Help the Aged), and Eleri Price.

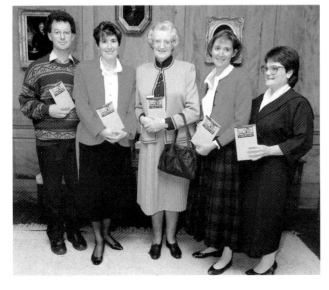

Plate 23 With (left to right) Robert Dunlop, Jacqui Field, Jo Hockley, and Judith Reddie at their book launch, 1990.

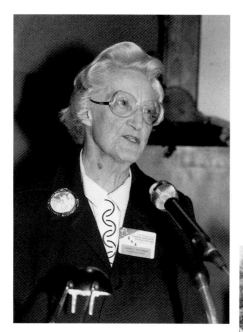

Plate 24 Speaking at the Second Congress of the European Association of Palliative Care, Brussels, 1992.

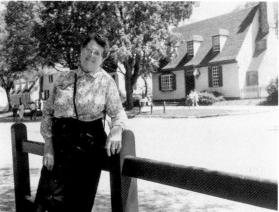

Plate 25 Grace Goldin – a friend for over thirty years, photographer, poet, and historian. Pictured outside her home in Swarthmore, Pennsylvania, USA.

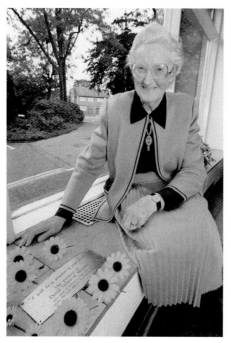

Plate 26 David Tasma's window.

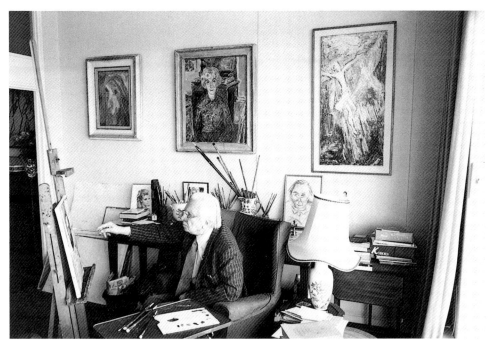

Plate 27 Despite periods of major illness in later life, Marian Bohusz-Szyszko was able to continue painting with vigour and enthusiasm.

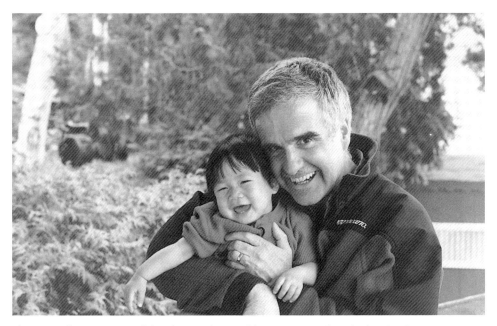

Plate 28 Balfour Mount and daughter Bethany, mid-1990s. It was he who in 1975 began to popularize the term 'palliative care'.

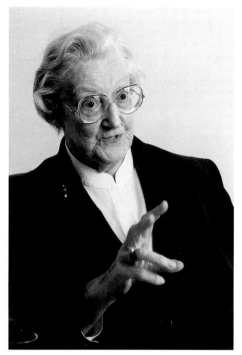

Plate 29 Making a clear point.

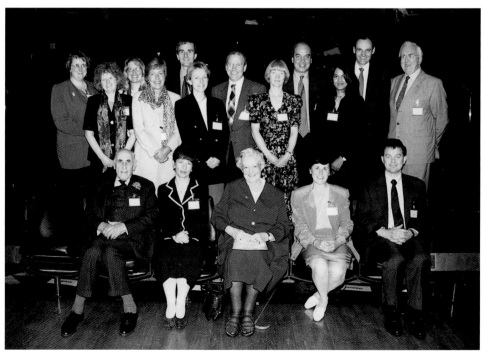

Plate 30 Surrounded by friends and colleagues at a conference to mark her eightieth birthday, Royal College of Physicians, June 1998.

I gather from Mary Baines there was a good article in the *Sunday Times* yesterday but other people have reservations about such words as 'private institutions'. Major Garnett is coming down to see me this afternoon as he rather wants to write a joint letter in answer to the report of comments made by Mr Sturgess of the Marie Curie Memorial Foundation which I expect you saw in the Guardian.

John Scott has just written to me from Canada saying, "I am pushing hard for the use of the word 'hospice', but Bal has done an incredible job of selling the term 'palliative' in Canada. Theologically and psychologically, I prefer the positive and community connotations in the word 'hospice'. The thrust in the word 'palliative' is far from ideal."

(Continuing is better I agree – but I still like Hospice best)

Dr Colin Murray Parkes
St Christopher's Hospice

3 April 1978 Ever since you spoke briefly to me about the possibility of some kind of central set up for your work I have been turning it over in my mind. I have also talked to Tom, Gill and Helen and the following thoughts come to my mind.

Individual Chairs are moderately common and I think becoming more so at a time of stringency in the National Health Service. Something in your field would be remarkably cheaper than for example a Chair in Oncology. I do not think there would be a great difficulty in finding the money for this. From some recent discussions, with more than one Trust, I would not anticipate any difficulty in interesting someone in funding a personal Chair.

Any Chair of course has to have an attachment to an academic department but surely this would logically be the London if Desmond likes the idea. This would be money apart from his budget and presumably he would then have another psychiatrist in your present place.

If you think the time is ripe I would very much like to talk with him about this. It would surely be a great addition to the field in general, to the links with the community around the London and St Joseph's and I cannot think of anyone I would rather see holding the first professorship in our field.

Sorry not to be seeing you this Thursday, I will be in Derby.

(Do lets have a go!)

Judith H. Quattlebaum
National Committee on the Treatment of Intractable Pain, Washington, USA

19 April 1978 Thank you for your Newsletter and the folder on the work of the National Committee on the Treatment of Intractable Pain which were brought back for me by Dr Twycross. He tells me he enjoyed meeting with you all and I am glad to have his talk in print.

When I read about cancer pain in your literature I think you are over-estimating when you say that cancer "causes chronic and intense pain to almost all sufferers". The studies I have read suggest that only about half the people who die of cancer will have this kind of pain, and I think in your eagerness to arouse public concern and pressure on the legislators you tend to over-state and so to arouse more fear than is really justified. If I may say so I think that this has been a problem for the American Cancer Society. So much of their public education programme seems to me to have increased fear. I was discussing this with a Professor involved in cancer education for medical students last week and it did seem that the withdrawal of students from patients with cancer – which I think is probably worse in America than in England – has the same kind of foundation.

I am enclosing a paper I wrote on Terminal Pain for presentation to our Medical Research Council. It is not really for reproduction – merely a discussion paper, but you might like to see it.

I know that you were disappointed that George Will did not mention heroin in his excellent hospice article! but it really is not the only answer to this problem. I am sure that he was right to emphasise the more general aspects. After all the great majority of doses given here are as morphine.

Christer Tovesson

Gothenburg, Sweden

17 May 1978 You are the second Swedish newspaper to write in the last few days and I am afraid I am going to write to you as I did to the other to say that it really is very difficult indeed for us to see you. However, as you are prepared to wait until September I suppose I cannot say a complete No at this point. I am leaving for the United States on 18th September and already have a fairly busy programme before then.

I need to have more details from you as to the kind of article you are thinking of writing and the reasons for your approaching us at St Christopher's. As you no doubt know, one or two nurses have visited here from Sweden and I feel that you would do better to talk with one of them. Ulla Quarnstrom was here on one of our courses and is publishing a thesis shortly, and Dr Loma Feigenberg of Karolinska Hospital also knows our work well.

I am sorry to sound so unwilling but we have many journalists asking to visit and we have to make certain that an article in a foreign language is going to present a responsibly accurate picture, and also it is time we should give to our patients rather than to you.

Kathleen Mavretich

Rosedale, New York, USA

18 May 1978 You are one of very many people who write to us about our drug regime. I am enclosing our latest literature and also a reprint of the work referred to in the Annual Report which you saw. We do not call our mixture by the name of the Brompton Hospital and, as you see, have simplified it considerably. We have not noticed a difference in the wards as a whole since we both changed the morphine and omitted the cocaine, but this was of course based on controlled clinical trials to back up this clinical impression.

I have been using a narcotic mixture since 1948 in various settings and am convinced that this is a very convenient way of giving strong analgesics – and very acceptable to patients. It is, however, much more the way you use your drugs and your total care of the patient which is of greater importance.

There is a great deal of work going on in this field in your country and I suggest that you get in touch with the Public Relations Officer, Hospice Inc, New Haven, Connecticut.

I would be very grateful for 3$ for these reprints plus the cost of postage as we are in fact a charity.

Professor Tadeusz Koszarowski

Instytut Onkologii im Marii Sklodowskiej-Curie, Warsaw, Poland

29 June 1978 I must thank you very much indeed for all the arrangements you made for my visit to Poland. Dr Zborzil looked after me beautifully from the moment I arrived to the time he saw me safely off to London.

I enjoyed all the visits and the responsiveness of the very varied audiences. It was particularly interesting to see the two Sue Ryder Homes and to make a ward round with Dr Zborzil.

The enormous strides that have been made in your country since 1962 are most impressive to a visitor and added greatly to the enjoyment of the trip. I see well that to build a unit such as St Christopher's Hospice would be well nigh impossible in view of the many demands and needs of acute medicine. However this is not the only way in which the principles of Hospice care can be interpreted. I hope that some development in pain control will take place. It seems to me that this would enable patients to be more active as well as more free from pain and would enable them to cope for longer in their own homes.

I am enclosing some reprints that will show you that the general wards in our country can be shown sadly inadequate in this field.

Our own text book[42] should be out in the autumn and I look forward to sending it to you as a small thank you for a very good trip.

Joanna Jasellarian

Ioana Sakellarios, Athens, Greece

7 July 1978 Thank you for your letter and donation for reprints. I am very interested to hear from you as we had some conversation with an oncologist from Athens at a conference in Amsterdam two years ago which interested me greatly. We understood from him that it was well nigh impossible to tell patients and even their families that they had cancer and that the psychiatric support needed was very different from our efforts in England as well as in the States.

This was just one person's view but I have heard it elsewhere and I wonder how you will find your work compares with ours which is illustrated in the enclosed reprints.

I will be very interested to hear how your work goes on.

---

[42] A reference to C. Saunders (ed.), *The management of terminal malignant disease* (London: Edward Arnold, 1978).

Dr Halina Iwanowska[43]

Department of Surgery, Gdansk, Poland

13 July 1978 I am glad to say that my picture of Gdansk with two rainbows over the airport has come out beautifully and I will be sending you one. It was a lovely few days and I really feel optimistic that something will happen in your city. I feel very strongly that although you really have little hope of a separate building this is far less important than developing teaching. Obviously the anaesthetists are going to need a lot of persuasion that the routine use of oral narcotics can give excellent pain control without blotting the patient out in any way. The more I talk with people in Poland the more I realise the situation is just the same as we found in Italy that people have no idea at all of the effectiveness of that kind of pain control. Consequently one hears of a lot of demanding techniques which will only be done by a few and only reach a few whereas I am quite sure those patients we saw together with unrelieved pain could be helped without any extra use of people or time.

If there is any chance of your being able to come over here we would welcome you and I know you appreciate how much time we will need to know in advance for making plans.

Best wishes to your student group and to everything else you are doing.

Reverend Edward F. Dobihal[44]

Hospice Inc., New Haven, Connecticut, USA

22 August 1978 Your letter of August 8th only arrived yesterday but I hasten to reply with my grateful thanks to you all for changing your dates. Tom joins me in our pleasure that we will have our holiday with a totally clear conscience and I am blocking out September at this point so there will be no problem with my coming. I take it that your big week will therefore begin on September 30th and I will want to get off as soon as it is over so that we can keep 3 weeks for our October holiday. I am delighted that we can work this out safely.

You surely have a problem in protecting the quality of hospice care in the States – rather different from our own. I think that for us both a careful statement of the basic essentials of any hospice programme or team needs to be talked round and illustrated and established in the same kind of way that the basic essentials of an intensive care unit are fairly well comprehended and established across many frontiers. I have been asked to speak to this kind of brief in Washington and I will as usual be illustrating it from St Christopher's and possibly from the old days of hospice development in St Joseph's. Time in Washington will be pressured but it would be very good to see you and Sylvia and perhaps we could plan something along these lines for your important Dedication week.

---

[43] The journalist, philosopher, and inspiration to hospice developments in Poland. This letter follows Cicely Saunders' visit to Poland in 1978 which included important meetings in Warsaw, Gdansk, and Krakow: see J. Luczak, Palliative care in Eastern Europe, in *New themes in palliative care* (ed. D. Clark, J. Hockley, and S. Ahmedzai), (Buckingham: Open University Press, 1997), pp. 170–94.

[44] The Reverend Ed Dobihal (d. 2001) was a member of the group at Yale who together established the Connecticut Hospice. He had first met Cicely Saunders in 1966 at the 'Institute' convened by Florence Wald and involving Colin Murray Parkes, Elisabeth Kübler-Ross, and others: see letter to Colin Murray Parkes, 24 March 1966, p. 103. He also spent time working as a chaplain at St Christopher's in 1970.

Everyone at St Christopher's is delighted to know that you are able to change and that I am going to be able to attend your Dedication.

Why were you laid up in the hospital? I hope it was just for a rest.

Professor Henryk Gaertner

Biernacki City Hospital, Krakow, Poland

24 October 1978 How wonderful to have a Pope from Krakow, it is a wonderful work of the Holy Spirit.

Is there any hope of your coming in December? I am sending another copy of the letter sent to Miss Bortnowska. This letter explains what we hope you will be able to do, could you let me know if there is any chance of this. I am sure we would be able to tuck your wife in too and you must not worry about money. I have very much that I owe to Poland, and I was fortunate in the honoraria I had recently in America.

Ulrike Goetzner

Wurzburg-Heidingsfeld, West Germany

7 December 1978 Thank you for your letter of the 9th November which has only just reached me. I am enclosing a copy of our Annual Report which answers many of your questions and gives a list of our reprints which you can send for.

I assure you that "hard" drugs as they are used here do not give us "drugged" patients. The patients, of whom we write in the Annual Report, when they are receiving them are fully able to write poetry, enjoy their families and behave as normal, though sick, people. Truth is a very relative term and being "sincere" as you state does not necessarily mean giving full medical information but trying to understand where the patient is in his understanding and fears and what help he needs at this stage of his journey.

We do not have dying children at St Christopher's although we have teenagers from time to time. One of our doctors is anxious to move into this field in her next post.

I am afraid that there is little possibility of our having a space available for you at St Christopher's. We have so many students from our own country to whom we have to give priority.

Dr C. D. T. James[45]

King's College Hospital, London

9 January 1979 Our best wishes for the New Year and thanks to you for your help in 1978.

Secondly, I wonder if I could prevail upon you to come to the next meeting of our Terminal Care Study Group on Wednesday the 31st January, at 10.30 am. This group has been going for about two years and works as a kind of "think tank" drawing in people on a regular basis and others from time to time. We would very much like to have a brief discussion of alternative methods of pain control. This is particularly stirred up by a letter from Mark Mehta a copy of which I enclose and partly by the fact that I have to write a chapter

---

45 Dr C. D. T. James (1921–2000), a consultant anaesthetist (and enthusiast for medical history) who founded the pain clinic at King's College Hospital, and who during the 1980s conducted sessions at St Christopher's.

for Mark Swerdlow next Summer and he too, has been prodding me to make more reference to blocks, stimulators and so on. I think it is true that in most articles and lectures, we do mention the activities of pain clinics such as yours, but I admit we probably give them no more than a fairly passing reference, as indeed we only refer a very limited number of patients. However, Professor Calman who is Secretary to the group thought it would be of great value if you, or your Registrar and probably both of you, could come to the meeting and be ready to speak to us very briefly and tell us if you too feel we do not look often enough at your scene.

I know this is very short notice and I apologise, and if you cannot manage this time, please will you come at our next meeting which will be in about three months time, and perhaps you would let me know which days of the week are best for you.

We usually have about fifteen people, and the meeting includes, as well as the people involved in Hospice care like Robert Twycross, Professor Calman who is in Oncology, Michael Williams and Professor John Hinton, a psychiatrist.

I enclose a copy of the Agenda and hope very much we might have the pleasure of welcoming you if possible to the whole meeting; lunch is on the house, and we usually finish at about 3.30 or 4.00 pm.

Alison Dunn

The Editor – The Nursing Times, London

15 January 1979 I enclose a copy of a letter I have just had from the Japanese Journal of Nursing. I would be grateful if you would give me permission for them to reprint the article they mention "Watch with Me". I will be sending them a copy of your answer and also of the booklet you produced of my "Care of the Dying" articles and will ask them to get in touch with you direct for any permission that is needed. So far as I am concerned, I am delighted for them to be reprinted.

Dr Robert Twycross

Sir Michael Sobell House, Oxford

29 January 1979 I would say that you were absolutely right to hold off the Western side of the USA for 1980/81. There is a great deal going on over there and they now have some people who have been caring for patients both in home care and within hospitals for some time now. I think we should limit our activities in the main to their big conferences where we have a chance of spreading the work very widely and to the occasional medical center where we have a chance to get a hearing from the Senior Doctors and may give a boost to a good local effort.

Tom is not thinking of the States apart from a brief visit to the International Institute of Health and St Luke's New York in February this year. I will be speaking at the big conference they are planning for the opening of the Branford Hospice and Sylvia tells me this will be a therapeutic type meeting comparable to the excellent show in Montreal in November last year. I will probably visit one or two other centers in which I have a personal interest on my way to the Branford Conference.

My only potential engagements in the West at the moment are the Catholic Hospital Association in San Diego at the beginning of this coming June with a week near the Hospice of Marin preceding that, which has a good programme at the moment and hopes for a building.

I think you can tell Mr Snapp that we are trying to help the major therapeutic discussions where we can and unless you have a personal desire to move around the very beautiful Western side of the United States, there is every reason for you to say "no". If you do want to do a trip of this kind I would keep a lot of the arrangements in your own hands and not be dependent on the Reverend Gentleman whose contacts may not be of the best and I do not think that you would in any way be merely providing an encore or stealing the thunder of any of the rest of us.

Dr Samuel C. Klagsbrun

Four Winds Hospital, Katonah, New York, USA

6 February 1979 Two splendid letters from you and I am really only going to write to you as briefly as I can this time! You do us so much good in all ways when you come.

We are fascinated by your thoughts about our Bar-Mitzvah. I am sure that you have put your finger on a most important spot and we may find ourselves coming back to ask you to speak at it yourself anyway!

I am somewhat concerned about the enclosed correspondence. I can never bring myself just to put letters like this in the bin. I wonder if you know this gentleman, and whether you think I ought to pursue the matter any further.

My next problem is the newsletter of Fall 1978 from "Concern for Dying". We kept up a sporadic correspondence with them but as far as I know the Hospice point of view has not appeared in their newsletter, although I may be mistaken in this. Two things concern me in this particular number. Firstly, the sad story of the gentleman with amyotrophic lateral sclerosis. Surely medicine in the USA is not so insensitively aggressive that one needs to have court orders and changes in the law to avoid this group of patients being put upon respirators. I am seriously thinking of bringing 80 patients with Motor Neurone disease to the International Conference and writing a paper on the terminal care of this disease which should appear in some reasonable medical journal. Is there any other way that I should try to put forward a far more sensitive solution with far fewer sinister implications?

Then secondly, in their questionnaire they say:-

> "In England, Dr John Goundry proposed that a 'death Pill' be made available to all individuals over 65, upon request."

The way it is put it sounds as if Dr John Goundry is a person of consequence and importance. The only thing that I can find out about him in our Medical Directory is that he qualified in 1959 and apparently works as a family doctor near London. The statement sounds as if it is representative of the National scene. Perhaps there is no need for me to be so sensitive about it, but it does seem to me a pity that what I thought was a responsible society should be campaigning in this way.

The part-time secretary who will be wholly concerned with our Bar-Mitzvah Conference starts today. We will soon be short listing those we intend to invite. I have gone some way towards ensuring that we will have sufficient funds to pay accommodation for everyone and travelling expenses for speakers.

Professor Julian Stolarczyk

Gdansk, Poland

13 February 1979 I am delighted to be able to send you a copy of the book. It should have reached you for Christmas, but St Christopher's seems to get busier all the time.

I hope very much that I will one day hear that something has happened in Gdansk in this field and because I think it may well be the best way of development, I am sending a copy of the first annual report of the support team at St Thomas' Hospital. This way of starting work is being developed in other Hospitals. The Royal Marsden which is the oncology centre has a doctor and a nurse. The Nurse is an ex-Senior nurse from St Christopher's and does a considerable amount of work carried out by the social worker and chaplain for St Thomas's. In the Brompton Chest Hospital there is a nurse acting as clinical specialist and counselling in the wards with the problems faced by patients with cystic fibrosis and emphysema, who are terminally ill as well as those with cancer.

I look forward to hearing of the Polish development in this field.

We were very excited to have visitors from the potential Hospice in Nova Huta, but that is another way of tackling the problem which I would not expect in Gdansk.

I hope that the information in this book might be a help in developing something in your part of Poland.

Dr Ronnie Fisher

Christchurch Hospital, Christchurch, Hampshire

15 February 1979 We have just published a text book which is being printed by Year Books, Chicago in the United States and the title is "The Management of Terminal Disease" edited by Dr Cicely M Saunders, No. 1 in the series "The Management of Malignant Disease". It is the first volume of a series on management of different forms of malignant disease. I think the fact that we are the first volume of this series emphasizes the important point that we are a thoroughly respectable part of medicine.

I hope you will be able to incorporate this information in any other presentation of the work of St Christopher's Hospice.

Patricia Parkes

American Hospital Association, Chicago, Illinois, USA

22 February 1979 I was interest to read your "Trends in Caring for the Dying" and found it a useful summary. However, if you are reprinting it I would be very grateful if you would update your information about St Christopher's which as far as I can see has been acquired from other people's writings about us.

The points I would particularly like to mention are that from the moment of our first planning (1959 onwards) the idea of the family as the unit of care began to invade our thinking. This was partly because of the lack of ability to do this adequately at St Joseph's at that time, and from Dr Colin Murray Parkes' presence in our planning meetings from 1965 onwards.

You will see from the enclosed reprints that we also planned "home care" from early on and the actual development of our home care service has been surprisingly like that of my application to the DHSS [Department of Health and Social Security] for support in the Fall of 1966 which was reprinted as this article.

We have not been using diamorphine for our oral narcotic mixture since May 1977 and we dropped both the alcohol and the cocaine at about the same time. We never used chlorpromazine syrup as a routine, but our choice has normally been the less sedative prochlorperazine (Compazine). It is now some time since our admissions have exceeded the 600 mark and two years since our costs became 50/60% of a teaching hospital and 60/70% of an ordinary general hospital.

Finally we have never said that we only work to give comfort. We have increasingly used cytotoxic chemotherapy over the years and you will see from the annual report that we feel it very important that the way back to the "acute care system" should always be open. We share care at times with radiotherapists and have several patients on regular treatment at this moment. We do not take this sort of decision lightly but I think it is extremely important that Hospice care should be integrated with medical care of other kinds and not just be seen as a "dead end".

Social Workers started writing in this field very early notably Ruth D Abrams whose book "Not alone with Cancer". A guide for those who care, what to expect, what to do" (published by Charles C Thomas, Springfield, Illinois, USA) would probably lead you into good references. I met her first in 1963 when she had been working in the field for many years.

Dr Balfour Mount
Royal Victoria Hospital, Montreal, Canada

11 April 1979 First of all I do hope that Faye is better and that the Masters Degree in Theology is coming along all right in spite of it. Lots of love and good wishes to her from the Professor and Tom and me.

I do hope you will get further beds. I think you really do need them and I hope the Committee takes some of the administration weight off your shoulders.

Certainly St Christopher's sends an anniversary card to all its bereaved families. The only thing we say on this is "we are remembering you at St Christopher's" and, as you may recall, their names are on the board outside chapel. Always one remembers somebody and indeed this week it is the three men of whom I wrote in the Annual Report last year.

I am afraid I would never consider using this as a fund raising activity and I see that you would be very careful about your wording. St Christopher's is really very slow in doing ordinary fund raising at all. This year we have had no particularly worded newsletters and no fund raising activities of our own (as usual) and £175,000 has come for the financial year, the total for which we were now and again remembering to pray.

The above was dictated before you 'phoned. I am delighted about Dr Leber and will have met him by the time you get this and will push him towards Professors Vere and Desmond Laurence. I enclose a copy of a letter I received when I was scouting around for our

Research Fellow and also a note of his Curriculum Vitae. I also enclose a copy of my most recent letter from the Medical Research Council.

I hope you had a marvellous holiday and that Faye feels better.

Dr Melvin J. Krant

University of Massachusetts Medical School, Worcester, Massachusetts, USA

24 April 1979 Thank you for taking it so well. I am very glad to be able to simplify my journey and to participate where I know I am needed.

The Hospice development in the United States is quite something and even we have a fair amount to do with it. I was not happy at some of the political overtones of the meeting of the National Hospice Organisation at which I spoke in Washington last October, but I appreciate that with your reimbursement problems this is probably unavoidable. I believe that people like Sylvia Lack and Janet Lunceford of the NCI are fighting for the right kind of standards in their different worlds. Somehow, in all this, people must have freedom to develop in a way appropriate to their own scene.

I cannot remember when I used the words 'special hospital' for St Christopher's. I tried to sum up what I thought about Hospice work in the enclosed Editorial which was commissioned by the American Journal of Medicine and also in the last chapter of our book which should by now be available to you.

I enclose a copy of the chapters and you will see that we have tried to cover the field fairly widely. Over the years I have felt more and more that we moved out in St Christopher's in order for the basic principles we could work out, in research and teaching, to be fed back into the health Service. I am happy at the current developments of support and symptom control teams working in the general teaching hospital and in the development of continuing or palliative care units on a hospital campus. We could not have done that when we began but I believe that our hospice has made it possible for them to develop. Somehow or other we have made this a very respectable part of medicine in the United Kingdom and here I must add that I have got rather a prestigious gold medal in therapeutics from the Society of Apothecaries coming this summer.

Of course there are people who do not think they will ever need to use our kind of skill or attitude but more and more among the younger groups of students and doctors they are asking for teaching.

Two other articles may interest you. Professor Hinton's who is an old friend and on our Research Committee and Dr Gill Ford's who is an even older friend on our Council and Chairman of our Education Committee. I think we would all define Hospice as being somewhat different from the general hospital but would not limit it to terminal care only. We carry out such care in the context of a mixed group of patients, some long stay, many at home and with our wing for elderly residents which is increasingly integrated into the House as a whole. It is difficult to make a neat definition, but I think a Hospice is a community offering skilled support to patients and their families when they are struggling with long term or mortal illness or disability. St Joseph's now has a long term rehabilitation wing. We are having more and more outpatients and if you omit the people who die within a week of admission, that is the group who come here as the family situation breaks down right at the end, then our discharge rate last year was 29% and we have some 20/30 people at home among our usual 650 or so. We are much cheaper than a general hospital as you will see from the enclosed newsletter. This is because of our much less complex overhead costs. We are still able to have a higher than normal nurse/patient ratio and an at least normal doctor/patient ratio.

I think attitude both grows out of and leads into function, and I hope the work of the support teams will make a major difference both to attitude and efficiency in the hospitals in which they work. England is more used to a discontinuous scene because patients leave the care of their own doctors at home and have a different set of doctors in hospital, returning back to their own doctors for outpatient care. The existence of somewhere like St Christopher's adds to continuity because we work alongside both groups of doctors and are very often the link and the best route for communication. I think we are rather more sophisticated about all this than we were when you came and we are certainly effectively integrated with the area from which the great majority of our patients come.

I think that we have to allow for a certain amount of teething troubles in each country, but the development as a whole gives plenty of cause for optimism.

Mr and Mrs J. Quinlan[46]

Landing, New Jersey, USA

18 June 1979 It was a great pleasure to meet you both in San Diego. I really appreciate the fact that you are using your own experience for helping so many other people not only in your courage in fighting for Karen's peace earlier, but also for people with different problems who need a Hospice. I hope you found the Marin literature useful and that you were even able to talk with or see them. I think that their Conferences or teaching sessions sound very valuable and there is nothing really quite like it anywhere else that I know of.

I hope we will meet again. My next trip to New York is already very full, but I will try and catch you on the telephone. I hope also that one day you will be able to visit us here.

Grace Goldin

Swarthmore, Pennsylvania, USA

18 June 1979 Thank you so much for the duplicate transparency. I will talk to the Printer about adjustment as well as cutting me down a little further as well. It certainly made me realise that I was right to join the Hospice Weight Watcher Team and I am happy to report that 14 lb is off now.

I am sorry you have been having so much trouble with your toes, but I am sure it will be right in the long run. I have always marvelled at the way you get around.

---

46 The parents of Karen Ann Quinlan, the twenty-one-year-old whose life was saved by doctors in 1975, but who then entered a persistent vegetative state. Her family campaigned for her life support systems to be removed, but when this was done she continued to breathe. Karen Ann Quinlan remained in a coma for almost ten years in a New Jersey nursing home until her death in 1985.

I did call 2 or 3 times and am sorry to have missed you. I am afraid there is no chance of vacation with you in the Fall because I already have five days in New Mexico with Sister Zita Marie and this has been promised for at least five years. The rest of the time will be very hectic.

St Luke's is not an easy set up to show off to visitors. A team wandering around the Hospital has to be careful not to impose too much on the wards and I quite understand that they find visitors difficult even allowing for the added problem of an awkward Senior Nurse. In my view this has not detracted from the value of their work and I still think it one of the most exciting Hospice developments. The St Thomas' Team which is a direct development from their protocol is an extremely vigorous off-shoot and I hope so much will be copied elsewhere.

The Degree was a Doctor of Law but living would have been a nice idea. It came from Columbia and there was quite a lot of splendour.

I am so glad you like the marantology enclosure. I am dashing down to do a quick meeting for him in Virginia on my way to New Mexico.

Professor David Allbrook[47]

Carmel, Western Australia

2 August 1979 Your letter arrived on the 30th July and I have discussed this and your telephone call with Tom.

We think the Summer of 1981 will be just as convenient for us and we really only have one query.

Are you going to do some general medical refresher as well as the time with us? If you are then three months here will be fine. If you are not, we suggest that you should do a month of general refresher and for this we suggest Professor Duncan Vere at the London Hospital with whom our Clinical Research Fellow works and with whom Dame Albertine spent a most helpful month before St Christopher's opened and she came as my Deputy. We have not asked him yet, but he is a good 'crusader' and would welcome you I am sure if he possibly could. A month with him followed by two months with us would I think give you an excellent clinical base.

I don't think we could offer you accommodation while you were working with him. If you could stay with your relatives in Southgate this would be easy.

Delighted to hear that moves go on for the Perth Hospice. That is most exciting news and if you are going to be the St Christopher's of Australia you will need, as we did, to move out to a separate institution. I think the alternative would be a Palliative Care Unit like Montreal which is part of the Royal Victoria Hospital, as you no doubt know.

[Dictated by Dr Saunders before retreat in the Country! and signed in her absence]

---

[47] Born in the UK, David Allbrook had been Professor in Anatomy at the University of Western Australia and at this time was making plans for a subsequent move into hospice medicine. He had first met Cicely Saunders in 1946, in Devon, at a guesthouse run by Madge Drake.

Professor D. Brigit van der Werf-Messing

Rotterdamsch Radio-Therapeutisch Instituut, Rotterdam, Holland

16 August 1979 Your letter did not reach us until the 7th August as we have had considerable trouble with our post. It is very kind of you to suggest that you might propose me as a candidate for the Kettering Prize. I enclose a short curriculum vitae and a photo-copy of my not very tidy list of publications.

In 1942 I was left £500 by a patient "to be a window in your home". I went as a volunteer SRN [State Registered Nurse] to a home to which I had been sending patients and found there that pain control was a great improvement on what I had seen in my teaching hospital. In 1951 the doctor with whom I was working encouraged me to begin in medical school. I qualified with honours in 1957 and in 1958 began to prepare for the work of St Christopher's by developing the work in St Joseph's Hospice.

We were registered as a charity in 1961 and through introductions to various people I mainly raised the money myself and we were able to build and open in 1967 as a Christian and Medical foundation outside the Health Service. We have strong links with the National Health Service as you will see and I enclose a brief description of the Hospice which we insert into our Annual Report.

Susan C. Jacobs

Orange, Connecticut, USA

23 August 1979 I am enclosing a copy of our Annual Report which I hope will show you that there is a considerable amount of work done in St Christopher's by people other than the Social Worker herself. We have just increased our establishment by one Senior Social Worker and have made the appointment but are currently waiting for this important new member of staff. Our part-time Social Worker's post will change to whole time in November.

I wonder if anything has come of the meeting on Terminal and Continuing Care, arranged through the Council of Europe? I seem to remember that you were continuing with this group but that you were not very sanguine about it producing anything constructive. If you have a moment, I would be most grateful if you would let me know how it has gone on and if it is going to produce anything in writing.

We are looking forward to a small International Conference at St Christopher's in the Summer of 1980. We hope to invite people from various parts of the world. Europe seems to be a fairly blank area. We have had many contacts with the Netherlands, but so far as I know, no one has actually established a Hospice of any kind. Our best link is with Miss Marlyn de Jong-Vekemaus who you may have met. In France we only know of the Dame de Calvaire who should have come to us for a visit before Christmas but failed to make it and Professor Jean Lassner, an Anaesthetist who must now be a fairly senior statesman. There is a Palliative Care Unit in Lausanne that we know of, a Home Care Team in Oslo and some individual people in Sweden and some contacts in Denmark. If you think of anyone who you feel we should be in touch with, I would be most grateful for their names and addresses. I cannot give you a date in 1980 yet, but obviously we will let you know as soon as we have one.

I hope all goes well with you. I thought that Dr Woodbine's report showed what an impact the unit was having, but I hope you are not running yourself into the ground.

Mr and Mrs Joseph Quinlan

Landing, New Jersey, USA

7 September 1979 Thank you so much for your letter and your own book[48] which arrived yesterday. I am delighted to have it although I have only had time to dip into it so far.

May I say again how delighted I have been to meet with you and how pleased I am to read now that you are already moving forward in establishing the Karen Ann Quinlan Center of Hope. I think it is wonderful that her memory is being set forward in this way but I am sure that there are many people who will not reach this comatose state because of the publicity which you were brave enough to undertake.

New York has got completely filled up, but I will certainly call you while I am there.

Professor Patrick Wall

University College London, London

10 September 1979 It was nice to hear from you as you had been in my mind ever since I read your John Bonica Lecture. It ties together with Buytendijk's book which impressed me so much when I started out at St Joseph's. I enjoyed yours very much.

I am trying to see where our kind of pain fits in. I suppose one has to say that when one thought of pain as a protective reflex etc etc, terminal pain was pointless and if one thinks of pain as leading to healing it is again frustrating and apparently meaningless, yet diversion and interest remain some of our best pain relievers of all and stillness is not what is really wanted. As we move on into looking at the tricyclics and pain with our apparently very satisfactory Research Fellow, perhaps more light will dawn. He is developing what should be very fruitful links and good relations with The London and Northwick Park, Dr Iverson and others.

Delighted to hear of Arnold Rosin's plans. I agree with you about his Paper after the first quick glance. I will talk with someone else about it and write to him soon. We would also love to have him here, I hope he writes soon – we get so booked up.

The Mother Superior General[49]

All Saints Convent, Oxford

13 November 1979 I was very interested in your letter and your nice brochure of the work. I love that quotation from T S Eliot which I think so often refers to dying patients.

On the whole I do not believe in Hospices for children but I may be wrong and there may really be a need in Oxford. When we began here Social Workers at Great Ormond Street thought they would be referring patients to us and we thought we might be able to help. In

---

48 Published as J. and J. Quinlan, with P. Bettelle, *The Quinlans tell their story* (New York: Doubleday, 1977).

49 Sister Frances Dominica, founder of the first hospice for children in the UK, which opened in Oxford in 1982. See J. Worswick, *A house called Helen,* 2nd edn (Oxford: Oxford University Press, 2000).

fact they never did and the one or two children we have had here made us realise that this was not right for them or for our own staff. I think children need to go back to the Doctors who have treated them before and the staff they know, or best of all to die in their own homes. We have combined with the local children's hospital and one of the paediatricians, to help with home support, knowing that the children would be admitted to the children's hospital if need arose but that is as far as I think we should ever go.

Some of what I say would not apply to a specifically children's hospice, but I think it is the long term disabled children with educational requirements who are probably in the greatest need.

Dorothy Sutherland told me how much she enjoyed being with you. I am so glad she is coming back again.

I am not taking you up on the suggestion of coming up to see me as this month is almost impossible as I am catching up on being away from the Hospice for some six weeks. A lecture tour followed by a holiday gave me a lovely break, but I am paying for it right at this moment. December looks easier but I do not think I am really going to be very helpful at this stage. You have, of course, Sir Michael Sobell House at the Churchill Hospital, and although they are not able to admit all the patients that they would like to I think it is totally impossible to think of the Area Health Authority donating any more beds.

Grace Goldin

Swarthmore, Pennsylvania, USA

28 November 1979 Your reprints from *Encyclopaedia Britannica* have just arrived and I have only had a chance to skim through it but I really am impressed by what you have achieved.[50] I hope your re-writing of the book goes well. I think putting it under subject rather than place is right but probably one would only do it having done the places separately as you did originally.

I have been very busy with lectures this month, in fact life has been pretty hectic ever since I got back from holiday. Each week I have been talking with medical students at various stages of their training. There is no doubt of their interest and I hope as you write about the English Hospices you will emphasise that even though nursing may be the cornerstone of hospice care it is a medical set up and unless we teach students even more widely than we are doing and continue battling away with those already trained, the patients will simply not get the quality of care they should receive. If nursing were enough I would never have had to plod through medicine in order to be a catalyst in this field.

You may be interested in a photocopy of something sent me from South Africa two days ago, jut in time to quote a bit from it in a BBC debate on Radio.

50 G. Goldin, British hospices, in *Encyclopaedia Britannica Medical and Health Annual* (1980), pp. 80–93.

Dr Zbigniew Zylicz[51]

Sopot, Poland

28 November 1979 Thank you very much for your long letter. It was very good to hear from you and to know that you have successfully defeated the examiners.

I am glad that you have your post organised and hope that you will soon be at work and that there will be a chance for you to come over to England and visit the Hospice.

Just for your reference in planning, I will be on duty the weekend of February 2nd/3rd, March 8th/9th and April 5th/6th and would love to take you round and talk with you then. Our Research Fellow comes in on Mondays and I think you would find it interesting to discuss his reading and his plans for looking at the use of psychotropic drugs in pain control. He also thinks that the role of morphine may need to be re-assessed in the future.

We really enjoyed having Joanna though I have not heard from her since she got back to Warsaw. I had a short note from her Professor and am encouraged to think that we know him already and that perhaps she may do some work in this field eventually.

Halina and the Doctor who spoke a little English were here about a year ago but I have hardly heard anything since then. She is, however, coming to our small International Conference next June and so are several other people including Dr. Zborzil.

It was lovely to have news of Stas.

I hope you all have a lovely Christmas and all you want in the New Year.

Marty Hermann

New York, USA

28 November 1979 I hope China was marvellous. Egypt certainly was.

I had a very nice letter from Dr Borowich with a generous honorarium of $500.00 so I think Mount Sinai did very well by me. I look forward to hearing that something has happened there.

We have been truly hectic since we came back but I am seeing my way to have a space over Christmas to get my writing done and that is a comfort. I enclose a reprint from Grace Goldin's contribution to *Encyclopaedia Britannica*. The patient standing by the bed in the window is one of ours and I think she has really done remarkably well in presenting the Hospice scene as it is at the moment. I hope there is enough emphasis on its continuing development as a medically respectable entity.

Great joy in that Marian is almost certainly giving up his car. It went wrong the moment we got back from Egypt and is still not mended which has made him realize how expensive it is and also that he can get around on public transport very cheaply as an old age pensioner. The thought of not having him on the road is marvellous to me. Mind you, I will believe this when I finally see it but the signs look good. He is very fit and very satisfactory.

---

[51] Trained in medicine in his native Poland, Zbigniew (Ben) Zylicz had visited St Christopher's Hospice as a medical student and was involved in Cicely Saunders' Polish visit in the previous year, 1978. He later moved to The Netherlands where he established Hospice Rozenheuvel, at Rozendaal, in 1994.

Dr David Fullerton

Hull

11 December 1979 Thank you for your letter. As far as I can see we do not have any information about your project in Hull and I would be grateful if you would let us know what has happened so far and send us any memorandum that you might have. If you have not committed yourself to paper as yet might I suggest that this is one way of clarifying your own mind and of helping you to present your project with clarity to other people.

I am afraid there is not much possibility of my coming to Hull as it is so far away and takes a great deal of time away from St Christopher's. However Dr Tom West my Deputy here is a most excellent speaker and also happens to have friends near Sheffield and would probably be able to combine a visit to you with a weekend with them. Perhaps you would write to him direct about this.

I have given your name to Miss Summers our Co-ordinator of Studies who organises our Conferences so you will be getting news about them. This year we have an International Conference in the Summer in place of one of our usual English ones and can only ask a limited number of people in this field from this country. The next after that will be a Therapeutics Conference in November 1980.

I have spoken to Dr West about your anaesthetist. We only have a very limited number of places on our courses here and he suggests that in the first instance he comes on a Friday day visit, details of which I enclose, with a view perhaps to coming as one of our locum doctors rather than on a course which is designed mainly for family doctors. When one of our team is on holiday we fit in experienced locums and I think this may well be the best answer.

Official support is always a problem and undoubtedly more difficult for revenue at the moment than it is for capital. At the moment it seems that the best way of beginning a Hospice is to think of a team either based in the community or in a general or teaching hospital on the pattern being pioneered by Dr Thelma Bates at St Thomas'. Maybe in a few years time when the team has established its credibility it will be easier to get contractual arrangements for patients.

In the meantime, I think it is unrealistic to plan for building unless you are particularly confident of funds in your own area. However, in any case I am sure it is important to be talking with someone in the Area Health Authority and your Community Physicians and possibly Nursing Officers as well.

You may not have seen our Annual Report and I enclose one or two reprints as well.

The Rt Hon Patrick Jenkin MP

Secretary of State for Social Services, Department of Health and Social Security, London

9 January 1980 Everyone you met at St Christopher's yesterday wishes me to write and thank you for making the visit so interesting to us and apparently enjoyable to you. Each of the patients was delighted to have a chance of meeting you.

I am glad you felt that it was not like the picture of a "Hospice for the dying" and that living seemed predominant. We are glad that as well as those who come at the very last stages because their families find they cannot manage those few days, there are so many who are given a new lease of life and who use it fully. Our greatest challenge at the moment is, I am sure, to continue teaching as widely as we can and to add to this a more academic dimension as Miss Summers was saying. This we are looking at just now. It is only when we do this that we will know best how to help the staff of future Hospices and Hospice Teams in other parts of the country and the individual people who come and work with us on the short term and then return to the National Health Service.

We hope very much that Parliamentary recesses will so organise themselves that you will be able to open our International Conference for us on June 2nd 1980.

Grace Goldin
Swarthmore, Pennsylvania, USA

21 January 1980 Just before Christmas the Mother of your rosy cheeked child[52] came in to pay one of her occasional visits to the ward. She was quite happy about your including the photograph but did not want to see it. She told me that they took a lot of photographs while they had that lovely holiday in Wales but that they had left the film in the camera until now as they could not bear to look at any of them. They are a strange family but so Welsh and so Celtic that I do not expect to understand them very easily.

The lovely Mrs M has left us. You remember she was the splendid old lady who you photographed finger painting a year before and then at a follow up with her daughter and husband this time. The daughter moved near another Hospice and we transferred Mrs M who spent a happy five days near her daughter's new home, visited her twice and then got an acute chest and died. We were sad that we did not have the last goodbye but what was really splendid was she so much wanted to see her daughter's new home. I had a very good photograph made of one of the slides and had a delightful letter from her daughter last week.

I must tell you that I am now Dame Cicely Saunders! This is really equivalent to a knighthood in this country but I do not know whether the correct word is Damehood or Dameship nor as far as I can find out does anybody else. Although I have not yet been dubbed by the Queen I am expected to use the title already. Letters should be addressed as below. Acquaintances and enemies should speak to me as Dame Cicely (not Dame Saunders[53]) but my friends address me as usual. I have managed to answer five hundred letters and am so delighted that everyone views it as a recognition of Hospice as a whole.

Dr Hendrik Venter
Tygerberg Hospital, Johannesburg, South Africa

22 January 1980 A very long time ago you asked me for a copy of the Crucifix picture that I showed. At the time I just gave you an Annual Report which had a black and white reproduction. I now have had some coloured reproductions made and am sending you one in the hope that you will find it as inspiring as I do.

It is an old crucifix which was shot at as well as being burnt and bombed during the Warsaw uprising and is a most precious symbol of God's sharing of our pain.

---

[52] A reference to the subject of a photograph taken by Grace Goldin.

[53] In fact many Americans did use this form of address.

I gather from Judith Van Hearden who has just been here for a week that you are developing some work in Tygerberg. I do hope this is so and would be delighted to hear a little more of what is happening.

Thank you so much for your hospitality last year and for the marvellous bottle you gave me which I greatly enjoyed during my trip and with the students.

Miss M. E. Sellick

Royal Perth Hospital, Perth, Western Australia

11 February 1980 Many thanks for your letter. I most heartily agree with you that there should not be a Hospice solely under the auspices of the Anglican Church. I enclose a copy of an envelope which arrived at St Christopher's last Friday which I think is a marvellous mishearing of the word Hospice but also underlines the only auspices we should be concerned with.

We are just having a most terrible battle in altering the Statutes of the Hostel of God which has such trouble in meeting regulations such as every member of Council having to be a communicant member of the Church of England. A nonsense anyway!

As St Christopher's has a Christian foundation with a Jewish founder patient and a Jewish Chairman and people from other denominations and several other affiliations and non-affiliations all deeply involved I believe in being as widely based as possible. The only thing we wrote in our Articles of Association about the foundation was "there shall be a chapel available for Christian worship". This has certainly been sufficient for us so far and after that one must simply look to the Holy Spirit.

The best developments are those that grow out of the local situation and I would have thought that Rosemary's present position and the development of the Oncology Department was one such point. You may need a separate building as we did but we would not have had that nor got the ideas right unless I had been working for seven years in St Joseph's. Now however, with twelve years of St Christopher's experience behind them, new people will start in many different ways drawing, we hope, on our experience.

You are absolutely correct, it has to be the right action for starting or everything will be hindered.

Best of luck to you all.

Wendy Burford

Brompton Hospital, London

13 February 1980 Thank you so much for your letter and your good wishes also for the good news that you are moving towards opening your own Unit. We wonder if you would think of calling it Palliative Care rather than Continuing Care. It is in the tradition of the Montreal Unit which chose that name and I enclose something that Dr Mount wrote about this particular choice of name.

Your Chaplain came to see us the other day. This is really the reason for my slowness in replying because I sent your letter straight down to our Chaplain. He is an extremely nice person but I think he really agreed with us it was very early in his time to be a whole time Chaplain and your own suggestion of a Parish with special responsibilities is much more likely. I am going to write to suggest that he might get in touch with two of the other Hospices, one of which I know will be looking for a part time Chaplain in the near future.

All good wishes for the work and also for more help and support for you and possibly a little holiday?

Grace Goldin

Swarthmore, Pennsylvania, USA

15 February 1980 Thank you so much for your lovely long letter. Your vitality has always beaten mine and I was tired to read your second paragraph but you must have enjoyed it.

I am delighted that you are writing again and I love the sea. I have not been to our poetry workshop for weeks. My mini-muse has died out for the moment but I have been really rather busy. Thank you so much for the slide of PH which I was delighted to have.

The little red cheeked one did not have Lupus or if she did, we never made the diagnosis but I am a little unhappy that somebody probably other than you is using that slide. Her father is a doctor and it is just possible that he will be travelling and suddenly see his daughter's picture without warning. I would be very grateful if you could ask Dr Joy not to use it in this way or at least not unless she is very certain that there are no people from England in the audience.

I am so glad that you liked Dr Barrett as well as I did.[54]

Here is another piece of private news and I really mean private, to be shared only with Judah. I acquired two titles in January. On the 31st January I married Marian my Polish Professor. So now I have a totally unpronounceable surname which I am not using and so far the news has not leaked out beyond the noble body of secretaries and special friends (if they are different). We had a most delightful mixed wedding for a mixed marriage with two young priests, one Anglican and one Roman Catholic and four friends only. It was very special. It makes more difference than you might think and is all together splendid. Once Marian has got over the idea of His Poles knowing he is married, and I give him about three months, it will become public, but at the moment only three others in the United States know and I would ask you not to guess who they are if you should happen to meet them. I will let you know when it is out.

Dr Richard Scheffer

Gray's Hospital, Pietermaritzburg, Republic of South Africa

19 February 1980 Thank you so much for your letter and thank you for your congratulations and good wishes. I actually go to the Palace on the 11th March but am officially Dame as from New Year's day.

I am glad you are enjoying your house jobs and also that you are getting round to a bit of conversion work among the others. There is no doubt that plenty needs to be done. By separate mail I am sending you a large paper which I have sent in as a chapter to a text book on various methods of pain therapy. It sums up quite a lot of work and might just be useful to

---

[54] See letter to Grace Goldin, 28 October 1980, p. 205.

you. At the moment our Research Fellow is doing a paper for American consumption on oral morphine and I will send that when I get a copy of it.

We were discussing the needs for previous jobs for those going into terminal care just recently and came to the conclusion that you really need just about everything apart from obstetrics and sports injuries. Seriously, I think you should go ahead and get the equivalent of MRCP [Membership of the Royal College of Physicians] before you specialise. This will be very important. We have an MRCGP here and that is considered another possibility. We all feel, however, that a proper background in general medicine is essential. Other needs that should be useful are Radiotherapy/Oncology, limited experience in Psychiatry or Geriatrics or an Anaesthetist running a pain clinic would be a bonus. Our present Registrar is going to stay in the field and he had his MRCP before coming and he, I know, would endorse what I say.

I know it sounds like a long trail but we are not going to get our colleagues to appreciate that we have special expertise unless we can meet them on their level.

Do keep in touch.

Dr Arnold Rosin
Shaare Zedek Hospital, Jerusalem, Israel

21 February 1980 I am terribly sorry but when Tom and I talked to you we neither of us was expecting that by the time we were due in Jerusalem we would both have got married to different people! We might have been able to have taken up our rooms in St George's for one of the two new partners but unfortunately my husband and Tom's fiancée both have commitments which are impossible to break in the second half of April. We are therefore cancelling our holiday and are letting you down for the promised lecture at Shaare Zedek Hospital and also for the wonderful Sabbath evening which you promised us. I am terribly sorry about this because I really do feel that an outside speaker sometimes helps a group of Consultants to realise that Palliative Care is an integral part of medicine and should be an essential part of any hospital's practice.

If I am invited for a trip to Jerusalem for any Conference I will of course remember and come but at the moment I regretfully have to say we simply cannot come.

Colonel O. C. S. Dobbie
The Garden Tomb, Jerusalem, Israel

4 March 1980 First of all, thank you so much for your congratulations. As you know this belongs to many people past and present who I will carry with me when I go to the Palace next week.

Sadly, because I will not see you, but gladly, because of the reason, we are not coming to Jerusalem after all. Tom and I have both got engaged, but not to each other! In fact I am already quietly and rather secretly married and very happily, too. This is a friend of many years standing, a Polish artist who does all our pictures. Tom is marrying someone he knew at CMS [Church Missionary Society] training college, so he too is crowning a long friendship.

I cannot persuade my husband to come to Jerusalem. He was in our party when we came 2 years ago and he thinks it is too soon to come back. But I have every intention of coming again.

I do hope Flo is now keeping well. We often think of you.

Dr Samuel C. Klagsbrun

Four Winds Hospital, Katonah, New York, USA

19 March 1980 Your letter this morning with the enclosed copy of your splendid letter to Year Book Publications prods me into saying first what I should have written to you a week or two back.

The sound of wedding bells is loud and clear in St Christopher's. Marian suddenly decided that we should get married and in a great rush we did so on 31st January. This is absolutely splendid, and he is going around looking very sleek, so no doubt am I. This came together with other things, including your proddings, to wake Tom up and he is now engaged to his Dorothy and getting married on April 19th. Meanwhile, our Registrar got married and our Clinical Research Fellow got engaged. To celebrate this splendid epidemic I sang "I attempt from love's sickness to fly" at the Hospice concert about 2 weeks ago and took the opportunity to make the general announcement. We then had a champagne party last week.

I wrote to Carleton [Sweetser] with deadly secrecy because Marian did not want it to get out among his Poles. Now he is doing it gradually I am free to tell others. I will shortly be writing to Marty [Hermann], Carleton and Grace Goldin who are the only ones who know.

John Fryer is going to come as a sabbatical from September for 6 or 9 months for us to try how a more academic person in the Study Centre will work out. He will be at the Bar Mitzvah and be discussing plans at that point. Colin is hoping to latch him into the Academic Department of Psychiatry at the London Hospital and in the process of so doing had an excellent letter of recommendation from his senior Professor. I think that Dot will find this development much more difficult than she envisages and a little moral support from you at the time of the Bar Mitzvah will, I think, be much needed.

The people who you helped us with in December went on, with some problems, but came safely to port. The last was JM who having been splendid painting, going for family weekends and very entertaining and nice to everyone, then got very frightened. After efforts by all of us he finally made a full confession to Father Larn and went to mass. After this he relaxed completely and quietly slipped away. I am sure he would not have been ready before.

Dr William D. Poe

Veterans Administration, Salem VA, USA

1 April 1980 Thank you so much for writing to congratulate me on becoming a Dame. You are the only person who has given me the full verse of "There is nothing like a Dame!"
I remember with great pleasure my visit to your home and the whole time with the Veterans Administration. We have some rather important personage coming to visit the Hospice in June who is involved with the development of Hospice in the Administration. This was at

the invitation of Professor Torrens of Los Angeles who felt this would be important and I hope very much that he will be proved right.

Mrs R. B. Holmes
Philadelphia, USA

3 April 1980 Many thanks indeed for your gift in memory of your Charles' death. Thank you also for the note about him and your intense experience of bereavement. I personally still believe that he lives on in far more than just your memory. To me, God is a great rememberer and he lives in Him and His love. I also have probably rather naïve beliefs in ways of meeting both here and there.

I am sorry you did not get the Hospice post after so long and hope you will find something that uses your experience. I am interested in the things you have done to fill in time and I also enjoy learning poetry, although I do not have enough to sustain myself through a period of solitary confinement, as some seem to do.

Please will you share with Ben the fact that I am now married to Marian Bohusz, our Polish artist. We have been friends for many years but we suddenly decided to marry and did so secretly in January. It is now public and everyone seems very full of rejoicing. We certainly are.

Marty Herrmann
New York, USA

10 April 1980 Thank you for sending on the note to Phoebe Stein. I had a sweet note back.

The news of our marriage is now fully public. Marian was so pleased with himself that he has now told all his Polish friends and been delighted with the reaction.

Plans for September are a little more definite and it looks as though I will fly from San Francisco to New York on Saturday, September 27th. I do hope this is a right date for you and that you will have left Belgrade Lakes by then. I ought to call at Boston but I am going to try and leave that out. I really should see the new hospice in Connecticut in time to go on to Montreal on Friday, 3rd October. It is a short visit this time but I am longing to see you. No hope of bringing Marian but I hope to do so again one day.

Dr Otto Neurath
Upper Montclair, New Jersey, USA

16 April 1980 The institution known as Exit was previously known as The Voluntary Euthanasia Society.

I enclose a copy of a recent reprint in the JAMA [Journal of the American Medical Association] and galley proofs of an article to be published in the 2nd Edition of the *Dictionary of Medical Ethics* which I hope will give you some background about hospice work and a few references to follow up.

Whereas I would not judge those who kill themselves, I know how great a trauma this is for nearly every family in which this happens and would like to quote a patient of ours whose comment on the Exit idea was "How could you take your life without making other people feel they have failed you?"

I am even more troubled with the social pressures that would encourage the frail and the disabled and elderly to take the quick way out. I feel that "the right to die would soon become a duty to die". Hospice is involved with the alternative of living until death comes in its time.

Dr Denis Rogers
Hamilton, New Zealand

16 April 1980 Thank you very much for your long letter about your friend, Mrs B. I understand your concern and also her longing to do something of this kind. All the same, I am afraid I cannot encourage you to apply for a Churchill Fellowship for her in order to come and work here. We believe that we have reached the stage in which people really must learn from the pioneers in their own countries and you already have a few concerned groups and at least one hospice already opened. I enclose a list of addresses of people whose names you may not know.

We also believe that to go somewhere that is, I am afraid, seen as a kind of Shangri-la by many people, though understandable, is not necessarily the best way to rebuild a life which has to be lived in one's own place. Will you please give Mrs B our very good wishes and hopes that she will find the right place to learn and thus develop this work. As Dr Parkes mentions in one of the enclosed reprints, St Christopher's itself has a lot of this kind of impetus behind it and very few people get to be involved in this work without having adjusted to a loss of some kind in their own lives. But it is important that the adjustment comes first.

I am sorry not to be more helpful but I think you will understand.

Posi Tucker
South Bend, Indiana, USA

21 May 1980 Thank you for your letter. I am very sorry but I am afraid there is no chance of my coming to talk in Indiana in the foreseeable future. I am turning down quite a number of such requests partly because I think that it is time that American Hospice people fulfilled these engagements themselves and partly because I have recently got married and am not going to be travelling so much.

Dr Paul D. Henteleff
St Boniface General Hospital, Winnipeg, Manitoba, Canada

16 June 1980 St Christopher's Hospice and a Trust of which I am a member is paying the fares and conference fees for two exceptional young nurses to come to Canada in October. They are Miss Wendy Burford, Clinical Nurse Specialist at the Brompton Chest Hospital, London and Miss Jo Hockley, Sister of Rugby Ward at St Christopher's.

We would be most grateful if you could arrange for them to spend two days or so in your Unit after the Montreal Conference. Perhaps you could let me know if there is any chance of these two girls, who should be travelling together, coming to visit your Unit say some time during the week beginning October 13th. I am writing to Dr John Scott with the same request.

Both these girls are contributing a great deal to this field and I know they would find it most stimulating to see what you are doing now.

Dr Hans Wollasch

Deutscher Caritasverband, Freiburg, Germany

25 June 1980 Mrs Margarete Zimmerer asked me to send you printed material concerning the work of St Christopher's Hospice saying that you would be interested in translating some of this into German. I am enclosing a copy of our book as I really think that the most constructive thing would be to look at the entire book and translate that, as has already been done in Sweden. I am also enclosing one or two reprints which I think would be the most suitable for the readership you have in mind.

I understand from Mrs Zimmerer that there is a very negative feeling about "Sterbeklinik". I hope that you will see, particularly from the commissioned article in the *Journal of the American Medical Association*, that this is not at all the attitude of most doctors in the United States as well as in our own country. This is an important part of our total treatment for a patient with a deteriorating illness and at no time does admission to a hospice mean no further discharge or the exploitation of any improvement that may happen. We are constantly referring patients back to other hospitals and work in close cooperation with them. They in turn feel we have something to offer which they cannot and which they want for a considerable number of their patients.

Dr E. Hall

Colchester, Essex

30 June 1980 Thank you so much for your full letter. I am really very grateful to you for setting out exactly what is going on in Colchester. You really are developing in the way that one hopes to see among the various people who are trying very hard to start hospice work around the country.

I wonder if you are in touch with the National Society for Cancer Relief because, as you no doubt know and Mrs Clench[55] probably told you, they will sometimes fund Macmillan nurses to start work in a community area. They like the nurses to be called for Douglas Macmillan who founded the Society but do not in fact have a supply of nurses of their own.

May I wish you good luck and perhaps we will see one or two of you at our next Hospice Conference. We will be sending you particulars of that nearer the time.

---

[55] A reference to Prue Clench (later Dufour) who established a hospice home care service under the auspices of the Dorothy House Foundation, in Bath, England, in 1977. Later she worked as a national adviser to the UK hospice movement and in particular undertook development work for the National Society for Cancer Relief. See the letter to Prue Clench, 27 March 1984, p. 247.

His Eminence the Cardinal Archbishop of Westminster
Westminster, London

3 September 1980 Father Larn, our parish priest and Catholic Chaplain for St Christopher's, has encouraged me to write to you and to ask whether you would think it appropriate to invite His Holiness Pope John Paul II to visit St Christopher's Hospice when he comes to this country in 1982.

We would not think of suggesting he should do so and not visit St Joseph's Hospice as well and there may be far too many pressures on his time for you to think that a visit to two different hospices was appropriate.

As you know, St Christopher's has a Polish link in that our founding patient was a Jew from the Warsaw ghetto and I had a very close relationship with a devout Roman Catholic from Wilno during the time that we were planning and his memory and that of other Poles is built into the bricks.

You may not know that I have now married Professor Marian Bohusz who has painted all the pictures which do so much to give the atmosphere of welcome and faith to the Hospice. His son is teaching in the University in Krakow and is a personal friend of Pope John Paul and we have been told that my husband may be asked to present a picture to His Holiness some time in the future.

I know that you believe that the only way we can combat the present campaign for euthanasia or assisted suicide is by the development of hospice care and hospice attitudes. I believe this must include, as St Joseph's and to a lesser extent St Christopher's does, help for the aged and disabled as well as for the acutely dying. I believe that His Holiness would agree that this is an important part of the work of the Church in this time.

If you think it appropriate we would very much like to write to the Pope directly in Polish.

Dr Balfour Mount
Royal Victoria Hospital, Montreal, Canada

14 October 1980 It is amazing to me that you manage to put on better and better conferences every time and that the unit continues to function as though it were only dealing with its ordinary day to day business. It was a marvellous conference and I enjoyed the whole thing and look forward to remembering it as I listen to the tapes. It was also a splendid visit to both units, the old one in very good heart and the new one with all its potentials.

I liked the balance of the nuts and bolts with the philosophical and I hope you will keep this up for the next conference. If you have the star turn you mentioned, that certainly would be an added dimension. I think you are right to go on being multi disciplinary but I wonder whether you ought to cut your numbers back to 700 to 800 and limit the number of people who are only planning. Perhaps we need a little more in the way of workshops and even some when we go off in our separate disciplines. I am not sure whether the lunch hour meetings were enough for the Medical Directors to get together, for example.

I have no great ideas of other speakers, apart from Dr de Souza to speak for the third world but I wonder whether the kind of challenge that Paul Torrens presented would not be timely and helpful.

If I have any other ideas about speakers I will write again.

Grace Goldin

Swarthmore, Pennsylvania, USA

28 October 1980 Many thanks indeed for your letter, your chapter,[56] and the slide. AW, who you photographed I think on your first visit, was a splendid person and very much part of the Hospice for over a year, so it is wonderfully suitable that she should be chosen to represent the Hospice.

I am fascinated that you picked up how much I owe to Dr Howard Barrett.[57] I am glad you have given this recognition because I certainly have not talked enough about him recently and perhaps not written enough either. The big difference between us and him, of course, is that we set out to teach and therefore to plan a research programme to give us the objective basis of the scientific foundations. I realise now why I felt slightly uneasy when you said or wrote that you could see how much I owed to the faith of St Joseph's. The back of my mind was evidently saying 'do not forget St Luke's'. Perhaps one reason for this was that after going as a volunteer for seven years, I finally went back as an official observer from St Mary's Hospital and got shoved out with contumely by one of the visiting doctors. The fact that I finally had an apology from the Chairman of the Medical Committee, neither brought me back nor really healed that wound for a long time. It did, however, enable me to concentrate on the work at St Joseph's. I do not think I would have managed two places at once, so it all worked out in the end and I am on good terms again with the doctor concerned.

What I have said over and over again is that there are not many original ideas in the world. One only brings together things culled from here and there, shakes the kaleidoscope and finds a new pattern. That I have said often enough and it is really my feeling about the originality or lack of it of St Christopher's.

Jean Ihli

West Hartford, Connecticut, USA

21 November 1980 You are quite right in that we have carried out work which has shown that we can use morphine as effectively as heroin. We certainly have patients on long term use of morphine who are alert and capable of living in their own homes and so on. In order to completely alleviate pain the patient does not have to be rendered unconscious if each area of pain, such as bone pain, is treated specifically and the patient is seen as a person with his mental, social and spiritual needs. I am enclosing two reprints from Canada. I think that you will find that the work in Montreal has proved useful. You know, of course, that Professor Melzack is one of the two describers of the Gate Theory of pain. We have literature here and I am enclosing something which may be of use.

---

[56] A reference in fact to a journal article: G. Goldin, A protohospice at the turn of the century: St Luke's House, London from 1893 to 1921, *Journal of the History of Medicine and Allied Sciences*, **36**(4), (1981): 383–415.

[57] The Medical Superintendent of the West London Mission and founder in 1893 of St Luke's House, the annual reports of which Cicely Saunders had read with great interest in the late 1950s.

Grace Goldin

Swarthmore, Pennsylvania, USA

8 January 1981 I must tell you how much we are enjoying that beautiful engagement calendar. I am keeping it at home to mark the evenings we are each out and I cannot keep it in the right place, as Marian is always stealing it. You have achieved a great thing in sending something which includes pictures that he has never seen and in some cases, never heard of.

Also, I must say how much I have loved reading *Ruth* slowly in bed at night. I am so glad your springs of poetry opened up again.

Some extremely inaccurate statements about hospice history from more than one American writer have finally prodded me into thinking that whatever you write, I have got to do something myself still, just on the story of St Christopher's and the early stirrings of the hospice movement. I do not think that we will clash or coincide but simply supplement and I hope you will agree. I am going to make this a fairly personal story, I think, fixed around a series of my own special people, like Mrs G and Louie as well as David and Antoni.[58] At the moment I am plodding through the original correspondence with the first pioneering group, sadly moved to do this by the fact that Jack Wallace died at the beginning of December suddenly after a minor operation. He was of enormous help when I was battling with the community idea and tackling the seemingly hopeless task of getting sufficient recognition to raise the money needed for a full blown hospice from scratch. Periodically as I look at this building I am astonished at the effrontery of thinking we could build such a place around the window for a start.

Meantime, I am keeping the dates you gave me in March from the 9th – 21st and look forward to hearing from you which day you think it likely you will be able to visit. I have been using some of your older slides recently once again. They are very special.

I have to come over to the States for two, and possibly three, honorary degrees. I have to be in Nebraska for the 23rd May and possibly in your area for the 29th before I go on to New York for something on June 3rd. Marian is coming with me and we will quickly dash to San Francisco for 2–3 days to see his daughter and granddaughter. He had a prostate operation in early December and is remarkably fit, dashing around at the moment getting his students' exhibition organised. He is 80 in February, which is hard to believe. We would obviously adore to see you but I am not sure how easy we would be as joint guests!

I am delighted to have an invitation to be a key speaker at a big conference at Youville Hospital, Cambridge, Mass, the former Home of the Holy Ghost and one of the early US Hospices. I will do that on the way home.

Dr D. O'Connell

Mount Miriam Hospital, Fettes Park, Penang

19 February 1981 I really am not going to give up! Diamorphine and morphine when used in equi-analgesic doses, individually titrated to the patient's need, are both excellent analgesics. Robert Twycross's study showed that given regularly by mouth with a phenothiazine

---

[58] She never in fact produced this full history, though she did refer to elements of it in several later articles.

there was no observable clinical difference either physically in the form of side effects or in the emotional state. If you have found it a poor analgesic or had to use another analgesic when giving a Brompton mixture then I am sure you must have been giving an inadequate dose. The majority of our patients do not need more than 30 mg morphine by mouth, the equivalent to which is 20 mg diamorphine but there is some 25–30% who may need doses up to 120 mg or more. However, as you readily say, many patients need something with aspirin or one of the other non-steroidal anti-inflammatory drugs in combination, especially for bone pain.

I enclose two reprints that I may not have sent you before. Obviously you are doing extremely well with your care of dying patients and I could not agree with you more that one needs to prevent pain rather than to relieve it once it has recurred. That has really been my theme song since the early days at St Joseph's. May be I will be able to visit with you one day. In the meantime I am always glad to hear from you.

Professor W. J. Rudowski

Warsaw, Poland

17 March 1981 Thank you very much indeed for your letter of the 12th March which reached me with unusual speed. I am really delighted with your good wishes for I treasure this link with you and Warsaw.

I have heard recently from Dr Joanna Pepke who tells me that she is responsible for a certain number of lectures on the nature and management of terminal pain and she remains anxious for any new literature we may produce. We have just been revising yet again our paper 'Drug Control of Common Symptoms' and when it is in print will be sending it around to those interested, among whom, of course, I include yourself.

The [Templeton] prize I have received will go towards our starting a Day Centre here at St Christopher's. We find ourselves increasingly involved with the elderly and lonely bereaved in our community and there are people with chronic diseases other than cancer near to the hospice who would, I think, benefit from attending any such centre with our other patients. There is plenty of money to be found before we can actually start building but I am hopeful about this.

Thank you again for writing.

Professor Sven Paleus

Stockholm, Sweden

25 March 1981 It was very nice to hear from you again and I hope you will get a positive review of the book in due course and that it is selling reasonably well.

I am interested in the comments of your clinical pharmacist and in fact I think they have arisen out of a misunderstanding. We normally make up our morphine solution separately from the phenothiazine syrup and they are put together in the same glass from their separate bottles at the patient's bedside from our drug trolley. Occasionally, when a patient has a suitable dose of morphine we give them a bottle with the full mixture at home, but as we are often changing the morphine dosage slightly, this is often not possible. The bottles are not so big that there can be any deterioration in the solution during the time that they are in use.

I enclose a copy of our latest bulletin on the 'Drug control of common symptoms', just taking the pages that are relevant to your question and you will see how we make up our solution.

Over the last months we have been continuing our practice of prescribing a phenothiazine (prochlorperazine) as we begin to give the morphine solution, bringing them to the bedside in separate bottles as I have described. We have tried removing the phenothiazine after a few days and have certainly found that with a small number of patients there has been a breakthrough of pain, so most patients in our hospice continue to receive both drugs together.

Dr R. Khoo

Queen Mary Hospital, Hong Kong

23 April 1981 Thank you for your letter. I am enclosing St Christopher's last Annual Report as it gives you some general idea of how widely hospice work is spreading. I also enclose an earlier newsletter and a small pamphlet about the Hospice.

You will see that this movement is developing in many different ways and the idea of having a separate ward in a hospital has been developed in Montreal by Professor Balfour Mount, of the Palliative Care Unit, Royal Victoria Hospital, as effectively as anywhere. I am sure he would be glad to give you information about his staffing patterns.

Our own is complicated by the fact that we are, as indeed they are as well, a very busy teaching unit and a considerable amount of our time is taken in our own conferences, in outside lectures and in teaching our many visitors of every discipline as well as our own staff, many of whom come for short periods for experience.

We find that a Consultant whole time can care for two wards if he has a whole time junior doctor working with him. This is a total of some 30 beds. One of our Consultants also carries the load of overseeing our home care team while the other has responsibility in teaching and administration. Our third Registrar mainly fills in for holidays, study leaves and all the other reasons that people are away from the Hospice.

Our home care has a much lower doctor input than that of some other hospice teams because we offer a consulting service mainly on the telephone to the local community physicians as well as our two or three clinics a week. My own work is almost entirely administration and teaching and a considerable amount of commitment to outside affairs.

An adequately staffed and active hospice has a median stay of 12–14 days only for its patients with a number being discharged but the majority dying in the Hospice. This means that with 62 beds we are admitting between 700–800 new patients and families a year. This is a very heavy load for the nursing team and we all find that one nurse on the establishment to one patient bed is not quite adequate to cover holidays and leave of all kinds. We really need something like 1.25 nurses on the establishment to one patient bed but, of course, you will appreciate this means night staff, teaching staff and that I am talking of whole time equivalents.

I know Dr Mount will tell you that he has managed to pay for the extra nurses he has by restraining himself from a number of irrelevant tests on his patients. The hospice is expensive in ward staff but has much lower overhead costs than the rest of an acute hospital and as it should be discharging an unexpectedly large number of patients and supporting them at home, the financial saving should be much greater than appears at first sight.

I would be very glad to know if this information is of help and how your plans go ahead.

Dr Halina Bortnowska

Krakow, Poland

6 May 1981 I was really delighted to have your letter and to hear about the progress of the Hospice. The arrangement sounds wise to me and I do wish you well and hope one day to see it.

We have got the catheter bags. I have a box of 25 being sent off this week. I am sorry for the delay but it took us a while to get them here.

I gather the post has been very bad from Poland so I hope they will reach you safely without too much customs to pay. You may be interested to see the enclosed brochure of St Christopher's. It was rather overdue for me to write a neat handout.

H. E. Edward Count Raczynski and Madame Aniela Mieczyslawska

London

12 May 1981 We were delighted to receive your letter of congratulations on the Templeton Award this morning. I have just returned from Buckingham Palace where I was given the magnificent cheque which will go towards starting a day centre at St Christopher's.

We are leaving for America this week for a five week trip but hope very much to have the pleasure of visiting you after our return.

With kindest regards from us both.

Reverend Carleton Sweetser[59]

St Luke's Hospital, New York, USA

23 June 1981 Sister Patrice has arrived safely and I met her at prayers yesterday morning. Helen is organising her programme and I hope she will get everything she needs. It is very good to have her here.

Thank you very much for having us both. We enjoyed you and Dieter enormously and really missed you when we left. You are a wonderful host. The only gift I was not too keen on was your cold, which flared up again when I got home and has left me with a splendid croaky voice at the moment. I only really felt ill like you did on the Saturday after I got home.

Everything is going on alright here and Tom and Dorothy had a marvellous holiday and look splendid. Helen, who carried all the weight while we were away, looks alright too, which is probably more to the point.

My father's estate has timed a legacy very well again for me to take on all the drinks on the holiday, which I will have great pleasure in doing and we can drink his health safely in Paradise.

---

[59] The Reverend Carleton J Sweetser (1921–96) was chaplain at St Luke's Hospital Center (later St Luke's/Roosevelt Hospital Center), New York. Cicely Saunders had met him at Memorial Sloan Kettering on her first visit to the USA in 1963 and they were good friends over many years.

Grace Goldin

Swarthmore, Pennsylvania, USA

1 July 1981 I am sending this home because I hope you will have got back from having done something to solve your very difficult problems in Tulsa. It does sound extremely difficult and I have no good advice to give except that may be the crisis will have helped to change minds a little bit to the point of accepting more help.

The batches of prints and the one of slides are absolutely marvellous. We are totally thrilled with them but have not settled down yet to choosing the perfect one for an enlargement. You are the world's photographer and I am going to have a huge album of Marian, which will be a delight for always.

The one thing I am still a little anxious for when you have a moment is the lady sitting by the curtain with her hand across it. Her daughter had asked us if we had a picture of her mother and the others that I had are simply not good enough to send her. That one which you had chosen as one of your specials is really delightful. I have, of course, got it among my duplicates but you did say it would print better from the original.

We have been terribly busy since we got back, Marian catching up with everybody and finishing the end of their academic year, and me with everything that seems to have piled up over weeks. Once we get through the next days, the pace should get quieter, but I seem to have been saying that for rather a long time!

Someone is after me for writing my biography.[60] She has done some extremely good television programmes with two of which I have been involved and I like her very much. She has not embarked on a biography before and she has been told that it is going to happen sooner or later. I too have that feeling, and I have at least some chance of seeing the story as more or less correct. What do you think?

Reverend Francis O'Leary

Jospice International, Liverpool

3 July 1981 Thank you very much for sending me a copy of your introductory pamphlet, which I was glad to see.

I brought it to our post meeting and we are all questioning exactly what you mean by saying that your two hospitals in Thornton and Ormskirk are the only 'FREE' hospitals in Great Britain. Practically none of the hospices gives a bill to its patients and in all the years that I have worked in St Christopher's and St Joseph's, we have never considered ourselves other than free, although we have been grateful when families or patients themselves have made a gift. Like St Joseph's, we have considerable help from the National Health Service, but there are other hospices now who have nothing. I wonder if you could explain to me exactly what you do mean by this statement because I am not sure it is really fair to quite a number of other people.

---

[60] A reference to Shirley du Boulay, Cicely Saunders' eventual biographer.

Miss M. H. Evans

Haverfordwest, Dyfed

22 July 1981 Thank you very much for your letter of the 13th July and your draft aims and objectives. I am very glad to know that you have got on so far and so well. I remember an early letter and referring the first founders to Mrs Barbara McNulty, one of our former staff who lives much nearer your part of the world than I do.

I like your draft aims and objectives because they are very straightforward and simple. I think, however, you need to emphasise that you are offering extra help alongside the work of the General Practitioner and his nurses and the rest of his team. At least I presume that is what you are going to do, it is the usual pattern. It is not quite clear from your statement number one. I really have no criticism of your other statements, although I think you might perhaps extend a little bit on number 4 in saying that whereas many people do have relatives and neighbours who could help them through this difficult time, there are others who need extra help and here too, you might need to emphasise in some way that this will be as a supplement to the ordinary community services.

You might also make a further statement to the effect that you will be working together with all those who are already in the community and in the local hospitals. You need to be very tactful when you offer a new service as by that very act you are in a sense criticising people who are there already and they can very easily find this a threat.

I enclose a statement that I prepared some years ago about starting a hospice. I would modify some of the things I said now, but I have not had time to do so nor have I felt the need. I would certainly not emphasise one needed a building now because I think so few people are going to obtain running costs from their area or districts that it is quite unrealistic to think of anything other than a home care team or possibly a team based within a hospital.

I wonder if you have been in touch with the National Society for Cancer Relief. They are funding a number of nurses around the country in hospice home care and they are also sometimes able to give very good advice to those who are starting out. The District Nurse, Mrs Prue Clench, who started the group in Bath with home care only, is on one of their central committees and has been advising local groups.

Finally, may I suggest that you might get in touch with Help the Aged. I enclose a copy of a letter that I had from them after I spoke to one of their committees. I do not know if you have a need yet, for funding for example your own work.

Do keep in touch with us. St Christopher's Information Service tries to keep people aware of what is going on and needs them to inform us. We could also invite you to our conferences, if you would like to come so far.

You probably know already that there is a Continuing Care Unit now opening at Ty Olwen, Morriston Hospital, Swansea. The Medical Director, Dr Peter Griffiths, was a Consultant here for two years and I am sure you will find him extremely helpful.

Kirstine Richards

Bendejuin, France

27 July 1981 Thank you very much indeed for your interesting letter. I agree with you on almost every point and I am glad that as you look at the death wish you are still saying an unequivocal no to legalising euthanasia. I feel it is most important that we should battle on to do what we can for as many as we can and that a positive answer is always better than a negative one.

I am glad to say the evening's discussion with Exit was much more pleasant than I had expected as it was not Mr Nicholas Reed but Miss Celia Fremlin. We had a full house and I think a good discussion with excellent comments from the floor, in the main on "my side". It is nice to be on good terms with a member of Exit and, in fact, Miss Fremlin came to our Open Day last weekend.

Timothy Buckley
Chelmsford, Essex

10 August 1981 Thank you very much for your letter asking if I would come to your Hospice for Chelmsford group. I am afraid there is no way in which you can persuade me to a public meeting with so little information about the group. I feel very strongly that there should not be a general growth of hospices that have not got a really good medical basis, have really looked at the needs of their own area and, if they are looking towards a building, have both researched the need for extra beds and have some assurance of running costs from the District in which they will be working.

Even if you tell me all these facts, I am afraid I am still going to say I cannot come up to Chelmsford. St Joseph's Hospice is very much nearer your part of the world and I feel you really should be asking for a speaker from there.

You probably know that Tom West has been up twice to the hospice group at Havering in Essex and that he is, I think, one of their Vice Presidents. This, however, was started some little time ago and the pressures on our time have got worse since then. I hope, however, you are in touch with this group because it seems to me that you are likely to overlap to some extent.

I am sorry to disappoint you but as we are trying to keep an information service here at St Christopher's I would be very grateful, in spite of the disappointment, to have as much information as you can give us at this stage.

Shirley du Boulay
Great Haseley, Oxfordshire

25 August 1981 Many thanks for your letter and distilling our conversation into four options. On the whole, however, I go for the fifth as suggested by Edward England. I have real confidence that we could work together and I would certainly leave you free to look at all the available material and probably sink back relieved that I don't have to do anything about a book myself, at least for the time being. I certainly may do an article about hospice beginnings but that would not, I think, in any way pre-empt what you are going to tackle.

Have a lovely time in France and do telephone me when you get back and we will make a date for the next move on.

Ted said "Yes you have got to do it".

Grace Goldin

Swarthmore, Pennsylvania, USA

26 August 1981 The beautiful enlargement arrived yesterday and I have taken it home to show Marian with your letter. He thanks you very much for your comments in the letter, likes to hear about the roses and says he will be writing himself.

I am just going off to television to read your poem. I am glad I am not reading the nice subconscious one which you sent because I could not do it justice. I am fascinated that you write in your sleep.

I cannot remember whether I sent you the Templeton Prize Address, anyway here it is with a few typing errors which I hope have been corrected in the edition which will go into the Annual Report.

I am glad you quite liked the television programme the recording of it went on forever, and although I liked the interviewer all right I found the producer and director uncongenial. I didn't press the important point about our bearing on what is done in hospitals and I agreed with the Talmudist that this needs a great deal of emphasis. I am delighted that as well as St Thomas', Guy's and Kings the other two teaching hospitals near are starting teams in close co-operation with us, as is Lewisham Hospital, the largest general hospital near us. How we will all sort out our home care areas remains to be seen but it is marvellous to have had this effect on those around. Incidentally, Colin Parkes, is completing his figures on the study of patterns of terminal care in this area from the memories of spouses. We did this ten years after the first survey with the same protocol and an observer who did most of the earlier interviews so we really have got a comparison study.

He says that so far as he has analysed the figures, the incidence of pain would appear to have gone down everywhere, but I am waiting for the final results.

Patricia E. Reinking

Mary Breckinridge Hospital, Hyden, Kentucky, USA

26 August 1981 Thank you for your letter of the 7th August. I am interested in your working in Hyden and looking at the need for a hospice in that area. When I was there I was very involved with a conference of hospice people who had come in over the mountains from rather scattered little hospice groups and did not have much chance to see how the hospital was working. However, I did visit the old one and I did stay in the Frontier Nursing Service House and had some chance of talking with them.

I would feel that they are probably doing most of the components of hospice care in their present situation and that it would be a pity to have anything wholly separate from them. Certainly there needs to be the things that you have itemised in the hospital, and my own feeling would be not to be so much concerned with the organised volunteer programme as with more confident and effective symptom control and skilled nursing support. It may be that they need one or two people with particular concern in this field as a reference point as I do not think there would be enough patients for them to need a whole symptom control team on the pattern of St Luke's Hospital in New York.

The English hospices do not have the same tremendous emphasis on a volunteer programme in home care as has grown up in the States. This is partly due I feel that our practical community services are more effective and partly because the English are a rather more private people, and would mostly not welcome a volunteer with counselling skills to their homes.

I did visit with the Central Committee in Kentucky at the McDowell Centre when Ann Blues was still there and I realised that it was wholly a volunteer programme, but that most of the volunteers were professionals, including doctors, that seemed to be excellent and probably well suited to the scattered nature of the Kentucky population.

I am saying all this very much from a distance but I would not myself think that there was a need for a formal hospice programme in Hyden, but there is probably a need for a further development of hospice skills in their own unique situation with its many years of Frontier Nursing Service behind it.

Mrs G. A. Pryce
Whitchurch, Shropshire

3 September 1981 Thank you for your letter. I will be in St Christopher's coming to chapel on the morning of the 8th November and could see you and your husband at that time. Perhaps you would like to come to chapel, which is a Eucharist at 11.00 am and is attended by patients and a few staff and volunteers. I would then be able to have a talk with you and take you round briefly afterwards. You could then perhaps stay for lunch in the hospice.

There is a new hospice which has just opened in the Cambridge area: Arthur Rank House. They are gradually filling up their beds and I was pleased to speak with some of the members of staff at a meeting with their Community Health Council. The nearest hospice to that is probably Priscilla Bacon Lodge, Norwich. There is some interest in the Ipswich area and the person to contact there is Mr T J Mott, Consultant in Radiotherapy, The Ipswich Hospital.

Shropshire seems to be one of the counties in England which has no prospective hospice. It is becoming almost too popular at the moment and I feel myself that we have reached the stage when one wants to have home care teams or one or two specialists being used in consultation in general hospitals.

Perhaps you would let me know if you can come. I enclose an older Annual Report which gives a map showing exactly where the Hospice is. Do not try to come by public transport which is extremely unreliable on Sundays. I really do recommend that you take the local car hire service.

David N. Stocks
Huddersfield

8 September 1981 Thank you very much for your letter of the 1st September. Everytime someone writes to us about setting up a new hospice, we feel we have to raise some of the doubts and difficulties. Above all, at the moment I think you should very seriously consider whether you actually need to add to the beds of your area. There are some parts of England where there is a definite shortage of beds but in most places I would agree with the conclusion of the Department of Health and Social Security Working Party on Terminal Care that we do not want a proliferation of hospice units, without very serious consideration.[61] In case you may not have seen it I enclose a copy of an article in the BMJ this year and I would suggest that if you have not already seen it, you should acquire a copy of the DHSS Report. People will raise these issues and you must have done your homework to find the need as well as the demand for a new hospice in your area.

We keep an information service at St Christopher's and I hope that if you do develop hospice work you will keep in touch with us and we would hope to invite you to our conferences. I also suggest that you should consider getting in touch with the National Society for Cancer Relief who, as you no doubt know, have funded a number of Continuing Care Units in the past but who now concentrate almost entirely on supporting home care nurses for a limited period until the District Health Authority will take them over. In some cases a home care team has shown the need in an area and gained such respect that they have been able to fund beds with Health Authority assistance in running costs. In one way or another I believe you have to earn your beds, as it were.

I also enclose a leaflet that I drew up a long time ago now with some suggestions as to areas that should be looked at as you set out to start a Hospice of any kind. What I do not have is any literature to be used specifically as publicity. Some of the Friends of St Christopher's have run fund raising activities and in the past we had two radio and two television Week's Good Cause appeals. Apart from that we have not carried on activities of this kind, as the work itself which has now been established for 14 years, is really the only fund raiser we have needed. Whether we will be able to go on like this in the present financial climate is a question that is coming into our minds but we really do not have experience of this kind of work to share with you. Very active fund raising is carried out at St Ann's Hospice, Manchester and St Columba's Hospice, Edinburgh and other hospices in the United Kingdom. I think their administrators would help you.

As to coming to Huddersfield, although I would very much like to meet you I really feel that there are many experienced Hospice people much nearer your part of the world. I limit my trips as far as I can and have some visits north planned which I cannot extend and which really constitute all I can do in that area in the foreseeable future. I would suggest that you ask whether a speaker, even Professor Eric Wilkes himself, might come to you from St Luke's Nursing Home, Sheffield. In any case I would strongly recommend you to talk to him about your plans.[62]

Do let me know how you get on.

Professor David Allbrook

The University of Western Australia, Nedlands, Western Australia

9 September 1981 Herewith a copy of my little effusion to the Cancer Council. We really did enjoy having you here. I meant what I said and I hope it may help.

---

[61] She is referring here to the findings of the 'Wilkes Report' which discouraged the proliferation of hospices in favour of broad dissemination of 'terminal care' principles throughout the health service, including acute hospital and community services: *Report of the Working Group on Terminal Care* (London: DHSS, 1980).

[62] Kirkwood Hospice, Huddersfield, commenced building work in October 1985 and was opened on 23 March 1987.

We had an excellent evening with all the doctors at my place recently when we spent some hours talking round some ethical problems of the increasing number of decisions about treatment which may prolong life. I do not know whether we reached any startling or surprising conclusions but we did move on to deciding once again to start the quiet hour on Fridays when we think together about the spiritual side of the work. This will begin again this week I hope and we will see how it goes. I am also starting a series of Any Questions/Any Answers with groups from all the staff on a series of Wednesday afternoons. That certainly needs prayer!

Grace Goldin

Swarthmore, Pennsylvania, USA

10 September 1981 First of all, thank you so much for doing my Christmas photographs, for yet another lovely one of Marian and for all those others that you have sent. The enclosed cheque is for the Christmas ones and a contribution for some of the others. I know you send them out of the kindness of your heart but it is a very expensive pastime to go on giving to your friends like this, so I hope you will accept this. Incidentally, it comes from St Christopher's dollar account out of my interest free loan to the Hospice. It is not that they are paying for my Christmas presents, though it may look like it.

Thank you so much for various letters. I am so glad the article on St Luke's is nearly ready and even more excited about the verse. I have ordered three copies from Melissa Hardie because that, too, will be a couple of Christmas presents.

I do think that what you say about writing verse rings a bell with me. Certainly one does turn to God without certainty of being answered and sometimes it is a very inexplicable answer anyway. Poems, like Marian's paintings, surely come from very deep in the sub-conscious and must be very different from the essays that come from the top part of one's mind. Hopefully, there is some communication between the two.

I would agree with you that the verse or the thoughts or the sudden flourish of understanding of God's presence should come spontaneously and certainly cannot be turned on like a tap. I like your small Allelujah and am taking it home for Marian.

Sad news in that poor Carleton has got rather badly burned by an explosion of the engine of his boat. He will be in the local hospital on City Island for about two months. His face was spared but his hands were quite badly burned. I am assured by his secretary he is in no danger but of course it is a very dreary process to go through and we shall miss him dreadfully on our holiday. Did you send him any of the photographs of himself? I have the one of the two of us together which I think is excellent but I wanted to keep it for myself I am afraid.

Dr D. Souliotis

Nicosia, Cyprus

27 October 1981 Thank you for your letter and your good wishes. I enclose a copy of our latest Annual Report which gives you the speech I gave at the Guildhall on receiving the prize and if anybody takes the trouble to read it they will find, I think, a good description of what hospice means as well as where it came from. I certainly would like to emphasise that the ideal of a hospice is that there should be no financial barrier between patients and the care they need. We have never had paying patients in St Christopher's although some patients have been able to give us money in gratitude. We never even think about money when we are planning our daily admissions.

The idea of separating the patients and having the rich in private rooms in order to pay for the poor is not in my view in the true nature of hospice and certainly any division between the two groups would be contrary to our principles of offering hospitality to all those in need.

Although we sometimes accept patients who are having modified anti cancer chemotherapy, we normally only admit people for whom the acute hospitals say there is no possibility of cure any longer. A small minority of our patients improve so much they are able to return to their acute hospitals for curative treatment, for the traffic of a hospice is not only one way.

We meet daily to decide on our admissions and for most of them it is a matter of emergency. Most families will try to manage at home as long as possible and only ask for help when they need it rather desperately. It is important that an admission should be arranged as quickly as possible, even on the same day.

Finally, I am sorry to say that I see no prospect of travelling near Cyprus at the moment. All our travelling and holidays for next year seems to be booked up already. Perhaps I will be able to come to your lovely island some time but I do not know when. I would like to help you but I do not see how I can do so at the moment.

Mr A. B. L. Clarke

Imperial Cancer Research Fund, London

[n.d.] December 1981 From time to time you have been able to suggest to prospective donors that perhaps the work of St Christopher's was more appropriate for their own particular aims in giving money than the work of your own fund. We are very grateful for this.

I am writing now because St Christopher's is facing a crisis and, like many other charities, a larger deficit than we can continue making. We have no endowments and because we have never employed fund raisers nor advertised our needs, a great many people think that we are in no financial trouble. Over the years the work itself has been our way of appealing and the consequent giving has been sufficient to fill the gap between our National Health Service support and our full costs. However, now these are escalating so fast, particularly in the area of salary increases, that the amount given by our most generous donors is falling behind.

We are cutting back on staff wherever we can but this is difficult to do as we are a research and teaching hospice.

If by any chance you are in touch with anyone who might be interested in our work rather than yours, we would be very grateful if you would remember us yet again. I enclose a new brochure about the work which you will find described more fully in the Annual Report.

Dr John E. Fryer

Germantown, Philadelphia, USA

2 December 1981 It seems a long time since I last wrote to you. Kerry [Bluglass][63] is now safely on board and we are looking forward to Sam's visit next week.

Kerry, of course, had to give the full 3 months' notice to her previous job so that, together with her husband's trip to the States made her start very slow after you left us. All the same, we kept going and she is now working first in gathering together the data in the centre and secondly in making her individual meeting point with the Deans of the Medical Schools and the Post Graduate centres. I think we will have an honorary but official link with Kings College Hospital Medical School which I am sure is right for her and good for us. It will not tie us up exclusively but in the long term is a logical development.

News of our financial plight has probably reached you. It is explained briefly in the enclosed Newsletter to the Friends. We are not doing emotive advertising nor employing fund raisers or starting a whole lot of fund raising activities off our own bats. We are, however, taking the opportunities of publicity which are coming our way anyway because of the publication of our book and a few other things. These are already bearing fruit. Meantime, the house as a whole is being kept well in the picture, is coming up with suggestions and is doing a good economic drive.

After a certain amount of unofficial to-ing and fro-ing I have put in an application to the King Edward Hospital Fund for London for your salary for your visits with us next year. I had to persuade them that this in fact would be for the good of London and not just for people across the world for the International Conference. This was not too difficult to do and I am reasonably hopeful that your trip will be covered. I thought you would be glad to know this. If they do by any chance turn us down I have another string to my bow so your trip will not come out of the depleted general coffers of the Hospice.

As Kerry will no doubt have told you, the Pastoral Care Conference simply did not come together and we all joined with her in feeling it was too soon after her arrival to do this. We have, however, gone along with her suggestion of tackling the Post Graduate Centres in and around London and having a Conference for those Deans. I am all in favour of this. I still think that our first commitment is to get awareness in the general field of the skills and attention needed by our patients and their families. You may be disappointed about this but I hope you will also agree with the priorities.

Mr M. A. Pointer

The Friends of St Francis Hospice, Brentwood, Essex

8 December 1981 I waited a few days before answering your letter because I wanted to discuss it with all the senior staff here.

Our general and considered opinion is that it is making Exit far too important to set up another group deliberately with such an obviously answering title. Incidentally, there is somebody trying to start something called Exist, a word I do not like very much either.

---

[63] A psychiatrist, Dr Bluglass was Director of Education at St Christopher's, 1981–4.

The 'Hospice Movement' is rightly, I think, a rather amorphous entity. The phrase was originally used in the United States where they have a fondness for such titles. When St Christopher's was founded as the first research and teaching hospice we moved out from the older charities and the National Health Service in order to define general principles and develop the scientific basis for them so that they could, as it were, move back all this and develop right across the general field as well as in other separate units. To try and set up a national body would go right against my fundamental principles in this matter. If you did form such a body I am afraid St Christopher's would not join but I hope you will agree that it is better not to confine ourselves to one set of principles and one way of developing them in this juncture.

I have considerable experience of the National Hospice Organisation in the United States where they had a far greater need to fight for reimbursement at a national level than is the case in this country. As one of our Council is in an important position in the Department of Health I know that this is the view there.[64] Monies have to be found at local level with contractual arrangements with the Area or District Health Authorities and the DHSS can do no more centrally than advise and write such articles as the enclosed. I think we would greatly harm the individual developments by having a central body which, like the American National Hospice Organisation, laid down rather rigid standards, helpful though it is in other ways.

To answer your questions in order:

1   It makes Exit more important. I had started on my seven years at St Joseph's Hospice and the development at St Christopher's well before I knew of the existence of the Euthanasia Society.

2   Although many hospices have Christian foundations, there are many others which do not state that they have Christian principles and, indeed, I was discussing the possible formation of a Jewish Hospice the other day and know some where the staff feel strongly they would not commit themselves in that way, but yet do excellent work.

To consider your idea of the functions:

1   Hospice care is not available to everybody now, nor does it at the moment tackle some of the most difficult problems such as those in psycho-geriatrics etc. See Katharine Whitehouse article enclosed.

2   I think people should do this as they feel inclined by letters to the press and so on at either local or national level.

3   I think we have had quite good media coverage and I do not think a central body would improve the situation.

4   I think the conference of Hospice Administrators should continue meeting as a kind of standing conference and that this, together with the work of our Information Office, and the National Society for Cancer Relief, and the individual links between hospice groups in the same area, should be sufficient.

5   The needs in this country have already been reviewed by Lunt and Hillier (BMJ, Vol 23, 29th August 1981). As it happens I have recently been in the northwest where very vig-

---

[64]   A reference to Gillian Ford.

orous groups are setting up quite different work. One a separate hospice, the other a hospital team such as St Thomas's and others.

6   The Information Office at St Christopher's covers this and lists of available hospices are sent to anyone who asks for them.

I do not agree with you that such a body would not take much time. I think if you really set out to do something like the National Hospice Organisation you would find it needed considerable resources and more than one person full time. I really believe that the situation as it is, if not ideal, is the best that can be done at the moment and the right way ahead.

I refer you to our book 'Hospice The Living Idea', edited by myself, Miss D Summers and Mr N Teller and published by Edward Arnold (Publishers) Ltd, and to the last chapter by Professor Paul Torrens. I think there will be a need for special units where they will undertake research and teaching but more and more I hope that this will become part of the general knowledge and wherever a patient is he can expect skill and understanding.

I certainly appreciate your concern and your readiness to be energetic in this area. I hope you will think that the service already offered by the NSCR and St Christopher's covers most of your points and that we will do best by letting things develop in a more varied and spontaneous fashion.

Miss C. Sampson

Casteau, Belgium

21 December 1981 Thank you for your second letter which I have discussed with Dr Therese Vanier[65] because she, I know, has been in touch with some people in Belgium, who were anxious to initiate some hospice work. I had to wait until she returned from a trip to Canada before I was able to discuss your letter with her.

The group whom she met at a conference at which she was speaking in French came from Louvain, where we also have a link with the American Theological Seminary. This in fact was not connected and it was a French/Flemish speaking hospice they were talking about.

I must confess I am extremely hesitant at recommending that you set-up as an English speaking group. I feel this could well arouse antagonism and be counter productive. I am sure the way ahead is to be diplomatic and slow.

As you are in touch with Paddy Moon I expect you have continued to receive up to date hospice information but perhaps the enclosed reprints may not have reached you. They talk of different ways of starting work in a general hospital.

Grace Goldin

Swarthmore, Pennsylvania, USA

25 January 1982 First of all, I am very sorry that the office made an error and sent the hospice addresses by Quinquireme. There was an amazing correspondence in The Times about

---

[65] French Canadian by origin and a former consultant in haematology at St Thomas's Hospital, London, Therese Vanier worked sessionally at St Christopher's and at the L'Arche Community in Canterbury – part of the organization of which her brother, Jean Vanier, was the founder.

these ships a few years ago with a great deal of argument about how many oars they had and how they could have ever stayed afloat anyway. Obviously this one took a fair time to get across the Atlantic.

I do congratulate you on getting them all off. You have done a great thing for the memory of dear Dr Howard Barrett.

The news here is that Marian had a very slight stroke two weeks ago today. It very neatly hit his speech centre and for a few days he found all talking very difficult. His GP came at once and was excellent and I have just got back from taking him to a really top neurologist whom I know well. His Polish is much improved although he could not yet lecture. His English is more difficult and is really rather like talking through treacle. Even that improves day by day and he looks much better in himself. It is to be no more driving and no air travel this year and possibly restricted after that. However, he has already, with the help of his Polish friends upstairs, got all his things out of the Polish YMCA and is tidying up his studio on the fourth floor here and he will carry on his work there and take a few pupils.

He has taken all this with great humour, laughing at his attempts to talk and apart from one or two days of depression, has done marvellously. He tried mathematics on the fourth day and that was no good but painting came back straight away and he started in his pyjamas and dressing gown.

I have been dodging about between home and here and thanking God that Wladek and Hanka live upstairs and that Wladek is home for most of the day.

This is going to mean one or two very quick trips for me with everything pared down to the shortest time possible away from home but unless anything happens, I do not think I ought to cancel them. It would only make him worry.

I love your verse about your aunt. I had a most special one. I do not remember if I told you about her.

Dr L. J. de Souza
Shanti Avedna Ashram, Chowpatty, Bombay, India

5 February 1982 Thank you for your letter. I hope your time in Perth went well.

Your two Sisters, who are at the moment in St Joseph's, have been to see us and we have arranged for them to stay and work here with us from the 27th March to the 1st July. This is really the longest time that we can offer accommodation and experience and we look forward to having them. We would love you to come as well in May and I have discussed your letter with Dr West who organises all the doctors' visits. He asks me to say that he would be grateful if you would write to him as soon as you can to give definite dates as we do get booked up and our accommodation is limited. Also, if we have too many doctors around this makes teaching less easy.

How I would love to lay your Foundation Stone but I have two very good reasons why I cannot. In the first place my husband has had a very slight stroke and I could not leave him and nor is he at the moment allowed to travel. He is going on well but I have as much travelling as I can possibly do already booked for this year. Secondly, however, I have a feeling that much as I would like to do this in the first purpose built hospice of this kind, I think that it really should be done by one of your own senior people. I think it must be very much your own Hospice developing in a specifically Indian way and I am sure you would find someone of the 'elder statesman' type who would do it for you.

Mr and Mrs Gustaf Fock

Helsinki, Finland

9 March 1982 Thank you very much for your letter which has come very quickly. It is very kind of you to be coming to the airport to meet me and I will look forward to seeing you again.

I am afraid I have had to write to Professor Kivalo to tell him that my husband is not able to travel with me after all. He had a slight stroke about seven weeks ago and although it has only affected his speech centre his neurologist has forbidden any flying for the next six to nine months. His ability to speak Polish recovered quickly but his English is coming more slowly as it was in fact the sixth language that he learned in his life. He continues to improve and having cut down on some of his rather frenetic activity, he in fact looks much better than he did before it happened, well enough for me to be leaving him with reasonable confidence as we share a house with Polish friends who are all set to keep an eye on him.

So, I would much like to come to supper with you on the 18th April. It is always nice to have that kind of welcome the first night in a new country.

Grace Goldin

Swarthmore, Pennsylvania, USA

15 March 1982 Many thanks for your letter and also for the Christmas book for Marian which arrived only a week or two ago. He is not finding it easy to write in English although his language improves all the time and I said I would convey his grateful thanks. He really is better and looks very well but he has certainly lost his confidence in speaking English until he forgets himself over something he is excited about.

I am delighted you have got the insane asylums done and also shipped off the large number of reprints of the St Luke's article. If you have any spares, St Christopher's would love a few and would willingly pay cost and postage out of the library funds.

August is delightfully free at the moment and it would be lovely to see you here. We have not got our weekends organised but I am thinking of opting for July 31st/August 1st so that I should have some patients I know in the second week of August. However, that is not so important as the thought of seeing you again and hearing all about Israel as well as about home.

I am very interested in all you say about hospices and the friend who is going to use the St Luke's piece. I like the pictures you have chosen and as I am collecting up some slides for illustrating the history of hospices or an historical introduction to a more general talk, I really would like to make some slides from them or from the Reports that I have myself. However, before I do this I thought I would ask whether in fact you took transparencies or black and white prints at the time you went through the books because you certainly seem to have some pictures which are not in the ones that I have. If you remember, I only have a few that I was able to get St Luke's to give me. I remember being so sad in collecting them on being told that they had thrown a whole lot out only recently. Miss Pipkin who was Matron when I first went always told me that she gave one to any prospective nurse and told her to go away and read it before she came back to apply.

Our overdraft is still a great anxiety as it is indeed a great overdraft, hovering around the £200,000 mark. Then one realises that this is in fact only 10% of our annual budget, it does not sound so much but it takes a lot of collecting. This is happening and we have recovered about £50,000 since the news of our financial state got publicity in November. Because we have always been so quiet (just too ladylike?) nobody has really realised that we have always lived from hand to mouth. We had a deficit of approximately £100,000 last year, which was really balanced by the Templeton Award so it was not until late summer when there was a tremendous drop in our donations and our legacies that the potential deficit of about £200,000 for this year loomed up at us. As it happened, we had a press conference for the new book and various papers picked it up. Since then it has snowballed and we have had a lot of press coverage and local people have really come along strongly and as I said, we have about £50,000 towards it. There is other monies due to come in from the Region which accounts for the remaining part of the overdraft.

We are much encouraged by the interest of people all around and are writing to local businesses and solicitors and have finally decided to set up a fund raising committee amongst ourselves and to look towards two or three volunteers to help us keep all this organised. We are not going into the pressurising fund raising scene but we certainly have to move into a new era if we are to keep pace with our ever increasing expenditure. The staff are being splendid and while we have let our nursing establishment down by 8 by natural wastage and the ward orderlies by two or three, some of the latter group are working slightly shorter hours but still getting the work done, entirely of their own volition. We have just put a large glass jar in the reception area so people can see their £1 notes floating in like pennies in a fountain and this seems to be all set to raise about £40 a day as our visitors walk in and out. I only hope it keeps us. These all seem rather simple measures and I am, of course, in touch with the larger Trusts who have helped us in the past and I am glad to say have got a Week's Good Cause television appeal given to us during August. I think we will manage but it is anxious at the moment.

Dr C. S. Babu Rajendra Prasad

Vianagar Colony, Andra Pradesh, India

2 April 1982 Thank you very much for your letter. I am enclosing two or three reprints and a small brochure about St Christopher's.

Because the Hospice has a mixed group of patients and a considerable discharge rate of people who have had their symptoms controlled, we are not viewed by most of the community around with too much alarm. Indeed, the response of grateful families to our present financial need has been remarkable and I think that probably says as much as anything of how patients and their families have regarded the Hospice. It is certainly not thought of only as a place to die and again and again it has in fact given people the will to live. In a recent survey we found that only about half of our admissions were fully aware that they had malignant disease and only about one third told us that they realised that the end of their life was approaching. This was a survey on admission and many more come to know about their illness and its prognosis while they are with us, but gently as we give them opportunity to talk and ask questions when they are ready.

Thank you so much for your good wishes. Perhaps you would care to be in touch with Dr de Souza, Shanti Avedna Ashram, 15 Dadyseth Road, Chowpatty, Bombay 400007, who is starting a modern hospice as part of the neurological centre there.

Mrs P. Auterinen

Helsingfors, Finland

29 April 1982 Thank you very much for your letter and for telling me how well Dr Kirkham[66] represented St Christopher's. He seems to have been given a marvellous time, and was only sorry that he could not bring everything back that you wanted to send to us.

The reason that I did not come was that I had an accident, having fallen and injured my back which really made it impossible for me to walk around. I am now improving and hope to get back and start work at the end of this week. Thank you for your thoughts.

I was very pleased to hear how seriously everybody had listened and I gather from Dr Kirkham that people are really thinking of setting up some kind of hospice work in different ways that are suited to Finland.

I was able to make pancakes last night and eat some of the cloudberries which had a delicious and most unusual taste. We will be tackling the reindeer meat next.

We will be sure and send you the next annual Report but in the meantime I send you a reprint about the principles of hospice care for a reminder.

Dr Cesar A. Pantoja

Academia Nacional de Medicina, Bogota, Colombia

20 May 1982 Thank you for your letter. I am glad to tell you that our research work here at St Christopher's has been able to show how effective the oral giving of narcotics is now and that our study showed that morphine is totally acceptable as a replacement for diamorphine, which is what we were using originally.

There are many different versions of the "Brompton Mixture" but you will find here in the enclosed reprint the prescription which we are using. Chloroform water is used as being bacteriostatic and as a help with the unpleasant taste of the narcotic.

If there is no way of making this available in your country you will also see in the reprint a number of alternative narcotic drugs with their equivalent dosage and dose intervals. It is not so much the drug you use as the way that you use it, although we ourselves find morphine the most flexible, especially when one is balancing the dose to the individual patient's need.

I would be very happy to have any information from you as to the work in this field in your country.

Mr R. V. Sutton

The Wellcome Research Laboratories, Beckenham, Kent

26 May 1982 Thank you so much for your letter of the 20th May which we have discussed in our Senior Staff Meeting. We are extremely grateful to you for this help and I hope you will pass our thanks to your Director for your generosity.

---

[66] Stephen Kirkham, a registrar at St Christopher's and subsequently editor of *Palliative Medicine.*

Our greatest need at the moment is patient care, for which we have to find nearly half the monies required. This is at the rate of £2.50 an hour at the moment and I hope your Director will agree for the money to go to this, our most urgent need.

The cheque should be made payable to St Christopher's Hospice. There has been a splendid local response to our appeal but I am afraid this is going to be a continuing process with the Hospice having to find something of the order of £50,000 from charitable sources of various kinds every month for the foreseeable future. The Regional Health Authority is sympathetic and has given us a one off grant towards our accumulated deficit but are not able in the present climate to increase their regular allocations.

So you will know how welcome every grant is to us all.

Professor Balfour Mount

Royal Victoria Hospital, Montreal, Canada

22 July 1982 Marian is no more fragile than he was when I wrote to you last but I really think the time has come for me to make a definite decision about October and to tell you that I ought not to come. I am extremely tempted because I always enjoy your conferences to the hilt because they bring such a unique collection of people together and there is always a splendid atmosphere of work and sharing. However, I see you have Derek Doyle[67] who hopefully will have recovered from the three months off I am told he is taking, and Robert Twycross as well as yourself, all of whom could certainly tackle Derek Humphry.[68] I have been taking his 'Hemlock Quarterly' ever since we met on an English television programme and I think that he is about the most powerful opponent we have and will need very serious tackling, not only on the subject of our work but looking much more widely at other medical issues. I think also we have to consider the question of freedom as it is presented in the play 'Whose Life is it Anyway?'[69] and the absence of common moral standards throughout the western world. We can certainly tell good stories of family reconciliations in the last weeks and days as he can tell bad stories of poor pain control, but I think we have to address ourselves to even more fundamental issues.

I think this is tackled well by Fletcher in the enclosed reprint and less well, I must admit, by Robert Twycross's answer in the photocopy from the Journal of Medical Ethics. I am certainly not telling you how I think Mr Humphries should be tackled, I am only passing on a few comments that have been mulling round in my sub-conscious as I have been thinking about it.

I am really sorry to let you down but I did warn you right at the beginning and I hoped there might be time to get my name off the programme, and if you remember, you asked me to leave it on. Marian in fact is far less breathless on walking than he was a month ago with only an increase in diuretics and has just completed a really excellent portrait, painted with

---

67 For more on Derek Doyle, see letter to him of 24 May 1984, p. 249.

68 Derek Humphry, the journalist, writer, campaigner, and founder in 1980 of the Hemlock Society. Born in England, he had moved to the USA in 1978. See also letter to him of 13 August 1982, p. 227.

69 The play by Brian Clark (b. 1932), which first appeared in 1978.

great vigour and enjoyment. I just wish to keep him this way and he feels so insecure when I am away that I hate to rock the boat for him.

If you do not take *Hemlock* I do recommend you to do so. I have never been able to bring myself to take Exit's publications but I believe that Hemlock is a far more serious challenge.

The Rt Hon Mr Francis Pym MP

Foreign Secretary, Foreign and Commonwealth Office, London

22 July 1982 You will probably know that not only in this country, but in many other parts of the world, the last decade has seen a great upsurge of interest in the needs of dying patients and their families, which has been matched by a considerable development in knowledge of how best to control symptoms of terminal disease. St Christopher's Hospice, as the first research and teaching Hospice, has been in part a catalyst for this movement, our main aims being to encourage other people to do this work in whatever way is most suited to their circumstances and to work on its suitable foundations.

In 1962 I travelled to Poland with Lady Sue Ryder and gave a lecture to the doctors in the Oncology Centre, the Marie Curie Sklodowska Hospital. In 1978 I was invited back as an official guest to lecture there again and in other oncology centres in the country. In the course of my travels I met a group who were trying to establish a hospice near the well known church of Nova Huta which was built after many years' effort by the workers of that steel city. They already had a group of volunteers and I went on rounds in a local fever hospital where some beds had been made available for patients dying from cancer. They were full of plans for their own Hospice and I spent an evening discussing this through my most able interpreter. This interpreter, Dr Halina Bortnowska, came to our International Conference two years ago and told us then that the pattern of hospice, so far as they were concerned, was to be a building to which they could invite families to bring their dying and distressed members where they would receive professional help but would continue to do the daily care themselves. This is very much on the missionary hospital pattern and Dr Bortnowska says the urgency arises in part from the cramped housing in which most of these people are living.

I understand permission has been given to construct this building but that there is now a hold up which is preventing them from going ahead with the monies already raised by the workers themselves. We have already had a doctor from this group to stay for two weeks in St Christopher's and had invited another to our International Conference in June followed by special experience in the Hospice. She did not obtain a passport.

We are most anxious to give all the help we can to this project and I hope you may be able to ask our Embassy in Warsaw to make enquiries as to what other ways we can be helpful.

We are not envisaging any efforts to raise money for such a project in this country. I am a Patron for Medical Aid for Poland and I know that all monies available have to go for basic foods and medical supplies. We have, however, a long association with Poland, not only through this group, but through several other doctors who are concerned about the pain control for the terminally ill.

I believe that the Nova Huta Hospice, which has strong links with the Oncology Centre in Krakow, would be an important supplementary service to that very busy hospital in an area where medical work has great demands upon it.

I understand that enquiries as to what has happened to the Hospice and what help might possibly be given have a chance of moving the authorities to look into this matter.

Derek Humphry

Santa Monica, California, USA

13 August 1982 Our planned meeting in Montreal is, I am afraid, not going to take place as my husband's health is somewhat frail and I have decided that my first responsibility is to him and I cannot travel so far from home at the moment. I warned Professor Mount about this a long time ago but he asked me to postpone my decision, which is now definite. I understand from him that you will be meeting with someone from Montreal in my place.

I am disappointed about this because I would have enjoyed meeting with you again and to have tried to follow on from our attempts at dialogue when we met for television. I have been reading your journal and other literature in this field and in the meantime, of course, developing our own side of the work of relieving suffering. There is plenty of encouragement in the way our experience is spreading in the general field. Last time I wrote to you about your book you put my letter into your journal somewhat to my surprise. I see no reason for you even to want to do so this time.

You may be interested to know, as an illustration of the spread of our side of the work, that the demand for articles and books continues unabated with good signs they have in fact got read as part of pre and post-graduate medical and other education. When I have the paperback which the Oxford University Press is printing at the moment, I will send you a copy.[70]

Shirley du Boulay

Great Haseley, Oxfordshire

1 September 1982 So glad you liked the book.[71] I think it is going to have to be split into two but I am discussing it with SPCK in a couple of weeks' time. Meantime I am making up my mind how to do this, which I think is what they want. The suggestion is that one volume will be mainly for the ill and dying and another, which I think on the whole more likely to be read, will be more specifically for the bereaved. Anyway, we shall see.

I must honestly say that I do not think you would really gain more from visiting America and Canada than you have already got from interviewing all those people at our International Conference.

The only thing I can suggest would be perhaps that you went to the Montreal Conference, for which I enclose a brochure. The last time I heard it was not fully booked. As you will

---

[70] A reference to C. Saunders and M. Baines, *Living with dying: the management of terminal disease,* 1st edn (Oxford: Oxford University Press, 1983).

[71] Later published as C. Saunders, *Beyond all pain: A companion for the suffering and bereaved* (London: SPCK, 1983), a personal collection of poems, prayers, and writings which she had found helpful over the years. It contained selections from Viktor Frankl, Teilhard de Chardin, John Bunyan, Olive Wyon, and others, as well as poems by patients cared for at St Christopher's.

see, my name is on the programme because they would not let me take it off, but I have finally decided not to leave Marian.

Elsa Perkins
London

2 September 1982 How nice to hear from you and of course I had heard that the North London Hospice was making progress, both through Harriet Copperman and also as a member of one of the Sainsbury Trusts.

It seems to be turning into a rather ambitious project but I hope that something really will get going in that part of the world. I have a very high regard for Harriet Copperman and I feel she will have excellent experience to bring to the development of home care, if that is how it begins.

Certainly I would like to see you again. My husband really does not like going out in the evenings so I have to say that it would be difficult for me to come up to you for a meal and I would really rather suggest that you come down to me here. This month really looks full and I am on holiday in October so might I suggest that you come along on the afternoon of Saturday, November 6th when I will be on duty but with a backup doctor so that I would have time available. This would be a much easier journey for you at a weekend than coming through London on a weekday. I do hope this will fit.

Ray Miller[72]
Washington DC, USA

6 September 1982 Thank you very much indeed for sending me the cutting from the Washington Post. I am really delighted that the Bill,[73] of which I had a lot of information last time I was over, has managed to go through. It is certainly a step forward for hospice work in your country.

At it happens, someone is writing my biography at the moment. I wonder whether you feel you could dictate a brief version of your story as I think the author would be delighted to have it. A lot of the people who remember those early days have died and I am very pleased to have first hand memories wherever possible.

Please do not make it too long because I do not want to make a great labour for you but I know Miss du Boulay would be glad to have something from you. I will, of course, pass it on to her if you send it to me.

---

[72] Raymond Miller, a writer, educator, and lecturer, was a family friend of the Saunders and former Harvard Business School tutor to Christopher Saunders in the late 1940s. They had remained in contact over many years.

[73] This is a reference to the creation of a federal benefit under the US Medicare scheme for patients with terminal disease and a prognosis of six months or less. Though later seen as having problematic implications (it tended to foster late entry into hospice programmes), it was viewed at the time as a triumphant landmark in hospice history, occurring just eight years after the first service had opened in the USA.

Grace Goldin

Swarthmore, Pennsylvania, USA

30 September 1982 Many thanks indeed for the photograph which I am really thrilled with and certainly hope to include in the limited number of photographs I am allowed for the biography. That, incidentally, is going along quite well. A lot of research has been done and the author is into St Joseph's by now. I have only seen 1_ chapters where she wanted to check on facts. I think it makes good reading although it is difficult for me to judge.

Her Agent likes it very well, and I want it to be a success for her. She has done a lot of work.

Marian loved your letter and his comment was "she has a gift to describe". I think that goes rather well together with the interesting critique. You have an unusual gift for description which, of course, shows in your photography as well as the poetry.

I was sad to read about the death of your teacher but I think it is very difficult indeed not to embark on all the technology which is needed to bring someone through a bad stroke and which sometimes succeeds. It is difficult to decide not to begin and then almost impossible to decide to stop. It really is a Catch 22 situation. However, you seem to have managed to glean, and helped her husband to glean, some treasure out of the darkness.

Delighted to hear about the grandchild and about their delight.

Marian has just had another mild transient ischaemic episode, that is a small area gets meagre circulation for a short time. This time it was just a few days of feeling weak on both his legs and really within a week he is almost fully recovered, but it does mean he and I feel slightly more precarious. I look forward tremendously, as he does, to some time with you both, but I will have a really good check with his doctor and his specialist before we embark on such a long travel. He really does feel safe as long as I am about but I was away one night 10 days ago and it was when I came back that I found a rather pathetic Professor saying he was 'very weak' and although the Polish couple upstairs had him up for supper both evenings, he had refused to eat, so I had to cancel the next trip and arrange someone else in my place. I have now made the decision never to spend a night away. However, he is now better and has just completed a very good pair of portraits.

Finally, I enclose an anthology I was asked to do by one of our religious publishing houses. In fact, it is really the first of two volumes, the second one to be more specifically for the bereaved. Originally it all came together as one, but obviously it was too long for what they wanted and in any case, I think the division would be wise. We worked on this as a group for some time but eventually I decided only one person could do an anthology, ditched almost everything that the others had done but drawing on many discussions and on my own collections over the years, produced this by myself. You will find 'Diminuendo' sitting there, I hope you will feel happily, with its companions.

Dr Harold Lyon

Strathcarron Hospice, Denny, Stirlingshire

1 October 1982 Many thanks indeed for your letter and once again most grateful thanks for having gone to the Shetlands. I am sure you gave them just what they really needed. I totally agree with the last sentence of your penultimate paragraph. We have to show that the ideas are valid and that the methods really work.

I take your point about mixing patients with the frail elderly or the long termers and I think this must have something to do with size as both St Joseph's and St Christopher's are bigger than any other hospice around at present. As of course you know, our frail elderly have their own Wing and know they are an important part of the community. Certainly very much part of my own support system now that I know the patients so much less well.

I think what I am looking at as well as some kind of mixed community done on the basis of local possibility and need, is the thought that there are other groups apart from those more acutely suffering from terminal malignancy who need the Hospice type of concern. I really would like the word not to mean merely the acutely dying and dying of cancer at that.

I am delighted that Strathcarron goes well and I do hope your finances are picking up. Ours are doing so at this precise moment but one can never be complacent.

Grace Goldin

Swarthmore, Pennsylvania, USA

28 October 1982 I fear that our really wonderful week with you before is going to be a one-off, because I saw Marian's Neurologist yesterday and in view of his minor episode a few weeks ago, and the way he does continue to get that little bit older, he has forbidden any long flight. We are very sad because it was such a lovely invitation and we looked forward to having quite a different winter time with you after our marvellous summer break last year. However, I am glad to have my mind made up for me so firmly and Marian, while he sends his love and disappointment to you, also says he might have found it rather exhausting to come so far. He does look rather frail some times and then picks up with renewed vigour to get on with some more painting but he is conscious that his speech is still an effort and is very dependent on me being around all the time. While we were in Norwich he went to the Catholic Cathedral and obviously met a splendid old priest in the confessional and this has done him the power of good.

I am just back from holiday and no time for more now but I wanted to let you know straight away that that lovely restful break in January is off and to send you both our grateful thanks again for the invitation.

Marty Herrmann

New York, USA

25 November 1982 Rosie Laxton came back really lit up by her trip to the States and immensely grateful to you for all your care and cosseting. I hope she was not a nuisance with endless telephone calls and changes of plans, although I strongly suspect she probably was. It made a huge difference and it was a very big gift from our Vice President to the Hospice, who of course funded her trip.

I am afraid overseas travel is off for Marian and therefore for me from now on. He had another slight episode in September with wobbly legs for a week or so and his neurologist says that air travel brings just that extra risk of a repeat, so we are not coming to Carleton and on to the Conference at which he was showing his film in California and back via Grace Goldin as we had arranged for January. His film will be shown anyway, which is good, but I am sad we will not be seeing so many friends.

He is alright again but more dependent on my being there, so I will not be staying away even for one night again. He is extremely happy and as long as I keep him feeling secure, looks well and paints well and enjoys himself.

St Christopher's has kept its finances together for the last 6 months but it needs a constant effort. I am enclosing a statement that our Bursar drew up for the local fund raising Action Committee which we have established. It shows how we have been going for the first 6 months of the financial year and as I think it is much clearer than the general accounts that you will be getting in the Annual Report, I thought you would like it.

Meantime, there are possibilities of increasing Rosie's side of the work if we after all manage to do a day or family centre and someone is also talking to us about extension of our Educational programme. If only we can keep the running costs going, we may move ahead again.

Dr J. Waller

Halifax, Nova Scotia, Canada

15 December 1982 Thank you for your letter. Of course it is often extremely difficult when you first meet a patient with severe illness to know whether in fact the present measures can bring them through to a point in which they can resume a normal life again or whether in fact they really are approaching death. Once the measures suited to the first situation are started, it is extremely difficult to withdraw them, even though they become less and less appropriate. However, we hope that an increasing awareness of the possibilities of good symptom control at least gives an alternative approach to treatment which is gradually becoming better known and appreciated.

Many people have found that financial circumstances have prevented the establishment of a separate hospice or even of a separate hospice ward and I am not surprised to hear that this has happened to you in Halifax. However, on many occasions a home care team or a "within hospital" team with no special beds is often able to give excellent care, even having a greater impact more widely than a separate building might have. So do not be too disheartened if there is to be some time and much persuasion before you can go further than the team you describe. I think it is true that whatever the circumstances, a hospice has to earn its beds one way or another.

I enclose one or two reprints which may be of interest and wish you the best of luck.

Miss L. Lewis Smith

Barnstaple, North Devon

20 December 1982 Many thanks for your letter and all of the news of the Hospice Care Trust. I think you are starting in the right way and I hope you will get help from NSCR and, almost above all, that as your nurses come on board and develop their work, they will have really suitable medical back-up. One group who seem to me of the more supported kind is the group in Eastbourne. Here they have a link with the doctors in the Pain clinic as well as with the family doctors involved with the patients referred to them. I had the impression that they much needed this.

As for your two questions, we thought of a Memorial Book but we have never managed to keep one. I think you would have to ask about it from another Hospice that has managed to do this. I do not know of one myself, although I think the American Hospices tend to do it, I am not sure whether any of the English do. Secondly, as to sending something on the first anniversary, we have always sent a card of one of our Resurrection pictures and I enclose one which shows what it is like. All we write on it is "We are remembering you at St Christopher's". We have had a tremendous amount of come-back from the people who have said we were the only ones to remember and it was such a help to them, or words to that effect. Your instinct and experience that led you to write on such occasions was, I am sure, completely right. If your members feel it is too painful to have a reminder, I think they are simply unaware of the real problem, which is that the date will be indelibly imprinted on their memories and comfort greatly needed.

We do not write again on the second anniversary or thereafter, but I am told by someone that in fact it is often even more difficult than the first. One simply cannot go on with numbers such as we have here.

We have the word "limited" and have not worried too much about it. It goes on a few official things and not elsewhere and seems to be perfectly in order but perhaps your Administrator would like to be in touch with our Bursar, Mr Frank Hill.

Dr Angelo Taranta

CMC and New York Medical College, New York, USA

6 January 1983 Your letter of December 23rd arrived. I am certainly much honoured by your suggestion that I should come to give your 1982 Cabrini Lecture and to receive the 1983 Cabrini Gold Medal Award.

I would really like to have accepted this most attractive invitation but I am afraid my husband is now elderly and has shown in the past year that his health is rather precarious. On two occasions when I have had just one night away he has been less well and I have a definite decision that I do not do any travelling from now on. I cannot bring him with me as his physician will not let him fly.

This means that there is no way that I can accept your most kind invitation and I hope you will pass on my regrets to the others who made the decision to honour me in this way.

Mona Mitchell

Private Secretary to HRH Princess Alexandra, the Hon Mrs Angus Ogilvy, London

21 January 1983 How tedious of the Christmas mail but how nice of you to tell us of the Princess's pleasure at receiving the card. I was on duty the weekend after she came to us and took the card round with me and indeed, practically every patient and every member of staff I could find then and again on Monday signed it with love and good wishes.

Do you think we could possibly think ahead for another pre-Christmas visit this year? We do not wish to be importunate but I cannot tell you what a difference it made to our Christmas here.

James McCann

Associates of St Margaret's Hospice, Clydebank

28 January 1983 Thank you for your letter. It is interesting to hear something from St Margaret's Hospice as I have been working with and for the Irish Sisters of Charity for many years and visited the Hospice about 10 years ago.

I am sure you will have a great deal of detail on fund raising from your own St Joseph's Hospice, which over the years has been much more vigorous in fund raising than St Christopher's, there is not much information I can give you.

We have had Friends of St Christopher's since we were first raising money back in the 1960s who have worked and prayed for us in a fairly quiet and personal way. Over the past 18 months we have had to do more public fund raising because of financial difficulties and now have a local Action Committee, which is probably similar to your associates. They were drawn from among people who were already carrying out various sponsored activities, fairs, sales, concerts and so on in aid of the Hospice, once they had heard of our needs through our most co-operative local press.

So far speakers and acceptors of gifts have been members of hospice staff or of our large group of working volunteers and we have not yet a group of volunteer speakers who take this as their first priority as do some other hospices.

Thank you very much for your recently printed brochure. I enclose the first specifically fund raising brochure that we have ever had which has done a great deal for us in the year that it has been in circulation.

Mrs L. S. Muffet Frost

Toronto, Canada

2 February 1983 Yes, indeed your Matron was my aunt and Godmother and much beloved.[74] She actually lived to her 80s for the last 10 years in an Old People's Home in Reigate run by friends of mine and when she became suddenly ill, I was able to drive her up to St Thomas's Hospital with a doctor friend of mine on a most cheerful and chatty journey and she then had another heart attack and died in casualty so never had to be admitted or spend a night out of her own bed. She had a marvellous life and thoroughly enjoyed her last years, first helping to look after my father and then teaching the au pair girls at her Old People's Home and getting them through their English examinations. I think she did this up to the last day of her life and was never an invalid in spite of her arthritis.

In spite of all this, however, I cannot welcome you to St Christopher's for a volunteer training programme as we do not have such a thing available for visitors either from this country or overseas. Our volunteers are local people whose training is mainly in the form of careful orientation and then experience in their own part of the hospice as a member of the team concerned. A lot of support is given by our Organiser of Volunteers who has been here since the beginning and who makes a very careful selection. It is unlike most volunteer

---

[74] For an account of 'Aunt Daisy', see Shirley du Boulay's biography, *Cicely Saunders*, pp. 29–30, 51–2.

training programmes in the United States as we do not use our volunteers for visiting in the homes except for our rather separate group of bereavement counsellors.

I am very sorry to disappoint you and suggest that you pursue your contacts with this sort of work in Canada. A good programme is starting in Calgary under the leadership of Dr William Lamers, as well as the two that you mentioned in Toronto, and of course the Royal Victoria Hospital in Montreal.

Eric Smith

Hemel Hempstead, Hertfordshire

15 February 1983 Thank you very much for your draft which I have now had time to read.

First of all, I must congratulate you on having producing something which is to my mind more readable as well as more accurate than several other surveys I have seen recently. One general comment I have is that the main characteristic of a truly Christian hospice should be not only its commitment to loving and competent care which is certainly matched by non-Christian hospices and workers throughout the field, but also its belief in the presence of the God who died and rose again. I know you mention this (omitting the resurrection, I think). I think you might have more emphasis on the different attitude which such a faith should give. Hope for our patients is based not only in the belief of a life beyond but also in the presence of God within and around them here and now.

Although I think you have emphasised that the right personality and competence is more important than overt Christian commitment, we ourselves would not appoint to a senior post somebody who did not have all of this to offer. This has been confirmed by one or two appointments where we did not fulfil this.

One implied inaccuracy of fact comes in 10.1. We are an exception in that we are not funded by the NSCR but it does seem to be implied that we do not have home care nurses. This, as I am sure you know, is not true as indeed we started the first hospice home care service in 1969.

Otherwise, I have no particular comments for you and I wish you and the project well. I enclose a photocopy of the last two pages of our textbook as I do not remember whether you saw this before and also a copy of a sermon I gave to the Goldsmiths Company last summer.

Sister Ann Grogan

St Anne's Canossian Convent, East Sheen, London

24 February 1983 Thank you for your letter on behalf of the people in Brescia planning what I would, I think, call a Hospice. I am sorry though I am afraid I am not able to see them on the mornings of either the 5th or 6th April, and I wonder if I might make another suggestion.

Professor Ventafridda and the Floriana Foundation in Milan have been looking at the possibilities of starting hospice work in Italy for some years, and I would suggest that a very good first step would be for the Religious Institute to get in touch with him as I am sure he would know not only of the progress they have made themselves, but also of any other people in Italy with similar interests. I will willingly see your friends in due course, with you as interpreter, but I think they will have a much better idea of the questions they wish to ask if they have a look at the very different circumstances of their own country first. I would also suggest that you should consider taking them to St Joseph's Hospice in Hackney or another hospice run by Catholic Orders while they are in England as, of course, they will have something in common.

Marty Herrmann

New York, USA

10 March 1983 Just had your letter and am hastening to re-assure you that Marian is fine but only so long as he has the constant attention of his wife. It really is intensive tender loving care and he looks fit, has just completed a magnificent Resurrection for the Vatican and is in the midst of a series of portraits. However, he really hates it when I am away, even for a day, although he does not come in and out of my office very much while he is painting upstairs, he likes to know I am about in a splendidly demanding way.

This really suits me and I think staying with you is the only thing that I am missing with a real pang. You really did a major blessing to me and a major work for hospice in America by making it so possible for me to keep coming over and meeting with the people who were starting it up.

I like to think about you with your family in and out and all the other things you do. I wish I could see you.

By the way, an extremely nice woman is writing my biography and is about to set out on the final chapter which is concerned with my travels overseas and the developments of the Hospice Movement. If you ever felt like writing a short note to Miss Shirley du Boulay with your comments on my trips to you, I think she would love to have a direct quote. Do not make a hassle of this, but although she has talked to Sam Klagsbrun, Florence Wald and others who were at the International Conference, the domestic side of my major support system would have escaped her.

Dr M. Rabinowitz

The Chaim Sheba Medical Center, Tel-Hashomer, Israel

12 March 1983 When you wrote to me last in April 1982 you hoped to be opening a hospice in a few months and also that you might be visiting England again. I have been hoping that we would hear from you since that time because I am most interested to know whether the hospice has in fact opened and how it is going.

If you have any literature about this and any news you can give me I would be delighted to hear. In the meantime, we send our very best wishes for its work.

I am glad to tell you that the work of St Christopher's goes on in spite of some financial concerns. We now have two consultants, Dr West and Dr Baines, Dr Griffiths having gone off to direct another Hospice. We changed our staffing in that we replaced him with a Senior Registrar and this means that we now have three clinical Registrars and two Research Registrars. This is very good at refreshing our brains, and I think the patients, the work of teaching and certainly the development of research are all benefiting greatly.

With kind regards and hoping to hear good news of the hospice and, of course, of your own centre.

Shirley du Boulay
Great Haseley, Oxfordshire

17 March 1983 Here are some random thoughts which have come to me as I have been thinking over your chapters. Firstly, though, I want to underline the fact that we really do think you have done a major effort and I hope it really will be a blow for all the right things about hospice. Secondly, the more I think of it the more ideal I think it is that you should be putting in Ramsey's diary. I think it will mean it is read far more widely than any other method of getting it produced. Much better than in my anthology where it really did not fit in the way it will for you.

I am not sure if I ever told you that the evening after David died I went to a prayer meeting in St Peter's, Vere Street, which is where All Souls was at that time. We started to sing "How sweet the name of Jesus Sounds" and I was just thinking that it did not and feeling very desolate for him when I had one of those firm statements I get from time to time saying "but he knows Him – far better than you do already". I have never felt I could worry about him ever again, nor indeed about anyone else who dies in St Christopher's or anyone else who dies in the world without apparently any knowledge of Christ.

When we were being brought up with our good times there was, as far as I recall, no social conscience at all in the household. We just did not look at people in that way and I was certainly very unaware of the problems of the Depression.

Aunt. It was dad who thought that a school matron's job would suit Aunt when she left when I was a baby and she did that all her life and innumerable lonely children were comforted by her.

All through the time I was on night duty we used to do 12 nights on and 2 off. That might get put in somewhere.

I sang a lot more than appears at the moment and incidentally there were other comments in the Thomas' Gazette before the one you quoted, but that does not matter. I used to sing solos in the Nativity Play every year and a number of concerts with Margaret Dyke as well as conducting the carols in the Royal Waterloo.

I have not got any splendid Marian statement for you except the other night "I am very happy, my life is now in order".

I am not sure that it comes across how much I in fact had to do for my mother in the first few years but the question of having her to live with me was somehow out of the question, I suppose because I was comfortably settled in the flat with the others. Anyway, my father was determined that I should not be stuck with it, just as he was determined I should not feel I should come home to look after him.

Finally, the night before I told my mother she really would have to leave, we had a long conversation in which he said that if he knew we would not refuse to see him, he could somehow make a break, but did not see how he could do it. I still think you have left it as though I took more initiative than in fact I really did.

Sister Mary Sloan
St Gemma's Hospice, Leeds

7 April 1983 I was very sorry to hear that your financial problems still continue and I hope that you may perhaps have had some better news since Frank Hill last spoke to you.

Obviously we are always concerned when we hear of a hospice with money troubles but feel fairly powerless to do very much about it other than keep you in our prayers. I am still hoping, however, for a meeting with the Minister for Health to talk not only about St Christopher's needs but about hospice needs as a whole and maybe something will come of this meeting for which I have been waiting for months already.

In the meantime I thought I would pass on to you the comment from one of the Deputy Chief Medical Officers in the Department who is a member of the Council and a very old friend. In our discussion about the needs of people such as St Gemma's she put forward the idea that perhaps you would consider asking your own District whether they would be interested in funding a number of beds for the mentally frail elderly for whom many Districts have a shortage of accommodation and for whom they might perhaps enter into statutory arrangements. I know these are not the patients for whom many of the smaller hospices considered as their vocation but there have always been a number at St Joseph's and a much smaller number at St Christopher's, and I personally think they both need and benefit from hospice attitudes. I know the skills are somewhat different but tender loving care is not, and rather than have closed beds in your beautiful building I wonder if you and your staff might not give this idea some consideration. My friend makes the comment that Leeds has always been rather well off for beds though not always beds of the right kind and this must have added to your difficulties in getting funds so one may have to think of another way round it.

Lucy Chung
Our Lady of Maryknoll Hospital Ltd, Won Tai Sin, Kowloon, Hong Kong

7 April 1983 Thank you very much for your letter. I was very interested to hear that you had a palliative care programme and hope it will go well and you will let us know how it develops. I enclose a copy of a memorandum prepared by our Department of Clinical Studies in answer to your letter and hope this will be helpful.

You may have some difficulty in persuading your doctors that morphine is of use when given by mouth. A considerable amount of work has been carried out by this department here showing by radioimmunoassay the drug's ability to work at therapeutic levels which have considerable individual variations, but which give good sustained pain control when the drug is given regularly. We can refer them to articles in the literature already out or in preparation if they so wish, but I hope they will accept the clinical experience not only in this hospice but in many others in this country, North America and elsewhere that this is so.

I also enclose a copy of our latest edition of Drug control of Common Symptoms which summarises our therapeutic regimes and one or two other reprints which you may find helpful.

Please let me know if there is any other way in which we can assist your work.

Dr Hilde Berenbrok

Dusseldorf, Germany

8 June 1983 My husband has asked me to write for both of us to thank you for your letter in May and for the copy of the article about his work. We were most interested in them both and very glad to have the article.

My husband has made a collection of various postcards and reproductions of his work and also of an exhibition, which was incidentally, the exhibition which I saw and from which I bought my first picture and the way we met. Plate 9 was in the window and that is what drew me in when I was going past.

The big Resurrection has only recently been painted and though he is now elderly, I think shows that my husband is painting with as great strength, conviction and creativity as ever.

Dr Ingrid Burger

Psychological Laboratorium, Montessorilaan, Netherlands

15 June 1983 In answer to your further questions:

Apart from a small group of patients with motor neurone disease, all our patients have advanced cancer at the stage when active treatment is no longer considered appropriate. Their prognosis can be measured in months or weeks, or on occasion only in days. The doctors around know well the kind of patients who need our care and we consider all applications every day at a multidisciplinary meeting.

Our discharge rate has continued to rise during the years we have been at the Hospice. The current overall percentage is 18.33%, in 1977 it was 11.6%. If we exclude those patients who die within 48 hours it is 23.7% and if we exclude those who die within 7 days it is 31.8%. A number of people are referred back to their previous hospitals for further radiotherapy and very occasionally, surgery and we ourselves institute modified cancer chemotherapy or hormone therapy in a minority of patients. Most of those who return home remain in contact with our Out Patient Department, coming up for visits and being visited in their own homes by our nurses and a considerable number have an unexpected time of good quality of life.

All our capital expenditure came from gifts and grants and roughly half of our yearly income comes from the same source and the rest from the National Health Service. Most gifts come without our doing active fund raising but we do work to encourage our local community to support their local hospice.

Your last question was I think covered in my first letter.

Grace Goldin

Swarthmore, Pennsylvania, USA

20 June 1983 Here is love from Marian and me and a good report of a happy holiday for which Carleton was able to join us for two weeks, both idling in the Isle of Wight in good weather and in London and having his portrait painted by Marian. This came out very well indeed with a cheerful contrast between a red blazer with a background of confusion in Marian's studio here and Carleton's kind and vulnerable face. He is delighted with it and returns to the States today taking it with him. Marian painted with tremendous vigour and completed it in four sittings and hopes that one day you will have a chance of seeing it. Carleton's Hospice Team seems to be going very well these days and I am delighted that it keeps its small size, no beds of its own and has reached its 10th Anniversary with a well attended conference and a number of people learning from them.

Looking again at your last letter, I am so delighted that your father got his own way at the end and I hope very much that your mother is finding things gathering round that inevitable gap in her heart and life. I imagine that she will not want to stay longer without him and while that is very hard for those around, it has comfort in it as well.

We have been choosing photographs for the biography with a rather interesting publishing manager from Hodder and Stoughton. Of all your portraits, she went for the one of me listening at the doctors' meeting and, of course, the one of Marian and me together. I hope she will also include one of Marian in the Philadelphia gallery and one of him talking after dinner. She did not choose any of your earlier portraits of me but went instead for action pictures in St Christopher's and of the opening with the Princess with the first patient ever to be admitted and one or two of the early days which you will not have seen. The final selection has not been made but she was so pleased with them that there may be more than she originally thought. Thank you once again for them, due acknowledgement will of course be given and I am glad in a way that she chose a different one from SPCK. That book will be out in the fall and will be posted over to you as soon as it arrives.

Marian, as you gather from the above, is keeping well these days. I have made the little toilet off what is now his study into a shower and he is delighted with this and splashes round like a duck every morning. It was becoming impossible for him to get in and out of the bath.

Incidentally, there is a line in the biography about the Jewish friends in America having something akin to the attraction of my Poles. I don't know how you will work this out!

Dr John Fryer

Germantown, Philadelphia, Pennsylvania, USA

7 July 1983 You are good at remembering birthdays and I was really delighted to have your card. I have, as you no doubt know, reached 65 but my Merit Award continues from the Regional Health Authority until I retire which, even in the NHS, consultants are not bound to do until they are 70. So I continue trying to keep the financial worries off the backs of the others and greatly enjoyed my last weekend on duty and everything else that goes on.

We are fairly patiently awaiting our new Sister Tutor and during this gap the Hospice has done well in giving a good course to our internal course members and we will be starting our next external course in November, when our new Tutor will have returned from doing the course herself in Oxford. Maybe you have heard all this from Kerry, who I heard from Sam performed very well at your meeting.

We have had some excellent conferences recently and I think Kerry does very well there and also in her outside links. The internal situation has always suffered from the part-time syndrome and people feeling that they never get any of her time. However, in spite of this we go ahead in developing a post-course programme for nurses which will be separately funded by the Lisa Sainsbury Foundation. I have an excellent Working Party, potential for a part-time organiser of them, separate from the ordinary course, and really unlimited funding once we show that the whole thing is taking off. The lawyer who helped draw up a number of the Sainsbury Trusts and who I know as a fellow Trustee of one of them, is a key person in the Working Party and I am really optimistic that this will start out from St Christopher's, move out into Regional centres in due course and be a new catalyst in following on not only for those people who have done the course but also for those interested nurses in the general field.

I am sure Kerry told you that we got her salary from the Leverhulme Trust and that we have costed our conferences etc to a break even point. The new Education Committee is coming along strongly at last and even if Kerry begins to find the commuting at such a distance is too much, I think we now have the right kind of momentum.

Sandol Stoddard

Vineyard Haven, Massachusetts, USA

24 August 1983 I was delighted to hear from you and very glad to share your letter with Chris and Tom, both of whom were anxious to know how things were going with you.

Congratulations on all the good news, the Doubleday Bible sounds superb and anyone would be delighted to have those comments.

I must say I think the idea of a huge book is a bit daunting and modern social science is certainly depressing. I have not read either of the books you mention and have not the slightest intention of doing so.

The idea of Hawaii would be wonderful but I am afraid Marian is not able to undertake flights of that kind on the advice of his doctor and I will not stay a night away from him now. He is really very good for his age and is painting remarkably well at the moment, but I like to be around so that he feels totally secure enough to concentrate on painting only and it gives me such a good excuse not to do some of the things I have been asked to do but I have to accept the loss of some of the things that I would dearly love.

The TV programme I have never actually seen but I believe it has been out more than once in the States. I think it was made about 3 years ago. We continue to have debates on this subject. I like the people on the Euthanasia Education Council but have very little time for any of the rest of them. I think what they are suggesting is very dangerous.

The Hospice is really all right. Money last year was better than the year before but we have to worry month by month.

Professor Balfour Mount

Royal Victoria Hospital, Montreal, Canada

25 August 1983 Tom and Mary have now got their invitations and are both very pleased so I hope you will be hearing from them shortly. Tom I know feels very honoured to be tackling that final session and I am sure will give you an excellent time. Thank you for still drawing so much upon St Christopher's.

I was just sharing with Tom Walsh your Editorial for the *Journal of Chronic Diseases*[75] and am looking forward to seeing this in print so that I can respond. I have also heard from Jo Magno with your concerns about the lack of physician and research and evaluation input to the US Hospice Movement. We are shortly going to write round to the Hospices of the UK to find out exactly what research is going on so that I can let her know. I am delighted with all the papers that Tom Walsh is producing and the new studies that are starting off but we have not yet identified a direct successor. However, Professor John Hinton will be coming on board in January, having retired early, and is going to look at families with patients at home and in some detail at what makes home care break down and whether or not admission solves these problems. At the same time another outside researcher from a well known centre is going to look at the nurses' view of the 6 weeks' course 'The Care of the Dying Patient and his Family' and what they see as the need for further education and development. Until we replace Tom Walsh directly, we are going to have some work done by his nurse research assistant and also time spent by a Senior Registrar coming on board in November and, of course, Mary's own studies in obstruction, which are continuing.

I am delighted with Mary's new chapter on symptom control for the second edition of our textbook and pleased that Saunders are going to publish it this time in the USA. It should go out next Spring and I hope might be available at Montreal. Also by then will be my biography, although we have not got an American publisher as yet. It is being published by a big house over here in February.

Finally, I enclose my little collection that I mentioned in my last letter. They have made it sound more for the bereaved than I wanted them to, as they took out two sections on that subject and I want to make a second booklet more specifically from that angle. However, I hope it will be useful to some people.

Marian Rabinowitz
The Chaim Sheba Medical Center, Tel–Hashomer, Israel

16 September 1983 I was really delighted to have your letter and to know that the Hospice is safely opened and I am sure you will be finding that the years of preparation were essential.

I am most interested in your idea of a study related to the book of Job. I am sure you have read Jung on the subject but I wonder if you have met a much more recent book on "When Bad Things Happen to Good People" by Rabbi Kushner[76] which is now published in paperback in this country and if you do not have it I would be delighted to send you a copy. Although he writes very simply, I think he is not at all superficial and his views come out of a profound experience. In the meantime I am sending you something which, although it does include, of course, a great many Christian comments, it also includes some from Jewish sources and also a number of poems and a meditation from our patients. I am

75 B. M. Mount and J. F. Scott, Whither hospice evaluation? *Journal of Chronic Diseases*, **6**(11), (1983): 731–6.

76 H. S. Kushner, *When bad things happen to good people* (New York: Schocken Books, 1981).

not too happy about the sub title which was the idea of the publisher, because there are many other things I want to include for the bereaved in a second book and I really planned this just for those facing suffering.

I am so glad that you are having seminars of that kind with your staff because I think the whole of the Hospice has to look continually at the meaning of what is going on, focused by their work but reflected in the world, as you say.

Monica Cunningham

Hodder and Stoughton, London

23 November 1983 Thank you for your letter. I am keeping the two dates that you mention and agree that it would be a good thing for journalists actually to visit the Hospice as the real background to the biography.

I have never been invited to either Desert Island Discs[77] or Pebble Mill, but not long ago I did a half hour interview with Judith Chalmers for ITV. I am not at all sure about Desert Island Discs as I know it is a fantasy but all the same, even being in the house at night on my own gives me the creeps and to even think about being alone on a desert island is most disturbing!

I wait to hear from you on that.

John Taylor

East Cheshire Hospice, Wilmslow, Cheshire

13 December 1983 Thank you for your letter asking me if I would come and help you at your Appeal launching next March.[78] I am very sorry but I am afraid I am already booked for a meeting on that day and will only just get back in time for an evening conference in our Study Centre.

I am very pleased to see from your letter that you are already negotiating with the District Health Authority for the acquisition of land or even a building for alteration as well as contractual arrangements. I think that it is most important that this sort of thing is clear very early on in Hospice planning, because as you probably know, there are some 19 independent hospices who have no statutory funding at all, several of whom have been open for a considerable time and see no prospect of this essential help. I wonder if you have also considered starting with something less ambitious in the form of home care, possibly with a day centre, as a way of helping people without such a great expenditure as a new building and also of gaining recognition and respect from local people. In some way or another, I find one has to 'earn' one's beds. St Christopher's were really 'earnt' by the 7 years work I did in St Joseph's Hospice and I think one has to be prepared to work for a considerable time before sums of the nature of which you talk are likely to come, or the means of continuing on into the future.

---

[77] In fact she later appeared on the BBC radio programme *Desert Island Discs* on 30 January 1994.

[78] A steering group for the East Cheshire Hospice was formed in Macclesfield in 1983, building work started in 1986, and the hospice opened in February 1988.

I am sure you will find someone else to come to your major launch, perhaps who is rather more local than St Christopher's, which is really rather a long way from you.

Mother Potier
Residence St Marie, St-Lo, France

22 December 1983 Thank you very much for your long letter and for telling me the history of the 'Dames du Calvaire'.[79] You certainly were the first of all of us I think. I am sorry it has taken me so long to find this out.

I am sorry to hear that you had to retire because of bad health. I hope very much that you are happy in your residence even though you have had to leave such rewarding work. As you obviously speak and read English so well, I thought you might be interested in the enclosed little book. It brings together some writings from our patients with various prose and poetry that has helped me over the years. I am so glad that we are now forging more links with France through Dr Vanier. We certainly will continue to respond to any requests we have from people who wish to visit and learn something here.

With very best wishes for the New Year and my most grateful thanks for all the history you sent me and our prayers and good wishes for the work that still continues.

Grace Goldin
Swarthmore, Pennsylvania, USA

22 December 1983 Bless you for sending the photographs, not in time for my Christmas presents but well in time for all my 'thank you' letters. Marian was so pleased with them he nearly walked off with the lot, repeats and all.

I do hope your time with your mother will not be too heavy and that you will enjoy every moment of the holiday with Judah.

We have just had yet another delightful visit from Princess Alexandra, who went round the whole Hospice and talked to everybody and then sat and talked round Hospice in general. She has a very real perception of people's needs and even on a visit like this, will pick out people who are specially stressed.

Marian remains really fit at the moment although even a minor tummy upset sends him into a Polish gloom. Recovery is quick, however, but re-affirms my decision to do less and less outside and concentrate on being here and with him.

Your real present will be the biography and I gather that I may get copies by the end of January. I could not mention everybody by name to my biographer, but the very special link with my Jewish friends in the States is recorded.

---

[79] As a young widow and bereaved mother, Jeanne Garnier (1811–53) formed L'Association des Dames du Calvaire in Lyon, France, in 1842. The association opened a home for the dying the following year and six others followed, from 1874 (Paris) to 1899 (New York). See D. Clark, Palliative care history: a ritual process, *European Journal of Palliative Care*, **7**(2), (2000): 50–5.

Reverend Carleton Sweetser

St Luke's Hospice Center, New York, USA

3 January 1984 I am delighted to enclose this and we are now looking forward all the more to the trip. I was talking to Rosetta last night and she is really feeling excited already. I also enclose the cabin plan and you will see that all your singles are down together but that Marian and I are up on the top deck, with I hope, room for you all to come in and have a drink if the lounge looks rather full.

You will be delighted to hear that Helen[80] has an MBE in the New Year Honours. We had hoped she might get one last June and are all the more delighted that she has it now. She will be back from a Christmas stay with her sister at the end of this week.

Her job with the local Rural Deanery is developing very well and we are all delighted that she has this extra boost to her retirement, which seems to be going very well anyway.

I do hope your Christmas was happy. We thought of you and will think of you especially at Epiphany.

Dr Samuel C. Klagsbrun

Four Winds Hospital, Katonah, New York, USA

23 January 1984 We all thought that you should know that SF died very quietly and peacefully the other day. She had been becoming increasingly gentle and sweet, smiling at all who came but not losing her inner toughness, although perhaps it may sound like that. We feel that once she has seen her husband safely away, she then quietly tidied things up and took her own departure without any fuss.

The ward really did very well with her and everyone found her much easier on her second admission, having really tried at home. When I went up to talk to the nurses the next day and to find out whether JA in the bed opposite was very sad and how the nurses themselves felt, I was told that J was a bit sad but was not talking about it, or I suppose I should say communicating as her talking is extremely limited, and the nurses themselves felt that this was so much what S wanted that they really could not feel sorry at all.

Tom and I have just had a very good meeting with Canon John White who organises the discussions at St. George's House, Windsor Castle. He is getting a good group together and I hope that you will be hearing from him. This confirms that your week with us is a bit earlier, starting on the 29th October and finishing up at Windsor but it does mean that we do not really complete that time until the Sunday morning. Would it be all right for you to fly back then? We can get you across from Windsor to Heathrow without too much difficulty.

This should be a discussion that ranges fairly widely, although I think Hospice needs seem to be so acute for some of the independent hospices at the moment that the Duchess of Norfolk will have set up her central 'Help the Hospices' well before then, both for raising money and for bringing political pressure. However, this will be nothing like the National Hospice Organisation and I think done by somebody so well outside the medical world, will be seen as an individual rather than a joint effort and probably be the better for that.

---

[80] Helen Willans was the sister in charge of the Drapers' Wing for older residents at St Christopher's and later Matron, 1971–83.

We had a good Christmas and the house is all right, although Lyn Hill is going to have a baby and this means some very hard thinking about staff.

Edward England

Edward England Books, Crowborough, East Sussex

30 January 1984 Shirley's book has just arrived as a pre-publication copy and several of us have had a chance to read it through. Those who had not read the story told me they found it compulsive reading and I certainly think Shirley has done a marvellous job, leaving me with the feeling that she knows me better than I know myself, but glad that this part of the story of St Christopher's has been so sympathetically told.

I hope you are being successful with your efforts on the American scene, because I am sure there will be many people in the Hospice world, which after all is now widespread throughout the States, who will want to read it. Indeed I hope they will as the spiritual side of the start of the Hospice Movement is to me as important as the medical side. I am sure Shirley has told you of such things as the National Hospice Organisation and some of the other people that we know over there, in case there should be any difficulty in finding an interested publisher. I do not expect she will get a sale like that of Elisabeth Kübler-Ross 'On Death and Dying' but there is no doubt there is a great deal of interest in this field.

The Most Reverend Metropolitan Anthony of Sourozh

The Russian Orthodox Church, London

2 February 1984 It is a long time now since you came to us before Christmas and gave us an afternoon which many people found very helpful. Thank you again for your willingness to come here and for all this means to us.

Now I am rather diffidently sending you a small anthology which SPCK asked me to do. I am not too happy about the sub-title which was their choice, as I really just wanted it for those facing loss and I have a number of other things which I would have put in for the bereaved had they not been so firm about size. Maybe there will be a companion volume.

I think you might be interested, particularly in our patients' contributions and there might be someone to whom you would like to pass it on.

Edward England

Edward England Books, Crowborough, East Sussex

6 February 1984 Thank you very much for your letter. I am glad you like Shirley's book so well. I am not sure that it matters that the book is "very British in certain aspects". I think if you went for the publishing houses of religious books, which I understand are fairly powerful and prosperous in the States, you might find an unexpectedly ready market. There are over 1,000 registered hospices and many other groups around the States interested in this field and I am afraid I have to say that the majority of them think they have some kind of inspiration from St Christopher's and indeed more particularly me. Added to this I gather from friends involved in different ways with the Movement that a high proportion of people working in the hospice field have, in fact, some kind of religious affiliation and would be all the more ready to acquire such a book. Let us hope that there are good reviews to encourage them.

It is not that I am that keen on having my own story around but it does put the story of St Christopher's in perspective and is become something of a 'Shangri-la' as our perpetual stream

of visitors constantly tell us. Also, of course, I want Shirley to do really well after all the enormous effort and skill she put into it.

Dr William Lamers

Tom Baker Cancer Centre, Calgary, Alberta, Canada

7 February 1984 Having the details about the IWG in February brought you strongly back to my mind. I am sorry that my inability to leave Marian these days means that there is no way that I can come to one of these meetings unless by chance it happens to be in London. I hope Kerry Bluglass will be able to come but I am afraid that will be the only representation from St Christopher's and I have not met anyone from the UK who is going.

We are very pleased with the initial information which is coming out of our last two controlled studies with the slow release morphine and with the tricyclic imipramine. This, together with all the other work Tom Walsh has completed and that his team is finishing off now he has left us, is going to amount to a considerable contribution to the field I think.[81] Is slow release morphine available for you and if so, how do you find it? With 30 within patient cross-overs we found there was no clinically observable difference, no break-through pain in the 12 hours nor any difference with the side effects. However, these were all patients who were stabilised as they went into the study and we still feel that the aqueous morphine gives one the greater flexibility both when establishing pain relief and in the last two or three days of life, if there is no change in need for analgesia.

Colin's latest study is really encouraging on the improvement of pain control in the local hospitals and now there seems to be scarcely a hospital that is not looking at a team on the St Luke's pattern, often growing out of the Pain Clinic. I am sure you must be having an even greater effect on the people around you and I look forward to any papers or reports that you may have.

Although I do not leave him, Marian is in good form, painting most vigorously and very happy, a most enchanting husband.

Major H. C. L. Garnett[82]

The National Society for Cancer Relief, London

26 March 1984 In spite of my reservations, which we have discussed together in the past, I have now been persuaded that the time has come for some kind of general hospice organi-

---

[81] See, for example, T. D. Walsh, Common misunderstandings about the use of morphine for chronic pain in advanced cancer, *CA – A Journal for Clinicians*, **35** (1985): 164–9.

[82] Senior Officer at the National Society for Cancer Relief (later Macmillan).

sation. I think that the initiative of the BMA [British Medical Association] has come together very well with the Duchess of Norfolk's enthusiasm for this and as you already know, Eric Wilkes and I have accepted positions with "Help the Hospices".[83]

Apparently, Andrew Hayes is also anxious to start something which he suggests calling "Last Rights" and I am sure this means that unless something of the calibre of "Help the Hospices" starts up quickly, we will have something less soundly based. I believe it is true that any fund raising tends to open up public awareness of a subject and I hope that your own efforts will be helped rather than hindered by this new body. In any case, I think the Duchess will be reaching in many ways a very different group.

I know that Professor Quilliam will be in touch with you and I hope very much we will see an observer from the NSCR and that we will be able to find that this initiative will eventually help patients on a considerable scale.

Prue Clench

London

27 March 1984 The Duchess of Norfolk brought your letter to her friend to the first Steering Committee of "Help the Hospices" and I proposed you as a possible nurse member of the Council.

I am just about to go on holiday but if you could let Chris know that you are willing to be put up she will send the message across to Professor Quilliam who is chairing things at the moment.

I am going to be President and Eric Wilkes and the Duchess are going to be Co-Chairmen and I think the time has really come for us to look at fund raising, secondly for some co-ordinating political pressure and finally, and after very due consideration, some kind of more centralised organisation.

This is really in place of meeting with you before the Administrators Conference which I really cannot do and because I have failed to get you on the telephone.

The Reverend Canon John White

St George's House, Windsor Castle, Berkshire

29 March 1984 Many thanks for your letter and also for the list which your secretary sent me of the response so far.

I am just off on holiday tomorrow and I will drop a note to Professor Eric Wilkes who I think is a wise person and who was also present at the meeting of the Steering Committee of "Help the Hospices" last week. They are moving so fast that I am sure that the fund raising aspect will have gone ahead by November. However, I sincerely hope that any thoughts of a National Organisation or some kind of Institute will still be a subject for discussion.[84]

---

[83] A reference to the charity, which was established to serve as an umbrella organization for hospices in the UK.

[84] She is referring here to a forthcoming high-level consultation at St George's House, Windsor, on the future strategic development of hospices in the UK.

The emphasis will therefore be more "how" any kind of central organisation should function rather than "whether" it should exist at all. I think there will be plenty to say about that.

I am writing to Professor Wilkes about this and I hope you may hear from him before I get back in two weeks' time.

Professor Kenneth Calman

Department of Clinical Oncology, Glasgow

26 April 1984 In case I do not reach you on the telephone I am putting this into the post. No doubt you have already seen Tony Smith's editorial, 'Problems of Hospices', in the BMJ of April 21.[85]

Although I agree with quite a number of things that are said there is one in particular that troubles me and, indeed, annoys me. They say: 'Several questions need to be answered at this stage if the era of well-intentioned amateurism is to be succeeded by hard headed professionalism'.

As the upsurge of the Hospice Movement started when St Christopher's tried to bring the model of care, research and teaching into the field of terminal care and as it included such people as Professor Eric Wilkes, Colin Murray-Parkes and now John Hinton, not to mention Robert Twycross et al, I feel this is a most uncalled for statement. You have always been a most helpful supporter, particularly Secretary to the Think Tank, and I wondered if you might feel called to take up your quill and write a short letter to the BMJ?

I feel it is more important for people to say this from outside the movement than for us to say how miffed we are from the inside.

Grace Goldin

Swarthmore, Pennsylvania, USA

4 May 1984 Our letters crossed and I hope by now you have had my last one with the news that sadly Tom will be on holiday but that we hope we may see you while you are in London. May I reiterate that I am free on the morning of the 14th and the evening of the 16th.

Incidentally, on Shirley's report on Antoni, she is right in taking it direct from my diary. I modified it in my TV script because that was the first time I had ever talked about him and I could not bring myself to use the real words.

I quite agree with you that she really could not get Marian across in his full glory but when she interviewed him it was not very long after his stroke and he was not able to talk as much as he was when he met you originally. He is happy about it.

I totally agree with you about the cover picture, which certainly will do for the next 10 years. I argued and argued with them because I wanted to have something of Marian's on the cover but I failed. Marian thinks it makes me look too old but on the whole people like it, particularly those who do not know me as well as you do.

---

[85] A. Smith, Editorial. Problems of hospices, *British Medical Journal*, **228** (1984): 1178–9.

Poles and Jews obviously are both important and I think the Jewish link does not come out enough and that is probably my fault. You must be very busy. We hope so much we will be able to see you.

Dr Asenath Petrie

Kiryat Moshe, Jerusalem, Israel

21 May 1984 How nice to hear from you and to have an address again after all these years. I have been in Israel three times in all and I am delighted that there is hospice work starting in various ways. Recently our Social Worker had a very interesting visit in Hadassah Hospital with the social workers and nurses and rather more doctors than we met on a visit there a few years ago.

Thank you for sending me the poems which I found very moving. I am sure you must know 'Man's Search for Meaning' by Viktor Frankl which has certainly been an important book for most of us in the hospice movement. You will also find several other Jewish writers in the enclosed little Anthology.

I also enclose two reprints. I will not bother you with all the research work that has gone on through our two excellent clinical Pharmacology Fellows but I think St Christopher's is maintaining its academic standards and has had an effect on the way people care for those in pain well beyond any hospice building.

I hope your wrist will soon be better.

Dr Derek Doyle[86]

St Columba's Hospice, Edinburgh

24 May 1984 I was not surprised to have a long letter from you nor to have another from Richard Hillier[87] the following day. I, too, have misgivings but was persuaded to join with Help the Hospices at the point when I felt the pro's finally outweighed the cons. The name and the terms of reference had already gone to the Charity Commissioners and there was nothing I could do to change that, although I tried. I think we can get round this by a repeated emphasis that Hospice means a team or a community, or even a small number of people doing hospice work, in the home, in hospital as well as in any kind of institution. Certainly the Americans have been saying this since 1974 and I have been doing so for quite a long time also.

---

[86] Derek Doyle, the Edinburgh doctor who had helped found St Columba's Hospice in the city in 1977. He subsequently had important roles in several national organizations concerned with hospice and palliative care and was the first editor of the journal *Palliative Medicine* and co-editor of *The Oxford textbook of palliative medicine*.

[87] Richard Hillier had been the Medical Director of Countess Mountbatten House, an NHS hospice in Southampton, since 1977 and, like Derek Doyle, had a close involvement in the formation of several key national organizations in the field during the 1980s.

Criteria for Aid Granting

I must have left by the time Dr Dawson[88] made his comment. I think the education of the BMA about hospices is a top priority and I am doing my best. Peter Quilliam has spent a day with us and I now have a date with John Dawson although I could not get him to come before the BMA Conference. I will, however, get something again to them in writing.

The problem of measuring good patient care remains with us and I am glad that John Hinton is working with us now and will be doing a study of home care with a particular eye on the use of the Spitzer Scale. I know this is not ideal but with his 20 years of work in the field I think we should get a helpful contribution from him.

National Hospice Organisation/Conference

Before I had your letter I had already rung Dr John Dawson to say that I felt very strongly that this should be a general coming-together on neutral ground. I gave him some suggestions of sufficiently large halls in London as used by the LMG [London Medical Group] and he thought the Senate House might help. I will continue to go on about this as I agree with you it is very important. I am afraid the Kings Fund Hall is not large enough.

Communications

I can only agree with you here and the telephone calls we had after the ITN News and some little confusion over the information we found being given out by the Help The Hospices office, confirmed it. I discussed it with John Dawson that afternoon as well as with the office itself.

As you no doubt know, Dr Gillian Ford, one of the DCMOs [Deputy Chief Medical Officers] in the DHSS is a good friend, a member of our Council and a volunteer weekend doctor. She was present at the meeting with the Minister and will, I think, be involved in decisions at that end. She is very well aware of all that is going on.

The main problem is I think the mistrust felt by people out in the field but I think if we can go as quietly as the BMA will let us, they will begin to take on board something of what has been achieved and are already becoming somewhat more educated about the hospice scene in general. I can see one is going to have to do this for the Officer for whom they advertised in The Guardian the other day and I see that as part of my responsibility.

I think the Duchess's fund raising will take some while and most of the publicity. Perhaps if we do not worry too much the other things will begin to work themselves out.

I have never sent you reprints but I thought you might be interested in the enclosed which I wrote by invitation and which tries to sum things up in general. I also thought you might be interested in the enclosed reprint of Sam Klagsbrun's who spends a week with us every year. When the time is right I will send it to the other people who think hospice is a rather light-weight part of medicine.

---

[88] Later head of the British Medical Association professional division.

The Duchess of Norfolk[89]

Help the Hospices, London

8 August 1984 Thank you very much for your letter of the 6th August and for bringing me up to date with the question of Royal Patronage. I understand the problem.

Although I know you are keen to get ahead with fund raising and that when this whole issue is resolved it will be a help, I think we have to be prepared not to be in too much of a hurry. We will do all the better in the long run if the various hesitations and uncertainties are resolved slowly and at reasonable depth, than if we paper over what may turn out later to be rather dangerous cracks. The October meeting may help to resolve some of this and so, too, may the much smaller and informal meeting at Windsor. I agree with Eric's latest comments and list of answers to likely questions and I hope that they will increase confidence and that we may go on from there.

I am glad to say that Brian Redhead[90] has agreed to Chair the meeting. He can only come in the morning and stay until about 2.00 pm but he has been involved with several other hospices in his part of the world around Manchester, in helping them with fund raising, so he will not be completely uninformed. He is also a lively Chairman and most obviously not belonging to any of the separate camps, although he did say on the telephone he felt it was time that some kind of separate body got its act together.

I look forward to seeing you next week. Perhaps you will have something to report from the Countess of Westmorland and NSCR but I still think we may have to be patient.

Professor Balfour Mount

Royal Victoria Hospital, Montreal, Canada

23 August 1984 I hope you had a good holiday and are enjoying your sabbatical. Marian and I had a marvellous time in Norway and are shortly to do 5 days in Rome to take part in a Conference on Therapeutic Communities in which I am presenting the Hospice as such. We are both taking part in a private audience with the Pope which is the main reason why I accepted, but Marian is now all right for a reasonably short journey and this will be a great moment for him.

When I telephoned your secretary to ask whether you still need table leaders I gathered the list was probably full. I was asking about Ella Hyde, our Home Care Nursing Officer. Now we have not heard I take it you are full, but in any case she feels that as she has so many changes in her department she really should not take time away so I am not now making the request.

Tom is working on his paper for you. I am sorry not to be hearing you all, but I am sure it will go well.

---

[89] The Duchess of Norfolk had first become involved with hospice activity when helping to raise funds for a teaching centre at St Joseph's, Hackney. In association with Eric Wilkes and others she went on to found Help the Hospices in 1984 and to serve as its Chairman.

[90] The broadcaster and journalist.

Dr L. L. de Veber

War Memorial Children's Hospital, London, Canada

18 September 1984 Thank you for letter of the 27th August, which only reached me yesterday. I think the enclosed article by Dr Walsh and letter that appeared in the New England Journal of Medicine from us both,[91] will answer most of your questions.

1 The position at St Christopher's is that, after Twycross's controlled double-blind study of oral morphine and diamorphine was completed in 1977, we changed to using oral morphine as our regular opiate. This includes year by year approximately 80% of all the doses we give. We have had no cause to regret that decision. Some Hospices in England have done the same, others maintain their use of oral diamorphine. So long as potency is taken account of, the two drugs are inter-changeable.

   However, most of our patients will need injections during the last 24 or 48 hours of their life. At this point, because of its solubility and therefore smaller volume, we changed to diamorphine. A small number of our patients (less than 20%) need fairly large doses and these might be difficult for cachetic patients. However, American Hospices who do not have diamorphine available use, I understand, hydromorphine or Dilaudid, which is also very soluble and as far as I am aware are not pressing for the introduction of diamorphine.

2 I think the point you raise may be a very valid one. The problem as we try to point out in our letter, is the overall attitude and education concerning the relief of terminal pain. Our work has shown that either narcotic can be used over months or even years, should this be necessary to relieve pain. They also show that where we control pain by other means, both these drugs can be withdrawn over a period of a week with no problems at all. Patients are not drug dependent in the usual sense of the term. It is this message that needs to be got across, not the thought that there is one wonder drug that will relieve uniquely all terminal pain.

3 I know of no such evidence. The answer to the practice of active euthanasia is better clinical judgement and education on the means available now for relieving pain in patients with terminal disease.

   St Christopher's main reason for changing to the use of morphine, was, as I have intimated, the importance of showing that good pain control could be achieved with the drugs available in the States. We do not currently have Dilaudid available here but I think you might find it helpful to be in touch with Dr Sylvia Lack who is Consultant in Hospice Care at St Mary's Hospital, Waterbury, Connecticut.

---

[91] T. D. Walsh and C. Saunders, Heroin and morphine in advanced cancer (letter), *New England Journal of Medicine*, **310**(9), (1984): 599.

Dr John Welsh[92]

Hunters Hill, Glasgow

4 October 1984 I hope Geoff Hanks' name is still on the Think Tank list as he does intend to come to the next meeting and as we were talking about something else yesterday, I got it into his diary.

Our discussion was about the rapid tolerance which patients develop to i.v. boluses[93] of opiates, a problem which he has referred to him from time to time at the Royal Marsden and which I happened to have as Housemen enquiries when I was on duty at a weekend recently. Geoff gave me some very helpful advice on how he has tackled this successfully and would be willing to use up a 10 minute or so slot on the subject at the Think Tank. As this seems to be increasing practice, I think it would be valuable.

I think it was a very good programme last time and although we did not have Pat Wall for that other discussion, we filled the day up well.

Many thanks for continuing to organise it.

Dr L. J. de Souza

Shanti Avedna Ashram, Chowpatty, Bombay, India

18 October 1984 It was such a pleasure to see you again and to meet your wife and I hope the rest of your trip went well and that you had a satisfactory answer from NAPP.[94] I really am very interested in your pursuit of adequate drugs for pain control in your country and I would be most grateful if you would keep us up to date with what happens, because we do get a number of enquiries on that subject.

I enclose Dr Baines' article for Professor Ventafridda and I am afraid my memory was wrong, in that it was symptoms other than pain with which she was concerned. I think if you want a copy of the chapter on Pain you would have to write to Professor Ventafridda at Istituto Nazionale, Per Lo Studio, E La Cura dei Tumori, 20133 Venezia, Italy.

The co-Editor who was dealing with Dr Baines was Dr Mark Swerdlow, who is now retired after running a Pain Clinic for a number of years but who is, I understand, particularly interested in pain control in the Third World. He is in fact the Consultant to the WHO Cancer Pain Relief Programme.

The Reverend Canon John White

St George's House, Windsor Castle, Berkshire

5 November 1984 It was really a most helpful weekend in a variety of ways and we are extremely grateful to you for all the trouble you took in putting it on and for your splendidly timed inputs.

---

[92] At this time working in the Hunters Hill Marie Curie Centre, later Olav Kerr Professor of Palliative Care at the University of Glasgow.

[93] Intravenous single injections.

[94] The pharmaceutical company.

I think that we still have some way to go to produce this common voice that the Hospice Movement as a whole really knows that it needs, but I think some important work was done. I am sure that I will have a certain amount of battle within Help the Hospices, though not I think with the Duchess herself, whose own role is rather clearer than some of the others. In the meantime I hope it will go on earning trust, which it has failed to acquire in some quarters, though not, I must say, in all.

The whole theological issue was fascinating and I am sorry we could not pursue that further. The enclosed is in no way an offering of theology but was written in an attempt to fulfil the Editor's demand.

Tom and I will very much look forward to having you here again and to continuing our discussions and I hope that it will not be too long before our PAs manage to sort out some dates.

Mary Johnson

Community Cancer Care, Aldham, Ipswich

9 November 1984 Thank you very much for sending back the photographs and all the other news you sent.

I am glad you have fixed your attention on your own situation and are concentrating on home care, at least for some time.

I am very concerned, however at the number of Hospices growing up all over the place and I hope you will not move towards your own bricks and mortar until you are assured of DHA [District Health Authority] support so that you would be a real link in a place where it has been proved such a link is needed.

Reverend Carleton Sweetser

St Luke's/Roosevelt Hospital Center, New York, USA

20 November 1984 I thought the enclosed might interest you and may be comfort you for another four years of Reagan. The writer is, in fact, the husband of my biographer, a former Jesuit.

We were all very sorry that there was no chance of your joining us for a holiday next year and I am letting you know now how our plans go because it would be easier for a sudden decision should you find that all is well with Helen Jane and you can think of travelling.

We have booked to go back to Peacock Vane on the Isle of Wight, Gill with her father, probably changing half way with her sister, while Marian and I stay the full 10 days. The dates are May 13th – 23rd and we have a nice letter welcoming us back.

I have just had a list of applicants for the British Council Course at St Christopher's at the end of February and see that Richard Geltman's name is not on it. Tom tells me that he was offered travelling expenses and that he thought he was making up his mind to come. I enclose the programme as we have now set it out and a further application form in case this has slipped his memory, as we hope very much that he will come.

I am sorry about that beautiful place on City Island but perhaps you will find something a little less luxurious and expensive. I would love to think of you being there.

We will telephone you some time soon but I wanted to get this in the post and also above all to let you know about the holiday.

We have gone ahead with organising four prints from Marian's pictures as suggested by your friend, whom I met in Rome and whose name now escapes me. If by any chance you can remember who it is, please let me know next time we are in contact, because obviously I must send him a leaflet announcing this, as the idea stemmed from him. He was, I think, at General Seminary with you and was working with therapeutic communities (mainly prisons) and I should be able to remember his name or get it from the programme, but we have mislaid it. It was rather an odd name, short and somewhat Scandinavian. Never mind if you cannot think about it.

Dr Derek Doyle
St Columba's Hospice, Edinburgh

30 November 1984 I am sorry to have been such a long time but I fell down some wet stairs last Sunday and had to retire to bed for a few days to recover and everything got somewhat held up. Now, however, I have a letter from Edward Arnold, of which I enclose a copy, which brings you up to date with their thinking and I would like to make some comments both on this and on your letter. Before I go on, however, in case you look straight at their papers, I must say that I never suggested that I should be the Editor[95] and we did not, indeed, discuss it, but I think as the initial move on their part about 2 years ago and again just before the HtH [Help the Hospices] meeting came from them, they assumed this. As our contact has been over our books, this is understandable, and not, I am sure, irrevocable. I am sure it is too late in the day for me to take over a major work like this but I think my name may be useful somewhere.

Trying to take things in some kind of order, I would say:

The title should, I think, be the Journal of Palliative Medicine. Care is a soft word and I think they are right in wanting some alteration in the title. I have also discussed this with one or two outside people and both Prebendary Ted Shotter and the Director of the King's Fund Centre, whom I happened to meet, felt that medicine was a better word. All the same, I think there should be perhaps some kind of sub-title such as "The treatment of advanced disease and hospice care". Tom and I would like to see the word 'hospice' somewhere in the sub-title but I think the emphasis should be on treatment as well as the wider word "care".

I take Thelma's point about a speciality because I think we have not sorted out whether we are a speciality, a sub-speciality or a general challenge. I would like to think that we were the last of these three, but a sub-speciality so far as training and the definition of a selected number of special units was concerned. I know Thelma uses the word 'Palliative' for a rather earlier stage of disease and feels that 'terminal' has to be used for doctors. There is certainly some sorting out to be done there.

I would like to think the readership would include a far wider circulation than Hospice/Continuing Care workers. This, I think, means that it would be dangerous to make it a multi-disciplinary journal overtly. Certainly, a multi-disciplinary meeting switches off a

---

[95] Cicely Saunders is referring here to the nascent journal *Palliative Medicine*, the first issue of which appeared in 1987.

great number of outside doctors. All the same, one would hope to have solid contributions from nurses, social workers and others from time to time.

I am sure that many articles ought to get into the BMJ and other wide circulating Journals, but surely this one could have a number of review articles or abstracts from such work as well as its own specific articles.

I do not think that this need make us into a speciality in the way Thelma fears if it is tackled properly. Surely, the Journal of Chronic Diseases, with its emphasis on research in that field, covers a whole lot of specialities, without necessarily running into this danger, though I would hope our readership would be somewhat wider.

Obviously, we must meet quickly and talk and I think the best plan would be for us to sort out some possible dates for Tom, Mary and I and possibly Professor John Hinton as well, to meet with you and then have my Personal Assistant ring yours to find when you would be free to come down to us.

Dr R. A. Oberfield

Lahey Clinic Medical Center, Burlington, Massachusetts, USA

20 December 1984 Thank you very much for writing and sending me your article, which I found very moving but also very sad.

Everything in my life and the things I have found in my reading has led me to a belief that there is meaning in our universe to be found beyond that which we impose upon it by the way we tackle our own situations. In the course of my reading I found Viktor Frankl's 'Man's Search for Meaning' very valuable from a Jewish point of view, as indeed was "When Bad Things Happen to Good People" by Harold Kushner. I remain convinced of a Christian answer and a life beyond this one. It seems to me against what we see to believe that there is nothing left of the energy of the loving mind. I also cannot find it possible to believe in a universe in which, although the minority battle their way through, the majority have no chance of a worthwhile life or death.

However, I am sure some people will be really stimulated by the way you have brought different strands of thought together. May I in exchange send you a little book of writings that I have found helpful and put together in a small anthology.

Margaret and Mary Scott

Arcadia, California, USA

8 January 1985 Thank you very much for your letter and for the good gift of dollars. I am sending some literature to Spain, which I hope will be helpful.

I am very sorry I was not around when you came. Any terseness in your welcome was, I am afraid, due to the number of Americans who arrive unannounced, swearing that they know me and being eventually revealed as seeing me on television or hearing me at a lecture once only. As I have always written to you personally, my Personal Assistant did not immediately bring your names to mind, as she normally does.

It is wonderful how Hospice is spreading and we have several links with Spain now, including a very nice group who came when we ran a Course at St Christopher's for the

British Council. When I write I will mention one or two names of people she might care to be in touch with.

I am not as busy as I was, as I have now turned into Chairman[96] and I am hoping to spend, very happily, a lot of time with my husband who has had several medical problems over the last months. The Hospice is well able to develop in its own way now, but I will still be about.

Dr Jack Kevorkian[97]

Long Beach, California, USA

13 January 1985 Thank you for your letter of the 4th January. I do not at the moment recall Rabbi Cohen, although he may have visited the Hospice. I think if he knew me better, he would not have suggested that I was the person to help you in your project.

The legal position in this country is summarised in the chapter in our textbook, which I enclose. I think Rabbi Cohen is quite wrong in suggesting that England offers an opportunity for the development of your ideas. There is a small vocal group which has been working towards legalising voluntary euthanasia since the 1930s and I have many times debated against them, both in open meetings and on radio and television. My own position is that good terminal care, which does not necessarily only have to be given in a hospice, but which is spreading, albeit slowly, through general medicine, is an infinitely better answer than a shortening of life. We know from many years of experience how important it is for the family not to be left with extra feelings of guilt as they are after a suicide and would be after active euthanasia. We know also how well they can use this time to find their own strengths while the patient is finding meaning in the time that is left. Of course, not everybody does this and there are sad stories, but I for one think that any law that gave the possibility of a hastened end, voluntary as well as involuntary, would detract immeasurably from our commitment to care for the weaker members of our society and to improve our means of controlling physical and mental distress, so that the patient can remain himself to the end.

Dr Derek Doyle

St Columba's Hospice, Edinburgh

4 February 1985 Many thanks for your good summary of our discussion of the 23rd January. I think it sums up well our deliberations. I agree with you that much more thought will have to be given to the lists but I think they would produce a good working start. Incidentally, Peter [Griffiths] will not be moving at the moment as the local candidate got the Cambridge job and we hope he will be staying here for a while, so he might well be in the running as Assistant Editor.[98] I am glad to hear Claud Regnard is enthusiastic. Your

---

96 It was a gradual process in the coming months; see letter to John Fryer, 27 August 1985, p. 261.

97 The advocate of 'medicide' and from 1990 responsible for assisting in the deaths of 120 individuals. He was imprisoned in 1999.

98 Again a reference to what became *Palliative Medicine*.

Personal Assistant has now let us have a few dates, so we are getting in touch with the others and will let you know when we have got a date.

Now that Robert Twycross is presumably back from his time off, I hope we will hear some more about an Association of Hospice Physicians. I think the time has come for this and I think it will be important that as the Administrators have theirs and the nurses and social workers have their Newsletter and get together regularly, that now the physicians should do likewise. I do not think we would run into the dangers that William Poe states in the enclosed reprint.

Incidentally, I read part of that out when I was talking to the group that met at Windsor Castle and Canon White from there and some movement in the DHSS are both talking about some kind of co-ordinating get together to give the common voice that is now thought to be needed. This does not seem to me to be the role of either NSCR or Help the Hospices or any of the bodies that exist at the moment. They seem to have their own separate functions and to combine fund raising with some kind of national voice does not seem right. After all, there is the National Heart Association and the British Cardiology Association looking at different areas of need in their own very different way. I do not think it is beyond the powers of any of us to sort out the fairly confusing scene at the moment. In the meantime, I think people should not feel too threatened by Help the Hospices which I think will settle down to its fund raising, which is going well, almost entirely outside the area already helping hospices, and which is going to concentrate on extra bursaries etc entirely supplementary to the ordinary fund raising for running costs which the Hospices do on their own. I think the Regional Representation is aimed at seeing that the money raised goes in the most equitable and agreed fashion possible and is not, so far as I know, aimed at being the National voice in spite of what sometimes gets said by the BMA at various conferences.

I hope by another year or so these various movements will be sorted out and will quietly be getting on with their own thing without more argument.

Mrs R. Dismore

Bath and District Cruse Branch, Bath

12 March 1985 Thank you for inviting me to add to your book on "starters and finishers".

My favourite starter, as I am married to a Polish gentleman who like all Poles adores mushrooms, is the enclosed which I culled from a book called "Super Suppers". I use it exactly as they say so you may feel this is too much of a direct crib for you to use. I leave that to you.

Professor Eric Wilkes

St Luke's Nursing Home, Sheffield

25 March 1985 Many thanks for your letter about AIDS. We had already been on to the RCN [Royal College of Nursing] and the DHSS about their guidelines for ourselves. We are thinking of looking at infectious patients of all kinds in basically the same way, for example those with infectious hepatitis, and Matron is leading our discussions on the subject. We also discussed this at our British Council Conference and it was interesting that nearly all the nurses who had any problems had in fact pricked themselves when putting a needle back into its holder (this from the USA).

I am not sure from your letter whether you think of a delegation from HtH or just Peter Quilliam, me and presumably yourself. I would like to suggest that Matron, Mrs Madeleine Duffield, took my place because I think it is principally a nursing problem.

By now you will no doubt have heard from Belfast that I have had to let them down for this coming Saturday as my husband has developed heart block and until he has been seen and hopefully treated, I just do not feel I can leave him for a whole day away even though the risk of being stuck in Belfast is obviously not great. I hope you are able to help and if you are I am extremely grateful for such a magnificent replacement.

Professor Balfour Mount
Royal Victoria Hospital, Montreal, Canada

26 March 1985 Many thanks for your long letter of March 5th which I have been doing some thinking about, although I am sorry it seems to have taken me rather a long time to come back with an answer.

I was glad to have the actual date of your 10th anniversary, as I have always been a little bit vague as to when you really took patients on board. It is interesting how near together New Haven, St Luke's New York, the first Continuing Care Unit over here and Montreal all had their opening dates.

Marian is a little under the weather at the moment having developed a degree of heart block. We are waiting to see a cardiologist and I hope very much that a pacemaker is on the cards. He is painting at this moment but I have to drive him in and he cannot manage stairs. We are hoping to have a trip to Grace Goldin in Philadelphia in September as I have invitations that will cover first class fare for us. I will let you know how he goes on. My fall was really carelessness on some wet steps but I am wearing very solid shoes these days.

In answer to your questions, the two people that I would suggest from Poland are Fr. Eugenius Dutkiewicz, Hospicum Pallottinum, Gdansk, a copy of whose last letter I enclose, from which I presume his English is as good as Dr Bortnowska who was involved with the other Hospice in Nowa Huta but who is now married and moved to Warsaw. The other possible speaker is Dr Joanna Pepke, Warsaw, who has worked here on several occasions, has tried to introduce better symptom control in a general hospital, but has not actually been in a Hospice programme. Her English is excellent.

I would be very interested to know who is your speaker from France. We have a number of contacts there. In particular Dr Michele Salamagne, Hopital Croix St Simon, Paris, who has been a link person discovered by Therese Vanier who has been over many times now and who runs French days here from time to time.

It is more difficult to suggest a British medical ethicist. Professor Gordon Dunstan is now well retired but remains an excellent speaker on his day. Paul Sieghart is an international lawyer and a most stimulating person whom I met at a conference and who I have watched on a very exciting discussion series recently on our television. He may remember me from a fascinating conference we took part in together in Sicily a few years ago. Finally, it might be worth your while writing to ask Prebendary Ted Shotter to see if he has any ideas.

Marty Herrmann

New York, USA

1 April 1985 This is just to let you know, in case the news filters through to you, that I have been offered an honorary degree in Philadelphia and two engagements which would make it possible for me to bring Marian with me, travelling first class. Grace and Judah Goldin's house is a perfect place for us to stay and we have had a welcome waiting for us ever since a last visit, so although I have been saying no to all overseas invitations, I accepted this one on condition that people realised that if Marian's health was less good (and he had a good checkup from his doctor as regards this trip) I would not go at all.

Now, however, he has just developed a fairly mild heart block and we are waiting to see a cardiologist and I hope they will think a pacemaker suitable, in which case we should still be able to come, I think.

I will, of course, let you know but I wanted you to realise that this was a really special invitation and very different from a trip to New York for Marian.

I have missed my visits to the USA and especially seeing you there.

Mrs A. Whitaker

Editor, Cruse Chronicle, Richmond, Surrey

11 April 1985 In your last Newsletter you quote "The dead are no further than God and God is very near" asking for the source. As it happens, I was sent a card at Easter with the words "Those who die in grace go no further from us than God and God is very near." The card was printed by Westbrook and is their number P7O6. It was sent to me by a very elderly Catholic friend who I do not think could give us any further information, but presumably you could track down Westbrook.

As a Christian who has great hopes of grace, even when very few signs are given, I like my own longer quote the better, but perhaps your shorter one may be more helpful to some people who have less hope of what "in grace" might mean.

Grace Goldin

Swarthmore, Pennsylvania, USA

2 May 1985 Our letters crossed and you will know already that we decided not to come. It was really Marian's decision in the end because when I asked him if he would be very disappointed if the doctor said that it would not be wise after all, he was obviously rather relieved at giving up the idea. I accordingly wrote off to everybody.

Things, however, have changed since the 17th April in that the Cardiologist telephoned me that very day to say that on checking through himself the whole 24 hour ECG, he thought the pacemaker should be done straight away and in fact Marian went into hospital three days later and had it done the following day. I had him home in four days and now nearly a week later he is already much improved. He is walking strongly into the Hospice and doing stairs again and when we go on holiday to the Isle of Wight in 10 days time, I think he will be ready to enjoy it to the full.

All the same, the decision about taking the trip, even to stay with someone who would look after him as well as I know you would, seems to be out of the questions and sadly, I reiterate that we will not be able to repeat our former stay with you.

I am sorry you had a germ after such enormous entertaining. I hope you are now quite better.

Mr H. Hassall
St Luke's (Cheshire) Hospice, Middlewich, Cheshire

5 July 1985 Thank you for your letter asking if I would help you in the launching of St Luke's (Cheshire) Hospice.

I am a little puzzled that there should be yet another Hospice setting out with a building programme in Cheshire when there are already Hospices and Macmillan Teams in action and, so far as our Information Service knows, another three projects. I hope you have seriously looked at the need for yet more beds and have at least some commitment from the District Health Authority for some running cost funding. I think if that is not so, you should very seriously think whether you should not be considering a Home Care Team with a possible Day Centre. There is no doubt that one has to, as it were, earn one's beds by careful evaluation and if possible by the practice of a Home Care Team which confirms the need of extra beds in a particular district.

I am writing all this because I feel somewhat alarmed at the number of Hospice units hoping to come into being who have not, as far as one can see, looked seriously at the questions I raise above and a number of others.

To add to all that I say above, I am afraid that I have to say that a trip to Cheshire to speak at an inaugural meeting is now impossible for me as my husband is too elderly for me ever to leave him overnight.

I am sorry to disappoint you and I do hope you have really considered the questions that I pose above.

Dr John Fryer
Germantown, Philadelphia, Pennsylvania, USA

27 August 1985 Quite a lot has been going on here since you saw us last, as you will no doubt have already noticed on the letter heading. There came a moment when it was right to go to Albertine and talk to her on the basis of a long discussion which Tom and I had with Sam while he was over, and indeed on the basis of what we have been thinking about over the past months. Albertine stepped down at a Council meeting she just managed to attend and handed straight over to me. Tom has moved his office next to me and Madeleine and her assistants have gone down to the back wing, taking over the Clinical Studies room as well. A third consultant will be appointed and hopefully be ready to begin in the New Year which will give Tom more time but he has already taken over Senior Staff, Diary and General Purposes and Finance Committee meetings as well as the new project, which was his anyway. I am realising from the comeback that I am getting that I will have a very interesting role as Chairman and the full changeover will happen on a gradual and already well accepted basis in the house in general.

Reverend Carleton Sweetser

St Luke's Hospital Center, New York, USA

28 August 1985 Gill told me that H had to go back for a full go of chemotherapy. I was very sorry to hear this but hope that it was only to prevent a small suspicious area from going further. How marvellous that she had that super holiday in London with you, but let us pray that this is only a temporary anxiety.

We have continued to pursue the idea of having Jim Smith as Chaplain here and Tom, who took this over straight away, is at the moment waiting to hear from his Bishop. If that is as good a reference as all the others we have had, we intend to go ahead and manoeuvre for him to come over in the New Year. I am told there should be no problem about work permits and that, indeed, for a priest doing pastoral care it is not really necessary.

The other piece of news are changes of roles which you will have already noticed at the top of the writing paper. This seems to be falling into place quite happily. Tom has moved into Madeleine's office next to me and Madeleine and her assistants are all down in the wing where clinical studies was, with of course Madeleine in Tom's old office. This symbolic move illustrates what is happening but Tom's full commitment will wait until we can take on the third consultant physician which we are in the process of doing.

The other change is the final retirement of Philip Edwards and the appointment of Sam as our Visitor. He really does act as a consultant and has done now for 10 years and we think it wholly appropriate that a Jewish psychiatrist with such an awareness of the Christian side of St Christopher's should become our Visitor. He sounds delighted and before this happened had already promised that if Tom and I started getting in each other's hair or other problems arose, he would always dash over.

Marian and I have had to cancel 12 days that we were going to have on Lake Maggiore with Rosetta because he has had a series of severe nose bleeds. These have now stopped but seem to be related to the aspirin he takes to prevent another stroke, so we have a problem of deciding what to do next. I am sorry about the holiday as I would love to have seen him sketching there, and could have done with a break myself. He himself is really rather relieved, I think.

Dr Derek Doyle

St Columba's Hospice, Edinburgh

15 October 1985 I am indeed sorry not to be able to come to your meeting as I am much in sympathy with the idea of an Association of Hospice Doctors.[99]

I agree that the time has come for us to begin sharing our common interests and demands, to set up a more structured way of spreading information and to look at the standards of our practice. I will look forward to hearing how this is going to be set up and to future meetings. This development should have important implications wherever Hospice work is being carried out.

---

[99] This later became the UK's Association of Palliative Medicine.

Catherine Musgrave

Jerusalem, Israel

17 October 1985 Thank you for your card which I am most happy to stick on the back of my office door with all my other cards.

I am enclosing two papers both of which are very definitely for private circulation only but when they were sent to me by the two separate authors, they were not marked as totally confidential. It is interesting that in both cases they give a very central place to the nurse as a manager and also that they come from experience in the smaller hospices, not one the size of St Christopher's.

Here we certainly think of our Matron as very involved with the day to day care of patients, their admission, the support and teaching of the nurses and many of the things that most closely affects the patients and families. The Medical Director has been seen as the one who has the ideas for development, maintains the essential clinical standards and in my case, this grew out of the fact that I actually founded the Hospice. The Administrator should make the ideas possible by good management and is much involved with drawing in the statutory monies but not very much in bringing in voluntary contributions, which have for historical reasons remained with the Medical Director. Dr West and I therefore feel that this is a stronger position than the "uncle" referred to by Desmond Graves.[100]

To sum up, I feel it is very important that there is doctor direction in the aims of the Hospice and that he is the one most likely to maintain the spirit of enquiry and keep up developing standards. A strong Matron is essential for a feeling of security in the house for patient, families and staff and a reasonably strong Administrator to make these two things possible by keeping a very close watch on the finances. How you would categorise these in the hospice "family" I am not quite sure. Perhaps I am not disagreeing quite so much as I think with Desmond Graves.

Dr E. S. Searle

South East Thames Regional Health Authority, Bexhill-on-Sea, East Sussex

24 October 1985 Thank you for your letter asking us if we have yet any plans in connection with patients with AIDS.

So far, led by our Matron, Mrs Madeleine Duffield, we have been gathering information from the nursing and community as well as the medical angle and have had several workshop meetings drawing on the expertise of experienced people, particularly from the team at St Mary's Hospital, Paddington.

We have made no firm decisions as yet and would obviously be thinking of the terminal stages of disease in patients who had malignant disease as a manifestation of AIDS.

We would be very interested in being involved with a Regional AIDS Working Party and I would like, if I may, to suggest that our recently appointed Medical Director, Dr Tom West as well as Mrs Madeleine Duffield, should be considered. As I am sure you know, Dr West is a member of the South East Thames Regional Health Authority Advisory Committee on Cancer Services.

I look forward to hearing from you.

[100] An adviser on hospice management issues.

Tasneem Kapadia

New Horizons of Oakland County Inc., Pontiac, USA

4 November 1985 Thank you for your letter asking if you could visit at St Christopher's between December 26th and January 2nd.

As you may perhaps not realise, the United Kingdom has a considerable number of public holidays during this period and the only visit that we can offer you would be for me to come in on Saturday, 28 December and take you round and discuss our work. It may be that other people will be making similar requests and I shall then put you together on the visit.

You are obviously aware that there is a major development of hospice work in your country but I do not know of any who specifically work with the mentally handicapped. We have the great good fortune of having Dr Therese Vanier working here as a part-time Consultant, who you may have heard of as the sister of Jean Vanier, who started the L'Arche communities some 20 years ago and which have now spread around the world. However, I am afraid she is not here on a Saturday and you will not have a chance of meeting her as well.

I enclose travelling instructions for the Hospice, and I would be very grateful if you would please confirm that you can come on 28th December, at 2.30 pm.

Dr L. J. de Souza

Shanti Avedna Ashram, Chowpatty, Bombay, India

20 December 1985 How lovely to have your letter which I have shared with the others. We are delighted with the news and congratulate you on having got this far after all your efforts. I hope very much that it will be ready in time for the Holy Father to bless it, but surely he could bless an unfinished building? We had several meetings in St Christopher's before we finally opened it.

I am so glad to hear about the MST supplies for clinical trials. It is really good news.

Thank you for asking me to send you a message to come at the beginning of your booklet. I will try and get this done in time to go with this letter but if not, it will follow shortly.

All good wishes for the New Year and for the exciting opening of your two hospices. I wish I could think of a time when I am likely to be able to visit you but I cannot now stay away from my husband overnight and he cannot travel, so I am afraid there is no chance of my being your side of the world.

Dr Michele H. Salamagne

Hôpital de la Croix Saint-Simon, Paris, France

31 December 1985 Thank you very much indeed for sending me the copy of "La Vie Aidant la Mort".[101] Therese had told me about it and quoted to me the lines that you have printed on the back.

---

[101] C. Saunders and M. Baines, *La vie aidant la mort: thérapeutiques antalgiques soins palliatifs en phase terminale* (trans. M. Salamagne) (Paris: Medisi, 1986). With a preface to the French edition by Patrick Vesperien, this book had originally appeared as *Living with dying*; see letter to Derek Humphry of 13 August 1982, p. 227.

I am delighted to see this in French now and hope very much that it will, as you say, help people in France to have a better understanding of palliative care.

You, with Therese, have done a wonderful job in France and now that she is going to travel less often, I am sure you have reached the stage of independence. As you know, Therese has given herself extensively to this work over the past 10 years but I think now the constant travelling has become too much and even she will have to do less. You can imagine how wonderful it is for us to have her in the Hospice for two whole days a week.

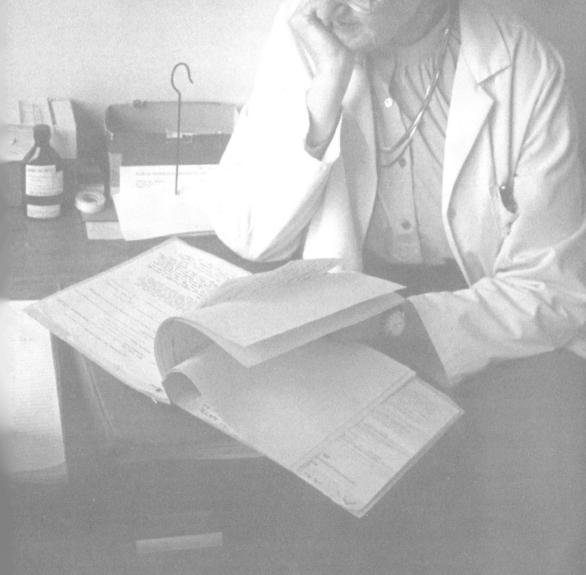

Part 3

An exacting joy (1986–1999)

In their early decades of growth modern hospice and palliative care in the west had many of the qualities of a social movement. This movement seems to have contributed to a new openness about death and bereavement in the late twentieth century. In Britain, for example, the first person ever to be seen to die on television was in the care of a hospice. Inspired by the charismatic leadership of Cicely Saunders and her colleagues, it was a movement which condemned the neglect of the dying in society; called for high-quality pain and symptom management for all who needed it; sought to reconstruct death as a natural phenomenon, rather than a clinical failure; and marshalled practical and moral argument to oppose those in favour of euthanasia. Indeed, for Cicely Saunders such work served as a measure of the very worth of our culture. As she had first observed in the early 1960s: 'A society which shuns the dying must have an incomplete philosophy.' By the mid-1980s, when she stepped down as Medical Director of St Christopher's Hospice to become its Chairman, she could reflect on much that had been achieved. Yet the years which followed also contained major development and consolidation and it was her pleasure and duty to continue to engage with such matters. There was still a great deal to be done and new energy to be found, but there was also a satisfaction to be taken in things achieved, time to be spent with her husband, and new insights to be discovered in both the routines of domesticity and the widening field of her spiritual vision. The line from Ann Ridler's (1994) poem 'Christmas and common birth' seems to sum up so many of these life experiences and qualities: an exacting joy.

The movement matures

In the years 1986–99 around 120 new hospices came into operation in Britain and Ireland, taking the total to well over 200. In the British context these were years of considerable challenge and growth. The hospice and palliative care movement began to enjoy the sense of recognition which it had been seeking for some time. Local interest grew, but so too did that of professionals who were willing to concentrate their working lives in the field of caring for extremely sick and dying people. At the same time policy makers began to take notice and there was an acknowledgement that the rapidly expanding world of the UK's voluntary hospices must be linked in some way to the structure, organization, and funding of the National Health Service. By the middle of the period there was also a growing debate about assessing the effectiveness of hospice and palliative care. In an environment which sought to give greater attention to costs and outcomes, palliative care providers were challenged to show greater evidence of the benefits of their activities. At times it was as if the hospice and palliative care movement was becoming a victim of its own success. Secondary commentators began to suggest that unintended and unwelcome processes were at work. There was talk of the 'routinization', 'secularization', even the 'bureaucratization' of hospice (see Clark and Seymour 1999). Put differently, hospice was coming of age; but with recognition came new responsibilities.

As we have already observed, the mid-1980s saw discussions in the UK about two key national bodies in the world of hospice and palliative care. In 1984 an umbrella organization, Help the Hospices, had been founded to promote the interests of the hospice movement. Cicely Saunders was closely involved in the discussions which preceded its formation and which accompanied its initial endeavours. At times there were tensions and concerns about how such a national body might relate to the many local hospices which it sought to assist. Some judicious lobbying and behind-the-scenes discussions were in evidence. The following year, 1985, had also seen the foundation of the Association of Hospice Doctors, soon renamed the Association of Palliative Medicine. Here Cicely Saunders seems to have been less directly involved, though she corresponded with its founders and took a close interest in its development. Indeed the St Christopher's 'think tank', an informal meeting of physicians in palliative care which ran for several years during the period, might well be seen as the direct source of the idea that the UK should have a national association of doctors working in this field. A third body emerged on to the scene rather later, in 1991. This was the National Council for Hospice and Specialist Palliative Care Services. Again there was some heated discussion: about representation, about the Council's role as an advocate and conduit to government, and about the relative weighting of different organizations and professions within the Council's structure. As with Help the Hospices, Cicely Saunders tended to take the view that the disadvantages of such a grouping were outweighed by its merits. In both cases she therefore accepted positions as honorary office holder, in which role she was seen as a source of inspiration and as a catalyst to development.

Up to now the emerging knowledge base of hospice and palliative care had been demonstrated through mainstream medical, nursing, and other professional journals. The year 1987 saw the launch of the first British journal to be concerned solely with palliative care. Again, there was discussion about its name and focus and eventually it appeared as *Palliative Medicine*, but with the suffix *a multiprofessional journal*. Certainly its existence went some way in supporting the case for recognition of the medical specialty in the UK in 1987, when close friends and colleagues of Cicely Saunders, Dr Gillian Ford in particular, were involved in detailed discussion with the Royal Colleges of Physicians and of General Practitioners. Elsewhere, other specialist hospice and palliative care journals were being established in this period, in Canada, the United States, and Europe. They were accompanied by others which took a wider view of thanatological matters, with contributions from the social and clinical sciences as well as the arts and humanities. As they appeared, Cicely Saunders not only read them all with great interest, but was also a regular contributor of articles, editorials, and letters.

Within this wider culture of recognition, important developments were taking place internationally. In 1986 the World Health Organization published its guidelines on cancer pain control, introducing the three-step analgesic ladder, and going on to an extremely influential definition of palliative care. There was a growing recognition that the benefits of good palliative care should not be confined to those in the affluent nations of the world, but that the epidemic of cancer in the developing countries also required attention. Gradually interest in these issues was spreading to many societies and cultures. Often the key players in development around the world would consult back to St Christopher's, seeking advice and information. Through the establishment in 1977 of the Hospice Information Service, much of this work was taken up by others, though Cicely Saunders continued to be the main point of contact for many and showed a keen interest in local developments in several countries, perhaps especially so in Poland and eastern Europe.

Many issues in palliative care were seen to cross national borders, and this led to the foundation of international groupings, such as the European Association of Palliative Care, which was formed in Milan in 1988 by forty-two members from nine countries, and which ten years later had almost 9000 members from over fifty countries. Moreover, by the end of the twentieth century numerous countries had a national palliative care association of some kind. Such organizations tended to have a common core of concerns: influencing government policy; promoting public understanding and professional education; developing guidelines for service development and clinical practice; promoting and disseminating research. Indeed it was now estimated that some form of specialist palliative care existed in around ninety countries of the world; and there was clear evidence of continuing expansion – in Asia, eastern Europe, Africa, and Latin America. In 1993 the first edition of *The Oxford textbook of palliative medicine* (Doyle, Hanks, and Macdonald 1993) was published to extraordinary recognition and acclaim. In a different vein, Cicely Saunders' edited volume with Robert Kastenbaum, *Hospice care on the international scene*, seemed to capture much that had been achieved (Saunders and Kastenbaum 1997).

Within the professional lifetime of the founders of the modern hospice movement, and that of Cicely Saunders in particular, a remarkable proliferation had occurred. At the same time the *definition* of hospice and palliative care had come into sharper focus. The debates and discussions which followed saw palliative care preoccupied with many of the wider questions relating to the work of healthcare systems in the modern world: costs, benefits, access, equity. Its ability to do so required greater conceptual clarification and a sharper focus on where its boundaries began and ended. Cicely Saunders' original clarity of purpose now became part of wider debates on the goals of palliative care, some of which generated more heat than light.

Professional changes

Meanwhile the founder of St Christopher's continued to receive numerous personal honours and prizes. Among these were the Aristotelis Prize for Man and Society and in one year, 1986, honorary degrees from both Oxford and Cambridge (though she was more impressed with the oration from the latter than with that from her own university). In 1989 her entry into the Order of Merit saw her achieve the highest honour within the UK system, joining just twenty-four members at any one time, each personally selected by Her Majesty the Queen.

At the same time that the level of public recognition was maintained, the period also saw her move out of the role of Medical Director at St Christopher's and into that of Chairman of Council. She was succeeded by a long-time close friend since medical school, Dr Tom West. Although the move to the position of Chairman was not straightforward at first, it was an opportunity to strengthen the Council of St Christopher's and also to forge new links with the outside world. It was also a position from which she could reflect on and at times take issue with ideas and debates to be found in the growing palliative care literature. So in the 1990s we see numerous letters to journal editors commenting on recently published articles as well as several prefaces, forewords, and introductions to the works of others.

Tom West was followed in turn by Dr Robert Dunlop, who in 1992 took up the position of Medical Director and Chief Executive. These were years of considerable expansion in the range of St Christopher's clinical service and in its academic commitments. The hospice continued to identify unmet need and responded with several service developments, including greatly expanded home care services. An academic chair of palliative care and policy was established jointly with King's College, London. There were major refurbishments to the education centre and to the grounds surrounding the hospice. Such developments were costly and were not always matched by increases in revenue income. By 1999, major financial problems were again looming. The hospice had of course experienced these before, but never on such a scale and with such serious consequences. The storms which swept through St Christopher's in the year 2000 are beyond the chronological scope of this book, but their consequences for Cicely Saunders, for her colleagues, and for the entire hospice were far-reaching.

The later years covered here were also a time when Cicely Saunders' private and professional life were opened up to unprecedented public scrutiny. The first major step in this direction had been in 1976 with the BBC television programme *In the Light of Experience*. Here she had talked openly for the first time about Antoni Michniewicz. In 1984 her biography had appeared, and as it became widely known she encountered the unnerving experience of meeting those who knew her far better than she would ever know them, not least as it was translated into other languages, including Dutch and Japanese. Her life and work were helping to shape the iconography of the modern hospice movement. Mostly she enjoyed this and delighted in the fame and recognition, often with a girlish pleasure in the treats and luxuries which they brought in their wake. Yet she was also uneasy about this. She knew that 'public speaking is a drug of addiction' and was wary of its aftermath. She took trouble to promote the recognition of her colleagues at the hospice, many of whom became its international ambassadors in these years. St Christopher's had now become the training ground for a whole cohort of healthcare workers who went on to forge the expansion of the modern discipline of palliative care, and this owed much to a determination that her charismatic leadership would foster able and free-thinking successors.

Cherished values

Relinquishing the duties of Medical Director created a space for further spiritual and philosophical reflection. We can see during these years a deepening and a broadening of her perspective on the nature of spirituality and the basis of Christian faith. She continued to read *Daily Light*, but also drew much from the writings of Julian of Norwich as well as many theologians, ethicists, and philosophers. There was also now more time and opportunity to reflect on the wider nature of human suffering as revealed in art, poetry, and literature. These influences contributed to the expansion in her notion of spiritual pain, first presented at St Christopher's international conference in 1988.

During the course of these years a small group at the hospice again met and reconsidered the original document known as the 'Aim and Basis' of St Christopher's. There was a growing sense of broadening the spiritual care of the hospice to incorporate those of other faiths – and those of no faith at all. Reflecting her admiration for Jewish friends and their ideas, Dr Sam Klagsbrun was appointed as Visitor in 1986, after having spent one week each year for the previous decade at St Christopher's.

Throughout this time there was a continuing willingness to engage with the proponents of euthanasia and to participate in public debate and lobbying. This was also coupled to a wider involvement in matters of ethics. Cicely Saunders took a particular interest in the deliberations of the House of Lords' Select Committee on Medical Ethics led by Lord Walton and was delighted with its conclusions, in 1994. She continued to take the view that less than 5 per cent of dying patients have pain which does not respond to treatment and that here the problems can be resolved if a certain level of sedation is accepted.

As some of the letters reproduced here make clear, these years were characterized by continuing attention to longstanding friendships. With those in America particularly, she emerges as an assiduous and attentive correspondent and there is a sustained and warm flow of letters with, for example, Marty Herrmann in New York, whom she had met on her first visit to the United States in 1963. Similarly there was a steady exchange of letters, poems, and photographs with the photographer and historian Grace Goldin. Closer to home, although not captured in correspondence, there are enduring friendships: with Gillian Ford, known since medical school; with surviving members of her nursing 'set' at St Thomas's Hospital; as well as with early supporters of the St Christopher's cause.

Cicely Saunders also took the time in these years to develop an extensive interest in the history of the hospice idea and its underlying philosophy, going back to earliest times. In this way she perhaps also took opportunities to cultivate the mythology of David Tasma as St Christopher's founding patient, of St Christopher's as the fountainhead of the modern hospice movement, and of her own place as its founder. Linking all of these has been her continued commitment to St Christopher's as a community, albeit increasingly of the 'unalike': a place of difference and diversity grouped around a common activity. The continued link with the sisters at the religious community in Grandchamp, Switzerland, is evidence of a longstanding preoccupation with notions of community, faith, and servanthood.

At the same time some of these years were also ones of unprecedented domesticity in Cicely Saunders' life. By the second half of the 1980s, Marian her husband was becoming more frail. There were scares and worries, tests and investigations. She took the decision to travel a great deal less and eventually not at all. She remained at home with him, encouraging his painting, warmed by his pride and dignity in advanced years, and caring for him with help from her neighbour as his needs increased. When his death came on 28 January 1995 it was appropriate that he was at St Christopher's in the care of her colleagues and friends.

Afterwards there was a new opening up of interests. She travelled again, accepted speaking engagements around the world, and gave numerous interviews. Each morning she was at the hospice in time for chapel at 8.45. She received visitors in her office, dealt with constant enquiries, and even indulged the requests of historians and archivists. Her eightieth birthday in 1998 was celebrated with private parties, but also with a major international conference at the Royal College of Physicians, in London. Characteristically, and at her own insistence, it was an event which celebrated what had been achieved in the modern history of hospice and palliative care. More importantly for Cicely Saunders, it concentrated in the main upon the work still to be done.

References

Clark, D. and Seymour, J. (1999) *Reflections on palliative care*. Buckingham: Open University Press.

Doyle, D., Hanks, G., and Macdonald, N. (ed.) (1993) *The Oxford textbook of palliative medicine*. Oxford: Oxford University Press.

Ridler, A.. (1994) Christmas and common birth. In *Collected Poems*. Manchester: Carcenet Press.

Saunders, C. and Kastenbaum, R. (ed.) (1997) *Hospice care on the international scene*. New York: Springer.

Letters, 1986–1999

Dr Austin H. Kutscher

Columbia-Presbyterian Medical Center, New York, USA

28 January 1986 I was very interested to see your programme for the symposium in April and I am only sorry that I am not able to think of travelling these days because of my husband's health. I am delighted to see that you are working together with Sam Klagsbrun of Four Winds Hospital in sponsoring this.

You may not know but St Christopher's has appointed him as our Visitor. He has been coming to spend a week with us for over 10 years now, once at least every year and so instead of appointing a Bishop or some similar person, we felt this time we would show how much we felt these visits help us in the way that the English custom of having a Visitor is expected to function. Sam is a great friend who helps us to see what we are really doing here and where we should be looking next.

So much has happened since you first started the Foundation of Thanatology and I am wondering if you have any literature about the Foundation that tells the story of its beginnings. I am very interested in hospice evolution in different parts of the world and your work is obviously part of the whole development of interest in this field. Of course I should know this, as I visited with you in the very early days, but I am afraid I do not always keep all the literature I should.

I think you would find that the hospice movement in England is much more medically founded than many of the groups in the States and I am sure you would have a big response to this particular symposium. All the same, our ethics in this area are rather different and I think some of the cases that we have reported in our press about people in your country who have every last piece of technology used that would be appropriate to an acute illness, but is totally inappropriate to terminal illness, would be very unlikely to happen here.

Grace Goldin

Swarthmore, Pennsylvania, USA

30 January 1986 You must have thought you were never going to get these back but it has taken the Royal Society of Medicine a long time to do black and white prints of the photograph of me and of the one which Tom chose of himself. Thank you very much for trusting us with them. Chris has just used up the last of my penultimate black and whites and I am very glad to have this now to take its place. We will duly acknowledge where it comes from.

I am delighted to tell you that a few days ago Marian felt strongly enough to embark on an oil portrait. He has had two sittings of about an hour in length each and has already got an exciting composition and an excellent likeness of one of his very interesting pupils. She in her turn is, I hope, going to paint him, but he felt well enough to do it in this order.

After a quite incredibly slow convalescence, a very traumatic time in at last locating the source of the nose bleeds and having it cauterized and two minor flare ups both of his gall bladder and his nose, I have now had him home for about a month and he has come back almost to being himself again. He is just a bit slower but he has the sparkle back. I do a bit of surreptitious help in dressing and undressing and other things that take a toll of energy because I have been determined that he keeps all he has for his art and his enjoyment of people, including me of course. This has really paid off. We have framed some 60 pastel drawings and he will be having an exhibition at the end of April. As the products of his illness and convalescence they are quite amazing. Many are more abstract than usual, but they are full of joy and lightness.

I wish you were not so far away, I would love you to see him looking so much better than when you took those photographs when he had so far to go and I would love you to see what he has been doing. When they have been exhibited they will be scattered round St Christopher's, Rugby Ward, the Study Centre, rooms and people who have helped and who want them. All the same, I think your drawing done when he was so happy in your home, will still be top of all for you.

Dr Ina Ajemian

Palliative Care Service, Royal Victoria Hospital, Montreal, Canada

17 February 1986 Your letter or February 12th has just arrived telling me of the changes in the Palliative Care Service. First of all, congratulations to you on being the Director, which I know you will do superbly. I am not surprised at Bal's change of role, which I suppose in some ways is not unlike my own change into being Chairman and handing over all the day to day administration to Tom.

I will put my wishes to Bal on a separate sheet for you to read out if you like.

Changing roles is not easy and we are benefiting very much from Sam Klagsbrun's readiness to come over and help us look at our roles and try to stop us getting across each other. I hope that you may perhaps have someone who will help you in some way because it is a much more difficult change than the retiring member disappearing completely. I am sure the patient care, with your immensely varied population continues as well as ever. Please give my special good wishes to everyone who remembers me.

Dr Robert Twycross

St Michael Sobell House, Oxford

19 February 1986 Many thanks indeed for your letter of 14th February with your good wishes on my somewhat surprising double.[1] I am, of course, delighted about this.

Thank you for your offer of assistance, but I think I will probably be staying with Bishop and Mrs John Taylor with my husband. He is very fond of them and I am hoping that his health will be good enough for us to spend 2–3 nights together there, although of course I have been offered accommodation by the University. I imagine that they will deal with my transport, but if not perhaps I might call on you for that.

I was sorry not to get to the Leeds meeting but it has really not been possible for me to travel any distance away from home this winter and in any case, I was already speaking at the Royal Society of Medicine. I gather you had quite a lively meeting and I hope some real sense and accreditation will eventually come out of the various efforts.

Recently I have found myself referring more than once to the WHO statement on pain control. The one reprint I have appears only to quote from it and I wonder if you could possibly let me have a copy of the full statement or give me the right address and reference

---

[1] She is referring to honorary degrees in the same year from both Oxford University and Cambridge University.

number so that I can get one. It would be of value for some of our overseas visitors as well as of interest for reference here.

Dr Oscar A. Throup Jr

University of Virginia, Charlottesville, Virginia, USA

25 February 1986 Thank you for your letter regarding Ms Maria Britto, which I am sorry to have to say is unlikely to be successful. However, I am passing it on to our new Consultant, Dr Michael Kearney, who is dealing with all applications of this kind and who I am sure will send other suggestions. St Christopher's programme is now so packed with new developments it is impossible for us to welcome students as we did a few years ago.

I am sorry that there has been a certain amount of trouble in the Hospice area in your country. We heard quite a lot about this from our American speakers at our International Conference last summer. The emphasis on hospice as a cheaper form of care and the terms of the legislation and insurance guidelines seem to add so much bureaucracy that I gather many individual hospices are still functioning on a voluntary basis in order to avoid it.

I think the major problem has been that hospice has grown up as a consumer drive rather than a development from within the traditional medicine and nursing fields as it has largely in this country. The emphasis here is on collaboration with a great deal of independence for the voluntary sector and although the finances of the National Health Service have prevented many Health Authorities from much in the way of financial support, I think the signs are that this is greatly improving. St Christopher's itself has to find more than half its monies from charitable giving and has a constant struggle, but in spite of that I am really encouraged by the medical drive of our younger Consultants and Registrars. I hope we will continue to keep the balance.

I am sorry I cannot come to your country now but my husband is much in need of my being here all the time for it enables him to continue as creatively as ever with his painting in spite of precarious health.

Dr Robert Twycross

Sir Michael Sobell House, Oxford

27 February 1986 Thank you very much for your letter. I know you will assume my arrangements are water tight but I hope to see you somewhere or other during the course of the day.

I am interested in what happened to the WHO Technical Report and I certainly will write to Dr Stjernsward.

As it happens, I was looking through the first copy of the *Journal of Pain and Symptom Management* yesterday and although I presume you have already received it I am photocopying their Information Exchange pages about the Pain Relief Programme. Let us hope progress will be made.

I think the idea of "pushing morphine" is almost ineradicable and I do hope that the subtle re-writing will get around this. I was aware of how much this was a problem in Ireland when being interviewed by an Irish television crew on behalf of Our Lady's Hospice,

Harold's Cross and their new drive. Education is a sadly slow process and so often deeply ingrained prejudices have to be tackled as well.

Dr Jan Stjernsward

WHO, Geneva, Switzerland

27 February 1986 St Christopher's Hospice has a considerable number of visitors from overseas and I am much looking forward to having the WHO Technical Report on the comprehensive management of cancer pain to pass on to them.[2] There is no doubt that, in places such as South America, ideas concerning pain relief condemn a great many patients to suffering and such a Report will, we hope, eventually be of major help.

When this is finally published I hope you will let us know so that our Study Centre may buy a number for our technical bookshop.

If you could at least give me a date when it is likely to be published, I would be grateful.

Dr Derek Doyle

St Columba's Hospice, Edinburgh

28 February 1986 What a splendid set of questions to spur me into writing an article for the first issue of the journal.[3] I will certainly have a go, particularly on the question of standards. The possible title "Just Good Medicine?" comes to my mind but, obviously, there is a lot of thinking to be done.

I will have a go for the end of May but as you have given me a rather flexible deadline, I know from experience I am likely to wait until the pistol is absolutely at my head before I do the final draft.

I have just received the first issue of the Journal of Pain and Symptom Management from the USA. You probably know this, it is the inheritor of the PRN News-sheet and because I have always taken it and thought well of it, I agreed to be on the Advisory Board, something I never do lightly for overseas requests. Obviously, it is not looking as widely as our journal will but there are certainly some interesting articles in the first issue and if you do not have a copy I will write to the Board and ask them to send you one.

Somebody mentioned to me that you are going to Australia. I am very impressed by how the whole of Perth is covered by the team there but I know less about the other parts of the country, apart from Dr Jocelyn Kramer and the team in Sydney. She was a Registrar here and works with Dr Dwyer at St Vincent's Hospital. If they are not on your itinerary, I do recommend a visit there.

Please do not run yourself into the ground with all these activities!

---

[2] Published as *Cancer pain relief* (Geneva: WHO, 1986).

[3] The journal in question is *Palliative Medicine*, of which Derek Doyle was the first editor; volume 1, issue 1 appeared in January 1987 and contained the article by Cicely Saunders, What's in a name? (pp. 57–61).

Sister M. Greaney

Ruttonjee Sanatorium, Hong Kong

4 March 1986 It is nice to hear from you again and I am very interested in all that you told me. I am glad that you are in contact with Wendy Burford who I am sure will have good suggestions as to starting out with a specialist nurse and then turning to the small special unit in the hospital. The other person who I am sure you should be in contact with is Dr James Hanratty, Medical Director, St Joseph's Hospice, Mare Street, Hackney, London E8 who you may well have met when he spent two weeks in Hong Kong about a year ago. I spoke to him after I got your letter and he tells me that he visited a number of people and thinks he must have met the doctors and nursing officers who you mention in your letter, although he did not remember the name of your Sanatorium off hand. He said he went to so many places that, although he has literature from them all, he could not immediately call them to mind. He would be happy to give you any details of people he feels you should be in touch with in Hong Kong if you would write to him telling him the people who are on your committee already.

I think that every place that sets out to start hospice work has to find its own best way and I think there are strong points in favour of both the separate ward unit such as was started in the Royal Victoria Hospital, Montreal back in 1975 and also in having the peripatetic multi-disciplinary team with no beds of its own, acting as a consulting service, as was started in St Luke's, New York in 1975 and again in St Thomas' Hospital, London at the very beginning of 1978. I think you would have extremely good advice from Sister Patrice, the Nurse Co-Ordinator of the St Luke's Team, at St Luke's Hospital Center, New York.[4]

Of all these, however, I think probably Wendy Burford's set-up at the Brompton Hospital would be the most like yours and I think I would put her comments high on any list you might make.

So far as material on education is concerned, I am sending you under separate cover a copy of our textbook as I think whatever else you have you must have something serious to show your doctors. Our *Drug Control of Common Symptoms*, which I enclose, is being updated at the moment and I will send you the new edition when it arrives. So far as education is concerned, I think you will all have to get together from your different settings and see how you can bring important ways of communication both with patients and families among yourselves, better symptom control and better appropriate family support in your own place. Our Study Centre would be very happy to answer specific questions and I think you should write to Mrs S Hawkett at this address, who runs our Courses, which are a mixture of external visitors and members of our own staff. We make our Doctors' Weeks overlap with this Course and bring in social workers as well so we have a truly multi-disciplinary approach which I would most heartily recommend you should try to develop, although it sounds as if you are moving towards that already.

Finally, I enclose a small book (*Living with Dying*) which was developed from my chapter in the *Oxford Textbook of Medicine*, which is easier to hand around than the larger textbook.

---

[4] See letter to Patrice O'Connor of 8 November 1989, p. 314.

Do let us know how you get on and also give us names of people who we should be asking to our International Conference which will be from Monday, 28th September – Friday 2nd October 1987. This is a long way for one of you to travel but I hope it would be worthwhile, not least for the opportunity of meeting people from all around the world who are practising hospice care in their different ways.

Mrs P. Mason

Community Services Unit, Brighton Health Authority, Brighton

19 March 1986 Thank you for your letter asking for a copy of our "operational policy".

When St Christopher's opened 18 years ago, we had worked as a very small group and did not have any large committee to which we had to be responsible with an operational policy. Consequently, such a thing does not exist. The nearest approach to such a policy was my application to the DHSS for a research and development grant for setting up the Hospice Home Care Team and initiating our research into the control of terminal pain. The enclosed reprint was developed, with very little change, from that (successful) application. I thought it might interest you as a piece of history, although it is not at all what I think you want now.

I also enclose a paper by Mr Derek Spooner[5] which you may not have had and which I think you will find helpful.

I remember visiting the Tarner Home even before Copper Cliff was opened. There was a very home-like feeling about it and I know from members of the staff who have come up here for conferences that good care continues. I hope you will be fortunate as you plan new accommodation for a modern service.

You do not mention what size you are thinking of and, of course, St Christopher's with its 78 beds in all must be much larger than you envisage for your area. Of the small hospices that I have visited, I would strongly recommend the Wisdom Hospice, St William's Way, Rochester, Kent as being an imaginative plan on a rather difficult site, with, so far as I can tell, an excellent working policy.

Cynthia G. Kelley

Hospice of Middletown Inc., Middletown, Ohio, USA

1 April 1986 Thank you for your letter asking if you could come and visit St Christopher's. We are not tired of Americans but we are fairly pressured by them and the multi-disciplinary day visit on June 6th to which I would have invited you is already booked up. The Friday during the May week you suggest is a French speaking day and so no good to you either.

We are short of a Social Worker at the moment and one of the remaining two is on holiday. I really do not think I can commit them to even an hour of their time. However, I would be willing to see you myself and our Volunteer Organiser can spend a short time with you. The best time for us is during the afternoon of May 21st and I suggest you arrive at the

---

5 Working for the Macmillan charity as a consultant in hospice and palliative care unit design and management.

Hospice at around 2.30 pm and ask for Mrs Marilyn Sumner, our Organiser of Volunteers. I will join you at about 3.00 pm. I can describe our work with families and give you some literature on our Bereavement Service.

The best way to get to the Hospice is to use the car hire service as described on the enclosed travelling instructions.

Please could you confirm that you can come on May 21st at 2.30 pm.

Dr Sam Klagsbrun

Four Winds Hospital, Katonah, New York, USA

14 April 1986 Carleton may not have managed to get hold of you to let you know that he has accepted with pleasure our request to join St Christopher's Foundation in New York as a Trustee. Our links with him, as with you, have always been so constructive that I am sure this is going to yield good fortune.

I was asked by Jo Magno to take some position in her International Hospice Institute. I am not sure how much you know about this but she started it on a shoe-string a few years ago with encouragement from Bal Mount and also positive letters from me. She was setting out to emphasise the need for medical input to hospice work in the USA and also to encourage research in clinical pharmacology and symptom control as well as the number of psycho-somatic studies which seem to be springing up. Her international connections were extremely slender and have remained so, partly from lack of money even for correspondence. I have now written to her as the copy enclosed. She was anxious for me to be Chairman of an international consultation group and I felt this was really going much further than I wished and would certainly be liable to confuse the issue. Being a President for one year and leaving it for her to pick up on links overseas for herself, does not I think present that danger. I hope I am right.

Mike Kearney is off on holiday this week so Tom has a white coat on and is doing his locum. He seems well and quite dominant and the group as a whole is functioning pretty well. The person who concerns me at the moment is W, who looks pressured and I think this is not only home, although that must have a certain amount to do with it. I think we have to work out ways in which the burdens of the Playgroup and Drapers' Wing are lifted from her because it does pull her energies in too many directions with all her commitment to the nursing. Tom tells me that Christopher Clark is ready to cope with the former together with the very good girl who runs it and we have to move slowly as we make plans for the Wing.

This is all the more so because dear ES finally reached the end of her 20 year battle with rheumatoid arthritis with a heart attack in which she died in seconds. As we had transferred her to the local hospital with another spontaneous fracture and other fractures as she had slowly slipped to the ground, this was a lovely way for her. Although she will leave such a gap, we are all comforting ourselves with the thought that nothing will hurt her again.

The nice counsellor I go and talk to is really helpful and Marian has gone on quietly improving. Between the two, I feel a lot better, but of course am aware that new problems may arise. At the moment, however, I am enjoying calmer waters and we hope to have Marian's delayed party tomorrow and his exhibition on Sunday.

Grace Goldin

Swarthmore, Pennsylvania, USA

30 April 1986 Many thanks for your letter. I had indeed been wondering why Judah was taking so very long to get well and had been wondering about radiotherapy. Depression is a very cruel illness and very hard indeed on the sufferer and those around. I pray that the MAOs[6] may help. We certainly had one patient here who totally failed on the other drugs and really emerged when we finally put her on an MAO. As far as I remember, the diet was not too bad once one got used to it and you are such an imaginative cook I am sure you will cope. Please give suitable messages of goodwill to Judah from us both. I shared the letter with Tom and Dorro and I know they will be writing.

I am so glad you have aides to help with your mother and I am sure it is very important for you to commit her to them and get down to work.

You will see from the enclosed photograph (which I know has too much leg to it), that Marian has put his weight back on and really looks well now. We even managed the exhibition last Sunday week, with him sitting in the middle of the room while four of us did the hanging and then, after a rest, entertaining the many friends who came flocking in. The pastels look marvellous and I will take one of the ones I especially like out of its frame, role it up and send it to you as soon as I can. Marian is delighted that you would like another. There are plenty of suns, some rather abstract, in the group and that is what comes to my mind. We are unpicking the exhibition this coming Saturday, so I will be able to get ahead with it soon.

Marian even went out with his secretary this week, the first time that he has been out and around without me with him. He still needs a stick outdoors but keeps saying his legs are getting better. We are thinking of planning a holiday later in the summer but we will have a few days in both Oxford and Cambridge for me to take Honorary Degrees in June, each time staying with friends or family and I will see how that goes.

After a somewhat up and down time I am now beginning to enjoy being Chairman and I am occupied in strengthening and enlightening the Council, not in competition with the Executive here, now led by Tom, but so that we can interact properly and regard the Council members more as the wise counsellors and bridge builders we need than perhaps we did in the past. At the moment I am just finishing a short paper I am giving on Friday from the point of view of a Medical Director still on "What I want and what I don't want from my Committee". I wrote round to the 55 Medical Directors we have on our list and had an 80% response with some fascinating letters and have tried to put them together. One Director simply sent my letter back with the two words "Support" and "Resources" on the top and that really sums up what they have been saying. A lot of them want clinical control and no interference and no worries about money without [missing from original] but I think just as the US told George III "No taxation without representation" we should say "No resources without some responsible budgeting". All the same, I am horrified at the groups where the Executive Officers have to report to the Committee and are then sent away while the final discussion goes on and decisions are made.

---

[6] Monoamine oxidase inhibitors, for the treatment of depression.

Hospices are gradually evolving good management practice and I am looking forward to a weekend for Chairmen which I hope our Management Consultant is going to put on in due course.

Yesterday, I sat in on a Staff Nurses' Study Day and of three good projects that were presented, one was titled "Hospice – Just a Place to Die?" It was extremely well done by a girl who looked at travelling and travelling on and all the other things that hospice does for living up until one dies. It was good to hear her.

Let me know if there is anything I can send which will help work when you get going again. I think you will get good comeback from Dr Naysmith when you write to her. I liked her very much when I met her at a Conference recently.

Dr Josefina Magno[7]

Southfield, Michigan, USA

21 May 1986 Thank you for your long letter of May 10th and also for your enthusiasm at my being prepared to accept the position of president of your Advisory Council. You did not mention that I am really only prepared to do this for a year and hope that you will have someone in mind to take my place then, so do not have too much writing paper printed in the first instance! I really do mean this because I think it is most important that if you are an International Institute you should cultivate other international links.

I have discussed your enthusiasm for our hoped for Institute with Dr Gillian Ford, who is, as I think I told you, seconded to us for three years from our Department of Health as Director of Studies. We both wish to warn you not to tell all your people that there are places available at St Christopher's at the moment. It is not all right for IHI to think of "recruiting and referring potential trainees for your Study Center". We move slowly in this country and it will certainly take years rather than months to get it fully established, even if it goes ahead smoothly. We would be sad if we got a lot of requests for positions here which we had no possibility of offering and I think the disappointments would not be good for either your Institute or our Study Centre. We hope there will be a very limited number of places but that is still well in the future as yet.

I am very interested in your work with Nursing Homes and delighted that you have got some funding for looking at the quality of life of their residents. I remember discussing a project that took place in the 1960s in New York but this is a long time ago now and their findings would be very out of date.

I thought you would be interested in the enclosed list of research projects going on in the UK at the moment. I seem to remember promising you I would try and send you results of a survey. I did not have the papers but I thought you would also be interested in the enclosed Abstract from our last major project in clinical pharmacology. It was presented in Los Angeles in March to the American Society of Clinical Oncologists and will be pub-

---

[7] Dr Josefina Magno qualified in medicine in her home country of the Philippines before moving to the USA in the 1940s. When, much later, she became interested in hospice, she visited St Christopher's and other centres in the USA and Canada. She went on to found various hospice programmes and umbrella organizations, including the International Hospice Institute (1984) which became the International Hospice Institute and College in 1996. She was also the first Executive Director of the National Hospice Organization of the United States.

lished. It has important implications for the understanding of pain chemistry generally and, of course, clinical implications for at least those patients who have opiate resistant pain.

Do not be too disappointed that we cannot accept your trainees straight away. Remember we have the rest of the world to think of as well and also that the English make haste slowly.

Finally, there is no way that my Professor is going to be able to cross the Atlantic in this world. I would not jeopardise his fragile health by such a manoeuvre so I am afraid the possibility of my coming to your Institute is no longer around. I am sure you will do fine with Tom West when he comes to you next year.

Catherine Musgrave

Clinical Nurse Specialist for the Hospice, Jerusalem, Israel

5 June 1986 Thank you for your note asking for help. I hope the enclosed will be of some use to you. I think Dr Cimino's paper covers well the problem from the American angle which may perhaps be more like the Israeli problems than our needs here in the UK. My own letter, which was printed in *The Tablet*, was kept deliberately short but summarises our own practice in that we never use tube feeding except in very rare circumstances and certainly never "force feed". We have, incidentally, only had two patients who said they were going on hunger strike, one of whom stopped and started again and was allowed both by St Christopher's and the National Hospital, with whom we shared his care, to continue in his chosen way of drinking but not eating. I think it probably hastened his death from motor neurone disease. The other changed his mind after a few days to the great relief of his wife but died not very long afterwards. He certainly did not die of lack of nutrition and nor did the rest of our patients. They died of their disease and to use words like starvation and dehydration are extremely misleading.

The last papers I enclose are a letter written by one of our Registrars in the *Lancet* which shows how remarkably normal blood levels are in most cases. The other comes from a book written by Lord Justice Devlin and that is referred to in the chapter from our Textbook by Ian Kennedy, which I also enclose. I hope all this will be enough.

About your dates, I am likely to be around during the times you mention and I think the best plan would be for you to telephone when you are in England and fix a date. It would be nice to hear how things are going.

Grace Goldin

Swarthmore, Pennsylvania, USA

3 July 1986 Bless you for your two letters. I was really delighted to know that Judah is really well at last. It is a convincing proof of the biochemical basis of depression when it responds to drugs like this, although I do not dispute that retiring is a very difficult experience and can somehow help to flip the switch. Give him my special greetings and I hope so much that you will be having a holiday and that we might even see him as well as you.

Marian continues on an even keel although the paintings are not coming out with quite such frequency. This means that I am a little doubtful as to whether I have exactly the right one for you yet. If you really are coming in September perhaps you would prefer to choose one anyway.

I am fascinated by your response to Florence's essays.[8] I agree with you about Carleton's and I am glad you like mine. Some of the others got into a really convoluted state and this showed up in very obscure English writing. However, I was interested in Inge Corless's who after being fairly muddled over her definitions, comes out with a very interesting statement about St Christopher's and the need for some kind of coming together in a ritual. I will have to pick up with her about her "state religion" because that is really not what the established church really is and in any case, we are right across the board of Christian denominations, as you know. All the same, I think it has given me a prod into writing some kind of article which I am thinking of calling "What's in a name?" for the first edition of the new *Palliative Medicine* Journal over here. I had originally done something about Hospice Management but they want that for a later number and want something on the spiritual side which they say "only you can say". That is not quite true but I think I have a right to try and produce something. I am thinking of picking up on some of the implications of Palliative/Continuing Care/Support Teams etc which of course have some international difficulties as I have always understood that Continuing Care meant Geriatric Care in the USA. I want to pick up something of the original meaning of Hospice or Hospital as I did in Florence's essay and try and bring it up to date as a very special contribution for which the word Hospice speaks in a way none of the other titles do – I want, of course, to give you credit in a reference here and will probably quote from your chapter 6 in your book with John Thompson. Do you think that it needs any kind of illustration? If so, would one of your black and whites speak to it? I know I have had one of a medieval hospice from you for which you gave me a very helpful note and that has been turned into a slide and I fear I do not have the original black and white any longer. You have done this so many times that I hope it might not be too much trouble for you to choose for me something that speaks to the original and then something to match it from your St Christopher's group. We have some nice new pictures taken for us recently but I would always have a yearning to use yours.

I thought you would be interested to see what Oxford and Cambridge said. In spite of my love for Oxford, I must admit that Cambridge did it much better.

Professor Patrick Wall

University College Hospital, London

25 July 1986 None of us who have heard you talking about mechanisms of pain ever forgot it and I would like same of the younger generation in hospice medicine and caring for dying patients in the NHS to have the privilege of hearing you too.

....

[8] On 3–4 May 1986 a colloquium took place at Yale University, convened by Florence Wald, Dean of Nursing and one of the founders of the Connecticut Hospice. The theme of the meeting was the spiritual care of dying people. Papers were presented by a variety of Cicely Saunders' associates including Herman Feifel, Sam Klagsbrun, Carleton Sweetser, Inge Corless, and Morris Wessel. Although she did not attend the meeting a paper was read on her behalf: C. Saunders, The modern hospice, in *In quest of the spiritual component of care for the terminally ill: proceedings of a colloquium* (ed. F. S. Wald) (Yale: Yale University Press, 1986), pp. 39–48. The colloquium is often referred to in later discussions of spiritual care at the end of life and set the tone for much subsequent debate.

The Study Centre here has even more conferences now and enclosed is a copy of this year's programme. The plans for next year include two advanced therapeutics conferences on February 20th and March 27th. These are essentially duplicates; our small lecture hall does not allow us to cope with demand in any other way. The opening session is entitled "Does Morphine Resistant Cancer Pain Exist?" and we wondered whether you would agree to come and speak on both days, or on one, on any relevant title you might like to choose. We hope to have two other speakers under this title, one tackling it from the pain clinic angle and exploring different modes of delivering narcotics and one taking the hospice approach and considering other possible drugs.

I do hope you will agree to join us.

Dr Halina Bortnowska

Warszawa, Poland

5 August 1986 Thank you very much for your long letter which I was very glad to have. I am delighted that your secretariat and the volunteers have a place to work in and I hope it will go on developing. One of my step-granddaughters, Alicja Szyszko-Bohusz, came as one of our summer volunteers last year and is now a Nowa Huta Hospice volunteer. She works extremely hard in teaching and with evening classes, so I hope she is really able to take the time.

We were delighted to have two students from the Gdansk group to our last International Conference and one of them gave an excellent description of their team. I am delighted with all this and particularly to know that you are bringing a group together in Warsaw.

Our various Polish summer volunteers have been a great success at St Christopher's but this year sadly only one out of the five who were trying to come managed to get both a passport and a visa. I rather think that the latter has been the main problem. We will still go on welcoming them and the plan is for us to make up our team very early in the New Year. I therefore suggest that your Tom should get in touch with us now and if possible come and see us while he is still in England. We do not make up our list until early next year so he would still have to write to confirm that he wanted to come and was able to get away from his medical studies. He would then, of course, have to cope with all the manoeuvres for special forms and everything else that has to be done. I hope it will come off. These visits are now six weeks long and usually begin in the middle of July.

Grace Goldin

Swarthmore, Pennsylvania, USA

11 August 1986 Many thanks indeed for sending the prints which I am returning as, after all your trouble, the Editor said no illustrations. I am very sorry that you had to go to all the bother and sorry not to be using them as I would like to have done so.

I tried to telephone you but obviously chose a time when you were all out for something or other and do hope you are going to get your plans sorted out and will have that holiday. We would so much like to see you.

Since I sent you the airletter about Marian's pictures on the way, he went through his collection and took out yet another sun for you. Please keep them all if you would like to. The one he chose especially after our original discussion is the one on top of the group of the sun coming through a rather abstract forest.

I am just embarking on my Chairman's Report for the next Annual Report and am probably going to do a little bit of a potted history in a paragraph or two, reflecting on the original commitment of hospice to the seven works of mercy. It reminds me of your criticism of some of the American Hospices for trying to show a direct line from the medieval hospices. I do not think this contradicts that at all but I think goes back to the original meaning without necessarily implying that there is a direct line. Obviously the medieval hospices/hospitals had an impossible mix of patients at times and we have been very selective as to who we set out to help. All the same, the development as suggested by Boros makes an interesting comparison. The article I have done for the *Palliative Medicine* Journal is much neater than the one I sent you before and I have cut Boros down to a much neater page and if I refer to it in our Annual Report, it will be cut down still further.

I wish one could do some research into why Mme Jeanne Garnier chose the word hospice for the dying specifically back in 1842 and why, with apparently no connection at all, Mother Mary Aikenhead did the same in 1879. It is not easy trying to research with the Irish Sisters of Charity and so far impossible with the Dames de Calvaire. You would be much better at that than I.

What you describe at the moment of your life makes me think you are running a very hospitable hospice around one person. Entertaining and wooing the staff is certainly part of the job and they must be having a lovely time with your cooking.

By the way, I apologise for being so slow in sending the enclosed figures. Our Information Officer went off to have a baby and the locum was rather swamped by the daily enquiries and got behind on queries such as yours. These figures refer to 1985/86 as they were compiled for our Annual Report which covers the financial year 31st March 1985 – 1st April 1986.

Apart from the day and half-day visits, we have a number of people who come for day conferences. I have not broken these down but they include doctors, nurses, social workers, pharmacists, clergy and recently school teachers tackling bereavement in local schools.

I will try and telephone you again. I love your letters but I think sometimes we might get into the habit of talking as well.

Ms C. Plunkett

Hodder and Stoughton Limited, London

18 August 1986 Thank you for sending me the proof of the jacket[9] which I agree is very nicely set out, and I cannot spot any "glaring errors".

My only comment is that in straightening the photograph up you have made me look much more direct and less inspirational. That may have been the idea, and I think I like the new one better. I certainly would not want you to change it; I only point it out.

For Shirley's sake I hope it goes really well, and also of course for yours. For my own, I still have not got over the somewhat uneasy feeling of perpetually meeting people who know me far better than I will ever know them.

---

[9] A reference to the paperback edition of Shirley du Boulay's biography, which had first appeared in 1984.

Professor Balfour Mount

Royal Victoria Hospital, Montreal, Canada

27 August 1986 Here is something that I hope will do for your programme. If you care to say so it is derived from an article I have done on the same title but much longer for the new *Journal of Palliative Medicine*. I enclose a flyer of that and I hope you will have others available. It is not in competition with the Canadian Journal but we felt it was important to have something from the UK to cover palliative medicine widely. You will see that for the Canadian representative we have Mary Vachon as we were rather short of nursing representation but we hope one day we will be welcoming an article from you.

I hope the enclosed is the right length – it certainly brings out your title of palliative care service as a strong contender for the right word and you must be amused when we finally chose it for the Journal.

I am only sorry that I cannot come these days. I do not at all grudge this in the context of Marian, who is as creative as ever in living as well as in painting, and a total joy, but I would have loved to have come to your conference and seen the services and Ina and everyone. Please give them special greetings.

Dr J. M. Gawel

University of Toronto, Toronto, Ontario, Canada

12 September 1986 Thank you for your letter which has been sent on by St Christopher's Hospital in Fareham.

I enclose the Review article which I wrote based on our experience here of our first 100 patients with motor neurone disease (ALS) which, although somewhat out of date, gives a reasonable overview. I also enclose a more recent article by a former Senior Registrar here, Dr David Oliver who I hope will be collaborating with me when we look together at our next 200 patients and copies of two articles by patients.

I should explain that our patients with motor neurone disease occupy up to 8 of our 62 in-patient beds while the remainder are patients with far advanced cancer receiving symptom control and support for themselves and their families. I enclose a leaflet about the Hospice which will give you a quick overview of our work. We have one or two patients who come in and out to relieve their families but we do not undertake home care unless we have a bed available should the need arise. This means that out of our normal number of some 50–60 out-patients, one or two at most will have motor neurone disease. We care for people in the locality, having a population of some 3 million within a 10 mile radius of the Hospice. Obviously if one is considering care for the whole family it is impossible to take people from a great distance.

I would be most interested to hear in the future how your own facility develops and also any articles that you may have written on the care of this group of patients.

His Grace the Archbishop of Canterbury

Lambeth Palace, London

11 November 1986 It was a great pleasure to hand over the Presidency of *Help the Hospices* to you at what I thought was a very good meeting. I think HtH really has a place as a forum and particularly in the teaching it is both doing and supporting. Relationships with the other charities are much improved as you may have gathered from their presence at the meeting. Although it is not doing quite what I think the Duchess had in mind originally, that is support in revenue, I think its present role is needed and it has certainly acted as a general catalyst.

I was rather concerned that, I suppose inevitably, *The Times* reporter picked up your comment about patients with AIDS. This is I think part of general pressure and some degree of panic but I am not sure how much the existing hospices have to be thought of as necessarily part of the solution. As I understand from one of the people who produced some notes for your background, he did not necessarily mean "challenge" in terms of beds but of the teaching and sharing of skills in counselling and symptom control. It is of course inevitably picked up by the media as meaning beds and this does rather concern me.

As I pointed out in my letter to *The Times* the last time there was a rather contentious article on the subject, over 130,000 people die in England and Wales of cancer and there are less than 2,000 hospice beds. We ourselves have constant pressure on our beds and have to keep people waiting and also have a long waiting list for our patients with motor neurone disease, for whom we can only offer 8 beds at a time. Our commitment and expertise and that of most hospices is to these patients in particular, although exceptions can of course be made. In some areas of the country, such as London, I think other arrangements should be made for the different needs of nearly all AIDS patients. Again, of course, some hospices will find a reason for making an exception. I am pleased to see that there are likely to be one or more specialist "hospices" especially for such patients and also interested to know that the NHS Hospice nearest to St Mary's Hospital, Paddington, is not being pressured to take these patients who either need acute care for their often unusual infections until they die or have a much longer term illness including dementia and need very different accommodation. I understand the Church of England is producing some comments on the subject and I hope it will take these sort of points on board.

As a matter of interest, St Christopher's carried out an experiment over some two years of admitting patients with Alzheimer's Disease while their carer had a holiday. We found that unless the patient was bedfast such a degree of dementia made them virtually impossible to care for in a hospice ward without great difficulties for other patients, their families and indeed, the staff. A representative of the Alzheimer's Disease Society has since written to me saying she appreciates that it is a different kind of accommodation that is needed for these patients.

This is rather a long explanation but whereas I think hospices may in time be able to look to the needs of other patients, I think our position at the moment in most of the hospices I know is one of great pressure from the patients we were nearly all set up to help in the first place. Where we should be looking at it, I am quite sure that your warning of ill-launched and inadequately prepared services has to be very carefully considered. Our own prolonged research into the matter has made this plain. Also that at the moment our main role is in teaching and training in skills that will be used elsewhere.

Helen Irwin

Social Services Committee, London

12 December 1986 Further to Dr Gillian Ford's telephone conversation with you, I enclose a memorandum which gives our present thoughts on the subject of the problems associated with AIDS.

I must emphasise that I do not speak for the whole Hospice Movement but I think what I say is fairly generally agreed, although I am sure that in some parts of the country where there may be less pressure on beds for the patients to whom we are already committed or where there is less possibility of other accommodation, a hospice might occasionally admit such a patient or, perhaps more frequently, add them to their Home Care patients.

If there are any further questions or comments that the Committee has, we would be very happy to respond.

Professor Douglas B. MacAdam
The University of Western Australia, Claremont, Western Australia

26 January 1987 Many thanks for your letter. I am really delighted that the Cottage Hospice will be officially opened on March 1st. I think your progress has been exemplary and I only wish I could come back to Perth again.

I hope the following message will do:

> "The news that the Cottage Hospice is to be opened as a further step in the provision of palliative care throughout Perth is most interesting. I remember with great pleasure all the people that I met when I spent that fascinating fortnight in your beautiful City in 1977. May I send my very best wishes for the future together with my congratulations on what has already been achieved."

I had heard from David and I hope he will find something else that really interests him. He still has a lot to give I am sure. I am interested to see that you are just Chairman but I am certain you are very busy behind the scenes. Speaking as another Chairman now, I am sure you are finding it as interesting as I do and I still carry on doing one weekend on duty each month.

The Rt Hon Norman Fowler MP
Department of Health and Social Security, London

27 January 1987 At St Christopher's we have, for some time, been debating in what ways we could properly contribute towards the care of patients suffering from AIDS. I feel that it is an opportune time to suggest ways in which we might help, and offer to discuss these further with you.

We believe that our home care services could be developed to provide symptom control, counselling and support, possibly throughout our catchment area of South East London – providing that close liaison can be arranged with local hospitals or specialist units. Such a service would lend itself particularly well to evaluation of the medical and social needs of patients and their families in the community, study of the appropriateness of community care, and definition of the type of in-patient support that is required.

I should explain that we have strong reservations about the use of our existing in-patient facilities for AIDS patients. We have difficulty in meeting the present demand from those suffering from terminal malignant disease and motor neurone disease in our wards.

Our present skills and experience in symptom control, family support and counselling are already available for teaching AIDS carers from within the NHS and, to a limited degree, have already been so used. We feel there is considerable scope for further development, possibly in collaboration with the NHS.

St Christopher's has an unique depth of experience and, as the pioneer of the modern hospice movement, founded the first teaching centre and both that and our research programmes have received considerable support from the DHSS. We currently have a research programme led by Professor Hinton assessing home care of the dying, funded by the DHSS.

In addition to our teaching and research we established the first Hospice Home Care Service in 1969, financed by a grant from your Department, and in 1971 started the first family and bereavement service. These have continued to grow and have formed the basis of developments seen throughout the UK, the USA and the world.

Last July I met the former Minister for Health and spoke of our existing financial difficulties. The prospect of further developments is, of course, daunting but, nevertheless, I would assure you of our willingness to help with this new and alarming disease. I and my colleagues at St Christopher's would be pleased to meet you or members of your Department to see how best this might be effected.

We have, in the past, received much support from the NHS Regions served by us, and I am also writing to Sir Peter Baldwin and Mr Driver to inform them of our willingness to collaborate with the NHS.

Marty Herrmann

New York, USA

27 January 1987 First of all, I must tell you that Marian, now we are sure that he only has tuberculosis glands is doing nicely. He has dressings to be done twice a day but they cause him no pain or trouble and it is nice to know that the original malignant diagnosis is right out of the picture. We are enjoying a rather quieter life.

The Hospice is going to make quite a lot of celebrating its 21st Birthday. The 14th July 1967 was the day we took our first patient and the 24th July the official opening by HRH Princess Alexandra. These are the key dates but we are really going to use the whole of the 21st year for a series of functions and efforts at publicity. We are making an international flavour of it because we want to develop an International Institute which will naturally have a considerable Anglo-American interchange. We will start with quite small things like bursaries and Fellowships and move into setting up residence for exchanges and so forth if and when we acquire sufficient monies. We have ourselves registered as a charity in New York and I enclose a note drawn up by our present Director of Studies of the way we are thinking around this.

I am writing to you now because we want to pick up on any links we have with your major networks and I hope you will remember that I was on a programme called, I think "60 minutes" which was a fairly long euthanasia discussion and I think it was repeated. I seem to remember your mentioning it in a letter. I hope I am right because we would very much like to know the name of the presenter and whether he is still doing this particular programme or something similar. There is just a chance that if I wrote to him he might turn up with some interest, such as comparing the American Hospice scene with ours, maybe and underlining our initial work.

I will try and call you but I thought I had better get this in the post as it really is easier than explaining it all on a transatlantic call.

Professor I. Tashma

Jerusalem, Israel

3 February 1987 Thank you very much for your letter which naturally interested me very much indeed. I hope the information I can give you may be a help because it would be wonderful to be in touch with someone who knew David.

His real name was Eli Majer but David was his nickname and the name he chose to use when I knew him. He was working as a waiter in London and I think he left Poland before the war and had been working in Paris but I do not know when he came to England, nor how long he had been here. What he told me about his family was that they had certainly lived in the Ghetto and that he was one of four sons. His mother died young and he was very involved with his grandfather, who was a Rabbi. The old man used to discuss the faith with him and I remember him telling me how he used to go upstairs and wake him up after he had gone to bed to continue their discussions. I believe that one or two of the brothers had also left Poland and I seem to remember that at least one went to South America, but here I may be wrong.

I am afraid this is not very much information for you but I only knew David for some two months and we were occupied in talking about where he was in his thinking and living rather than where he had come from. It was his need to find meaning in his life that led us on to talk about founding a special place for people like himself facing the end of their lives and the money he left me "to be a window in your Home" was in fact what was left over from his small life insurance after I had made gifts to his few friends.

I hope this is of interest to you and if it can help you make some connection with David Tasma, then your family has helped to found the hospice movement around the world and David's name has certainly been mentioned in many places. I am delighted to know that there are now two or three hospices in Israel and to have some connection with the people establishing the latest one in Hadassah.

Sir Peter Baldwin

Chairman, South East Thames Regional Health Authority, Bexhill-on-Sea, Sussex

5 February 1987 This is not a follow up of my last letter which I know is being considered, but a comment on another subject which we feel the Region will wish to know we are looking at.

Much of the recent publicity relating to possible hospice involvement in the care of AIDS patients has focussed on our in-patient facilities. You will know already from our Council members in the Authority that we have serious reservations concerning any displacement of our cancer and motor neurone patients, when demand for our beds is so high.[10]

Nevertheless, we have always believed we should be well integrated with the NHS, and have been examining how we might be of practical assistance with this new and alarming disease. In the knowledge that the Secretary of State will be approaching hospices, I have

---

[10] See C. Saunders, Hospice for AIDS patients. New teams should be developed for AIDS care, *American Journal of Hospice Care*, **4**(6), (Nov–Dec 1987): 7–8.

written to him suggesting that we might help in the areas of home care, teaching and research. I am enclosing a copy of that letter.

Although the medical problems presented by AIDS are in many ways dissimilar from those of terminal malignant disease, we believe that our Home Care Service could be expanded to provide support for AIDS patients with symptom control, counselling and in bereavement. It would however be essential that a close relationship be established with those hospitals or special units providing acute and terminal care if needed.

Additionally, the present lack of knowledge of the needs of these patients in the community, and what will be the most appropriate type of in-patient support, would make a service such as that proposed ideal for study and evaluation.

You will know that our teaching resources are available to the NHS, including those staff caring for AIDS patients and, to a limited extent, have already been so used. Although our teaching commitment is very full, we would of course be pleased to collaborate in any further programmes for AIDS carers.

The development of a home care programme will need considerable thought, for example regarding the catchment area, staffing and relationship with NHS Districts and hospitals. The Senior Staff of St Christopher's would be pleased to meet with any of your officers perhaps, initially, here informally and subsequently in a conference.

It will not, of course, come as a surprise to learn of our worry regarding the funding of this work, particularly when I have written so recently about our difficulty in meeting our present commitments. I, therefore, hope that we might look to the Region, if not the Department, for help.

Finally may I say how much we have valued the advice and encouragement given us by Joan Waters and Richard Hayllar in tackling this daunting subject. It really is of great help to have such support when facing the challenges ahead.

Sir James Gowans

Medical Research Council, London

5 February 1987 You will, I imagine, shortly be meeting with the Social Services Committee at the House of Commons in their discussions on the subject of AIDS.

There may be representatives from the hospice world there but we have not been invited from St Christopher's and I think that perhaps it might be helpful, in view of your interest in the Hospice and the enjoyable visit we had last time with you, for me to send you a copy of our recent letter to Mr Norman Fowler and add one or two more details.

The population of the South East Thames Region and part of the South West which we also serve means that we have a considerable proportion of the upwards of 140,000 people who die of cancer in this country each year and the pressure on our beds for these patients, for whom we were set up, is such that we continue sadly to fail to help a considerable number of those for whom application is made. Added to this, we have an increasing demand for our 8 beds for motor neurone disease. We believe that we have a unique capacity to meet the particularly difficult problems with which these patients are so often referred to us.

All the same, we wish to be helpful in whatever way we can and the suggestions of the enclosed letter developed from over a year of discussions and workshops here, visits to St. Mary's Hospital and a certain amount of upgrading of our capacity to deal with any infection. I still feel myself that while we would never close doors to new thinking, the suggestions in our letter to Mr Fowler are as far as we should go at the present moment.

The question may not come up in discussions but as you realise, I am thinking of you as in some way a possible spokesman for this particular research and teaching hospice.

Professor Balfour Mount
Royal Victoria Hospital, Montreal, Canada

12 February 1987 First of all. I must tell you that Marian is battling on through his slowly resolving tuberculosis glands of neck. He has two sinuses but they really cause him remarkably little trouble. His other problems of an ageing body are taken very lightly and although he is not in one of his really vigorous phases of painting, all the same he has been doing some very beautiful things. The ground floor of the new house for the Family Centre has a wonderful set of pastels done not long before Christmas, some of them during the time when the diagnosis was of malignancy. How we eventually arrived at the correct diagnosis is a long story with which I will not bother you. Thank you for your thoughts and prayers. We have been very well supported in every way.

My other reason for writing is that I have just had a letter right out of the blue from Israel from a Professor with the same name as 'my' David Tasma of the £500 for the window. He happened to see me mention David on a television programme when he was visiting in London and he has written to ask if I could help him with any news of what appears to be a long lost member of his family. I remembered that I had written rather fully about David in that article I did for you for Crux but when I went to get it out of my files I found that someone had torn out the first two pages and we do not appear to have another copy. Have you by any chance a spare copy left or could you send me a photocopy of my own article in it? That number was very well produced and I think the very telling photographs were your own, so if there is a spare available I would very much like to have it for the archives.

As you enjoy photography, I am enclosing two photographs. The one of me was on receiving an honorary degree at Oxford University.

I am not sure whether I wrote to congratulate you on your last honour, very well deserved and a great pleasure to all your friends.

Do you by any chance have an article or even an extract which sums up the relationship of the Palliative Care Movement in Canada with your National Health Scheme(s)? I happen to be taking part in a discussion in Cambridge in March in which the main lecturer is talking about the American medical scene in a way which somewhat horrifies me and I have been asked to be a responder. I always feel you fit rather well between our two countries and often have the best of both worlds, although I still would stand up for our NHS in spite of Mrs Thatcher's degradations. If I do go to Cambridge, Marian will come with me and we will stay with a Polish doctor friend of ours who will be delighted to look after him alongside her new baby. We are checking with both our doctors that there will be no problem with Marian's glands as he will have been on his drugs for three months by then.

Maaret Siitonen
Helsinki, Finland

18 February 1987 Thank you for your letter with all your questions about nursing in hospice work. You will see I have sent you a number of papers as well as our last Annual Report in answering.

All our nurses have the development programme which is described in the Report and the two projects that I have enclosed are part of that and I think they will tell you something about their job satisfaction together with what Matron has written in the Report.

We have nurses who have been here between 12 and 19 years as well as those who just stay the 2 years and go on to other work. Both groups would I think tell you that the major satisfaction is the reward of seeing a patient free of pain and other symptoms and of a family coming together. The major support is the ward group but we have a social psychiatrist who spends one day a week here which means a meeting a month in each of our four wards. However, he is not the main support. Everyone takes their part and we are small enough to know who is under particular stress. We do not have a "screaming room". That is an entirely American idea. We are much more ordinary than that although many of us have the support of Christian faith.

We do not have a few patients allotted to our nurses but rather work as a team so that everyone is the support of the rest of the group.

We have immensely rewarding letters from our families as well as very gentle thanks from our patients. I do not think that the people who live round here are any more frightened about coming into a hospice than they are about going into hospital and many of them, if they have had friends or family here, are not frightened at all.

Your questions about morphine are answered in one of the reprints enclosed.

If you have any more questions I will be delighted to try and answer them.

The Editor

The Tablet, London

18 February 1987 I was concerned at the comment in the article "The response of the Church to AIDS" in the 14th February issue, that "hospices will be able to extend the same care and love to AIDS sufferers" because I think it implies a misunderstanding about the establishment of a great number of hospices in this country at the moment. Most of them, like St Christopher's, were founded with a specific concern for patients dying of cancer and only a limited group of us care for a small number of patients with other diseases. At the present moment, some 150,000 people will die of cancer each year in this country – and for most of us the pressure on our beds for the patients for whom we were set up and for whom we have developed our expertise is so great that it is difficult for us to think of helping other patients.

However, some hospices are able to offer help in home care which I understand is likely to be the major demand and we are looking at extending our work in order to be available in this area. Many of us are also already involved in both discussion and teaching.

The fears about funds have, I am afraid, already been shown to be realistic but this is not in any way our primary concern. That is for those patients who have been needing our care over the past years and whose needs continue to escalate.

Mother Potier

Residence St Marie, St-Lo, France

18 February 1987 It was so good to have your Christmas card and to remember your visit.

I am happy to say that the Hospice continues as busy as ever and I think it continues to develop. We were very happy to have a visit from a volunteer from your Paris House last autumn, a Polish girl who is working as a pastoral helper. She did not meet you when you were working there so I imagine you will not know her.

I continue to talk of Mme Jeanne Garnier when I am talking of the evolution of the hospice movement because I still think that we should salute her as the first of us all.

I am also very happy to know how the group in France are coming together and developing this work and I hope very much that it will involve your House also.

Dennis P. Cullen

St Wilfrid's Hospice, Eastbourne, East Sussex

23 February 1987 Thank you for your letter. Although we have made a more positive response to the problem of patients with AIDS since I wrote the enclosed copy of my letter to The Times, I certainly stand by what I said about the pressure on our beds. Indeed, the numbers of cancer patients have escalated since the figure I gave and is probably over 150,000 now and the pressure for these patients and for those with motor neurone disease whom we also admit continues to escalate.

Where we have moved since the letter is in writing to Mr Norman Fowler to offer an extension of our Home Care to such patients with a built in evaluation of their needs and co-operation with a local special ward if and when admission became necessary. This is being discussed with the Chief Medical Officer later next month. We would also admit patients who we knew had AIDS if they also had cancer and not only, as suggested in the letter, those we discovered had it after admission.

If any of us are to do anything in this field, I think Home Care is the most needed and most suitable but I think we should stand out for 100% funding in view of the money that is being made available for this. The fact that our other funds may be affected by doing this work is, I fear, already being shown to be realistic. These may only be isolated instances but as so much of our monies often come in memory of patients who have died of cancer, I think we must not forget our responsibility to them.

Professor I. Ta-Shma

Jerusalem, Israel

6 March 1987 Thank you for your letter. I am glad mine reached you safely with what I could tell you about someone who surely must have been related to you.

David was buried in the Jewish part of Streatham Cemetery in South East London. I was his Executor and arranged this with the Orthodox Jewish Burial Service together with the employer for whom he had worked as a waiter. I went to his funeral and the part of it that I remember most vividly is that we said one of the Psalms, number 90 in our Bible, which starts "Lord thou hast been our dwelling place in all generations". I did not go back to see his tombstone but his employer sent me a photograph and it was very simple, giving just his name and the dates of his birth and death and the fact that it had been erected "by his friends".

As it happens, I have twice been asked to talk at a gathering of relatives of people who have been cremated at the Crematorium right next to Streatham burial ground. This includes many hundreds of relatives and is a very moving short ceremony. I have to confess that I did not try to find out exactly where David's grave was and go across to it but I did leave a stone to his memory in the garden nearby.

Dr Derek Doyle

St Columba's Hospice, Edinburgh

30 March 1987 I was so sorry not to come on the 20th March but would have said how much I appreciated the first issue of the Journal which I think is excellent, illustrating well the wide range of subjects which it will be tackling. I hope we can always produce a Review article of the calibre of Geoff Hanks, but that is asking rather a lot. I particularly liked the short Abstracts of articles one might wish to look at.

Thank you for letting me know dates so far ahead. My life is very dependent on my husband's health but I can tell you now that on Tuesdays I go to mass in St Christopher's with him and therefore I will not be able to get away and on Fridays we tend to have our whole day multi-disciplinary groups for whom I take the first hour at 11.00 am. Unless things change over the coming year, I am therefore really only happily free on Thursday mornings.

I was sorry that the active hospice world was rather poorly represented at Norman Fowler's Conference on AIDS and also that the rapporteur of our group was not in fact a hospice person. It seems to be difficult to get across to those we have met so far in the DHSS that most hospices are so fully committed to patients with malignant disease with the possible addition of patients with motor neurone disease, that they would find it very difficult to displace these patients. We have developed the expertise for their care and the job satisfaction that goes with it and apart from those patients with AIDS who also have malignant disease and who would fit easily somewhere where the average age is likely to be well into the 60s and the average length of stay about three weeks, we should not be thinking easily of opening our doors. Home Care is different, I think, and we are fortunate in that there is already a specialist unit nearby with whom we are co-operating in discussions and workshops and with whom we hope to work in the future in this area with the back-up beds being with them. This would seem to me a good pattern in one or two major centres where the largest number of AIDS patients are likely to be, at least for the time being. For the rest I think it may well be that the occasional patient would be possible to admit to a smaller hospice but, again, I am not at all sure that these patients should not go back to the unit that has been doing all the active investigation and treatment to which they are accustomed. Certainly it is going to be difficult for the average hospice to come near to being able to offer that. I have the impression that one or two people are saying yes, they would admit these patients, without having thought through the above or other things that will no doubt occur to you.

I presume this subject is likely to be discussed at the Association and I am sorry I can only come to London meetings but I would be very interested in any comments that you are ready to make at this stage. When Gill Ford and I went up to the Department we did not feel there was much meeting of minds.

Christopher Spence

London Lighthouse, London

8 April 1987 When I telephoned yesterday to find out if you would like to come and visit St Christopher's, I discovered that Dr Ford had already written to ask you if you would take part in a day conference here discussing the possibilities of our Home Care involvement of AIDS and other issues with representatives from the South East and South West Thames Regions on July 12th. Unfortunately, I have a long standing lecture engagement myself on that day and would miss seeing you.

However, we have a number of multi-disciplinary day visits on Fridays here and I understand that it is likely that you might be free on the 19th June and I hope you would be interested in coming to visit us then. I enclose a programme and would suggest that I take you round on the 12 o'clock slot and discuss things that might be relevant rather than that you should join one of the other rounds.

I do hope you may be able to do this. I would very much like you to see a hospice in action and follow on from our discussion the other day.

Dr Julian Ungar-Sargon
Spaulding Rehabilitation Hospital, Boston, Massachusetts, USA

11 June 1987 Your article in the May/June issue of the *American Journal of Hospice Care* was a pleasure to read. You may know that St Christopher's has had a link with Dr Sam Klagsbrun at Four Winds Hospital, New York, who has been visiting with us every year for a long time. He is particularly concerned with our management and teaching programmes and a great help to us in many ways.

You note that the Hospice movement has developed "without the sanction of the medical profession and, indeed, at times with its open hostility" but I have to point out that this has really not been the case in this country. When I first started in the field at one of the older hospices in 1958, this was thought of as dedicated custodial care and, indeed, it was virtually untouched by medical advance. However, with the opening of St Christopher's in 1967, a major change occurred and what was previously a certain amount of indifference has turned into an acceptance on the part of most people in the profession that this is a respectable part of medicine.

This has made it easier to point out that our care for dying people is still treatment and not suddenly a soft option called "care" or an abrogation of all medical responsibility. We have appropriate treatment to offer as well as psychological and spiritual support.

Two points are, I think, becoming clear and the first is that certainly with patients dying of malignant diseases and motor neurone disease (ALS) one does not "withdraw nutrition or hydration" one simply follows the needs and capabilities of the physiological process of dying. Patients lose their desire for food and are far better helped by the small normal drinks they can still take and good mouth care than they would ever be by i.v hydration or feeding. That would merely add to distress. Patients die of their disease and not of starvation and if any feelings of thirst or hunger tend to arise, they are well controlled by drugs given to control pain and other distress.

St Christopher's is holding an International Conference at the end of September this year and I enclose the flyer and full programme concerning this. We are trying to balance the intake from the various countries of the world who are interested, so this is certainly not a promise of a place but, you might be interested to know about it.

Dr Derek Doyle

Editor in Chief, Palliative Medicine, St Columba's Hospice, Edinburgh

23 July 1987 I very much like number 2 of *Palliative Medicine* and I congratulate you on the best of the "hospice" productions. In answer to your questions:

1 I think the idea of a symposium with different contributors is excellent and I wonder if you might get into the confusing subject of confusion. Among the writers, you might think of the psycho-geriatrician, Professor Elaine Murphy of Guy's Hospital who seems to be making an impact and have effective ideas. Averil Stedeford, of course, is a well known name in this field and has presented a structured way of looking at the problem at one or two of our conferences.

 Secondly, what about the challenges of neuropathic or morphine resistant or deafferentation pain, whichever you like to call it? Professor Patrick Wall, of course, is the basic researcher on that and he spoke at one of our Advanced Therapeutic Conferences recently. He is always extremely clear. However, he recommended a Dr A H Dickenson of the Department of Pharmacology, University College for our second Conference who gave us an excellent session and you might get something out of him more quickly. Another contributor here might be Dr Robert Dunlop, the new Lecturer with the Support Team at St Bartholomew's Hospital.

2. I remember you saying that you had difficulty in getting some of your Council to accept that there should be any research in a hospice and I wonder whether a general discussion about research in this field might be indicated. When Tom Walsh[11] was here, he gave us an interesting list of the types of research that could be done and spoke to this at a British Council Conference here. However, he is now in the States and will be starting a new job this month and it is very difficult to get anything from him. His list is as follows:

 1. Case Reports
 2. Review Literature
 3. Statistics
 4. Symptoms
 5. Clinical Series
 6. Practice Reports
 7. Pharmacokinetics
 8. Controlled Studies

3 I know you find it difficult to understand why I like cartoons, but I must tell you that Sheila Cassidy has twice talked here with her own cartoons done on acetates which are really brilliant. For example, she presented one to a group of ENT Surgeons at a conference at which I was also speaking in which she started with the surgeon with all his paraphernalia, including his cosseting nurse, interviewing a patient. She then lifted away an acetate which removed the nurse and then finally removed a second acetate which removed his white coat, head mirror etc and left two naked people facing each other person to person. It made a considerable impact. She also produced several new ones when

---

[11] Declan (Tom) Walsh subsequently became Director of the Harry R. Horvitz Center for Palliative Medicine, The Cleveland Clinic, USA.

she talked at our Spiritual Needs Conference recently. I think you might lure her into writing with these as illustrations or into doing them on their own. As a suggestion as to how cartoons can be used, I enclose an American Journal which I am sent by the Editor whom I met once on a tour in the States and which, incidentally, includes some excellent articles. One in the last number by Albert R Jonsen on "What Does Life Support Support?" might well fit into *Palliative Medicine*.

Finally, I know Gill is going to mention the question of AIDS at the next Committee meeting. To sum up our own position and that which, so far as I can gather is reasonably fair to at least the majority of hospices, I enclose a paper that has just gone off as a Personal View to the *American Journal of Hospice Care*. This will be part of a series of articles each giving different points of view.

Dr David Allbrook

Mater Hospital, Newcastle, New South Wales, Australia

17 August 1987 Thank you for letting me know about your move. It certainly is a big change, but you are a glutton for punishment and I cannot see either of you being idle.

We continue to think that Perth has a particularly interesting programme and always look forward to hearing more of it. Now we will want to hear what happens at the Mater Hospital.

Life here is never dull. My husband has battled through some medical peculiarities and is very good for his age – now over 86. He has two portraits on the go at the moment, but is mainly working in oil pastels.

Tom and Mary and Mike Kearney are all functioning busily and I am happy with the way the Hospice goes in spite of money needs. I enjoy being Chairman, and I am occupied in helping the Council become a really good bridge builder with the outside world and sounding board for the insiders.

Professor Eric Wilkes

Curbar, Derbyshire

21 September 1987 Paul has just sent me your paper on AIDS but I understand it has not yet been circulated further.

I am sure that as you say, if we were to meet and discuss policy together, we would find much in common but having said that I must go on to say that I am at a loss when faced with your HtH paper on almost every point of which I would argue, or express a different opinion or a different way of putting your points and would certainly put them in a different order.

At St Christopher's we have been looking at our policy towards AIDS patients since early 1985. Far from being inhibited towards opening our doors because we have a definite role we have found ourselves constantly changing our policy towards AIDS patients as their needs become clearer and we try to see how this hospice can fit in with the NHS and other organisations who are primarily responsible. One definite point to emerge is that a policy which seems right in January 1987 may not be appropriate by January 1988.

Gill Ford has summarised our thinking in an article she wrote recently and I rather prefer the positive (and, I think, more succinct than either of us) way she covers various points. "Many hospices are under pressure to take patients who have AIDS and admission policies have had to be re-examined. As far as infection is concerned it seems that the presence of the AIDS virus in an individual should not cause more problems to other patients or staff than the presence of Hepatitis B and that ward procedures must be correct and safe for all. It follows that the acceptance of appropriate patients who happen to be sero-positive or have HIV induced end stage malignancies is thus likely to be the policy of many hospices. Reservations remain about taking patients with non-malignant manifestations which require vigorous investigations and prophylaxis, as well as treatment, for which hospices have neither the facilities nor the skills. Other problems connected with the admission of AIDS patients are emerging but are not necessarily insurmountable. They do include the difference in age groups – hospices can appear very fuddy duddy to lively gay groups – and difficulties in caring for demented patients in homely small wards open to gardens, court-yards and other wards. A less tangible problem relates to the mode of transmission of the disease. Understandably, because of discrimination suffered by people with AIDS, there is an insistence on absolute confidentiality up to, and including, the cause of death as stated on the certificate. Cancer also was once a dread word to be whispered or cloaked in euphe-mism and evasion. The Hospice Movement set out not to break confidentiality or to force hard and unwelcome facts on patients and families but to give 'opportunities to express deeper fears and encouragement to both patients and families to share as much of the truth as can safely be handled'. AIDS related secrecy might be difficult for hospices to handle. By no means all of these problems apply when considering home care for patients with AIDS. Hospice teams may develop this as a natural extension of their work in the community in conjunction with existing domiciliary services. But they might be likely, for the time being, to turn to a hospital unit for back-up beds rather than a hospice."

I know that the Association of Hospice Doctors is considering the matter at its Edinburgh Meeting on October 23rd helped by a draft statement from Derek Doyle and I think it is very important that medical staff give this subject careful thought.

I gather from Paul that the HtH afternoon is for the giving of information but I hope that that very multi-disciplinary group will not find itself trying to produce any kind of general policy, nor feel pressure by the advocacy of the speakers to feel guilty if they do not say they will take patients who may prove to be very inappropriately referred. I think that it would really be very important that HtH should not distribute any AIDS statement as such until the Association has had its whole day meeting and certainly not your statement as it stands at present.

I am not sure if you belong to the Association but in case you have not seen it, I enclose a copy of Derek Doyle's statement for discussion.

Dr and Mrs L. J. de Souza
Shanti Avedna Ashram, Chowpatty, Bombay, India

12 October 1987 I enclose a cheque which our Bank has converted from the money that was contributed at the end of the Service in Westminster Abbey. I am also enclosing a £10 note which I hope you will be able to change and which came too late. I think it will proba-bly be easier for you than a cheque.

We were so glad that Carmen was able to come and that she enjoyed the Conference.

Please keep us in touch with all your developments and let us know when you are able to open some more of your beds.

Shingo Nakatani

University College London, London

26 October 1987 Thank you for your letter about the interview with Mr Hidaka.

The answer to your question is as follows:

A few hospices ask patients for some contribution towards their cost of care but do not refuse admission to those who cannot afford it. St Christopher's itself does not send patients a bill except to the very small number who have private insurance. The families are aware that we need financial help from one or two notices that show the hospice's needs but they are never pressed to give anything.

Considering hospices in England as a whole, the principle is that the lack of money is not a barrier to admission and having money does not gain admission. The National Health Service contributes approximately one third of our needs and we estimate that their contribution to the whole of the 2,300 hospice beds in this country is about the same.

So far as other countries are concerned, I think everyone has to work out what is suitable and viable in their own situation. There is a strong tradition of voluntary giving in this country which so far has enabled hospice work to develop.

I hope this answers all your points.

Soeur Gilberte

Taizé Community, Saone et Loire, France

19 November 1987 It was lovely to see your writing and to hear from you again. I often think about Taizé and back to the times that I came to Grandchamp.

I have some quite vivid memories of my visit to Mother Geneviève in hospital and I hope they have not been coloured too much by my desire to be of help to you.

My impression was that it was a very good hospital in which she felt safe and that she had confidence in her doctor, although he was at that time being a little over optimistic about her possibilities of living for a while longer with her disease. I was very impressed by the Deaconess Sister who was in charge of the hospital which had a feeling of community although the Sisters were a comparatively small number of the actual working staff. The other thing that seemed important was that Mother Genevieve's family had arranged this and, indeed, for me to come over, and gave the impression of loving concern as well as a determination to do everything possible. Perhaps it was important for them to do this at the end of her life and it may have made a difference to the way they lived on afterwards. The whole thing reminded me of the time when our first Matron had advanced cancer. She went to another hospital and was still having active treatment when she took a sudden turn for the worse and died there. We felt badly at the time, although two of her nurses were with her the evening before she died and her husband was with her at the end, but as we thought about it afterwards we realised that so far as he was concerned, working at St Christopher's as he was, she did the right thing for him.

I do not think it is my imagination but as I try to think back on the way we talked together, thoughts of Mary, the mother of Christ came into my mind. I think her "Be it unto me according to Thy will" was there as her particular message. Otherwise I can only remember the usual feeling of confidence that she gave and the refusal to give the impression of her being at all sorry for herself or expecting you to be sorry for her.

This is not very much but if I go on I will think it is my imagination but those thoughts must have come from somewhere and I believe they are valid.

I remember very vividly coming to you. It was a feeling such as we have known many times in the Hospice since then and it goes together with what you say of her final arrival in her chapel.

Thank you for your good wishes. My husband has battled back to as good health as he can expect at his age. He is now nearly 87 but the enclosed photograph will show you how lively he is and he is still painting joyful and splendid pictures and also delicate drawings such as I enclose.

I am so glad that you have another Sister at Taizé with you and also that you will have a longer stay at Grandchamp over Christmas. I hope you will see our Annual Report and Newsletter which still go to them there.

Dr Marcel Boisvert

Royal Victoria Hospital, Montreal, Canada

4 January 1988 Greetings to you from us all and all good wishes for the New Year.

I have just been catching up with the *Journal of Palliative Care* and was very interested to find your paper "All things considered … then what?" I agree with you that these are very difficult problems and over the years I have met a very small number of patients with a consistent desire to have their lives ended before death comes in its own time. However, I have not come down as you have in thinking that we should go along with such a decision and help our patients in that way.

My main thoughts about this were summarised some years back in an article for a nursing journal, a copy of which I enclose but I think even more strongly than I did then that to allow any kind of legal freedom for doctors to take such an action would bring disastrous social consequences. The pressure on the dependent, or those who fear dependence, would undermine their acceptance of care from the rest of us. I do not think that the small minority, and at the moment it is very small, can have that freedom without taking away freedom of pressure from a great many more.

All the same, I am quite convinced that many doctors prolong lives far longer than their patients wish and without proper discussion with them. I also believe that some form of advanced declaration that a patient did not wish all prolongation possible to be carried out is a possible step in making right decisions for those already unconscious or confused. We are committed to appropriate care, not to every treatment possible.

Perhaps I misunderstood what you have written and if so, I hope you will correct me but in the meantime perhaps we could keep on discussing, as you suggest.

Mother Potier

Residence St Marie, St-Lo, France

8 January 1988 Thank you for your really beautiful Christmas card. It was a particularly fine reproduction of a picture of which I am very fond and do not see very often.

I thought the enclosed reprint from a Catholic Journal might interest you. It illustrates something of the story of two of our patients. We are publishing the stories of 21 patients to cover our 21 years of working, taken from our Annual Reports and other publications as they were written at the time. As so many of them have an awareness of the spiritual dimension of care and growth, it is going to be on the religious booklist of a well-known publishing house, although that will not stop it reaching the secular bookshops.

I am continually talking of Hospice Evolution to those who come for courses and workshops here and I am happy to have slides made of a leaflet from the Dames du Calvaire so that I can illustrate something of Mme Garnier's work and salute her as the first, who as far as I can tell, used the word hospice specifically for care of the dying. I know that the word calvary was probably used more often but one illustration I have gives the word hospice itself.

I hope you keep well and are enjoying your retirement. I also hope that the continuing work will go on developing. There is much more interest in hospice type care in France now as you may have heard and we are having a French speaking Conference this May which we could have filled twice over, there was so much interest.

Dr Josefina Magno

International Hospice Institute, Washington DC, USA

11 January 1988 I am writing back straight away to say that it is really totally unrealistic for me to think of travelling and just as unrealistic for the Professor. He is 87 in the next month and lives on the edge of his cardiac capacity. He would certainly adore the trip but I would never have a moment of peace, either on the plane or while he was there. I am sure nobody would ever insure him and it is really not a viable proposition.

I will pass your letter on to Gillian [Ford] but I have already had a word with her and she will ask our Information Service to send our mailing list. That will include people from last year's International and some others as well. It will come by separate mail.

Good news from here about accreditation.[12] Gillian has managed to get this through our Royal Colleges and be on the inspection team approving hospices for such experience. Meantime, our own Association of Hospice Physicians is making a solid base of getting together and sharing experience while we are encouraging small regional Think Tanks on our own pattern here. This is a sharing of problems and seems to be very supportive to often lonely physicians.

Sheila Hancock[13]

Chiswick, London

29 January 1988 Once again you have done the most telling Appeal for St Christopher's and we are all most grateful. Money is coming in well and topped £14,000 at lunchtime

---

12 This refers to the accreditation of palliative medicine as a specialty by the Royal College of Physicians and of General Practitioners. Dr Gillian Ford, a long-time friend of Cicely Saunders, did much of the work to bring this about.

13 The well-known actress who had been a supporter of St Christopher's since the early 1970s, when her first husband had been helped by the home care team after a short admission.

today. It includes, as usual, some delightful letters to which I am replying as many of them have particular questions or are written about people who were in St Christopher's.

It is all marvellously timed with our "Songs of Praise" transmission on Sunday and we have got a local and national appeal happening in the press as well. However, the way you make your appeal and the last comment with your thanks was from the heart of St Christopher's.

I thought you looked absolutely smashing on Wogan and I also saw you with the group speaking against Section 28 of the Education Bill. We have cared for a patient with AIDS in the community and we will certainly take anyone who has AIDS related cancer. At the moment we just do not have enough beds for expanding our work more generally although several of us have been involved with those who are setting up Units or Teams.

Mrs A. Barends

Amsterdam, Holland

7 March 1988 Thank you so much for your letter. I am sorry life is so difficult at the moment.

I am not a very good person at suggesting works on prayer as I never find them terribly easy. I seem to have to find a way much more directly.

However, two books recently have been a great help to me. One is "A Matter of Life and Death" by Bishop John Taylor which is very cheap and of which I enclose a copy and the other, a new book by Father Gerald Hughes which has recently won a prize in this country. Its title is "God of Surprises" and it is published by Darton, Longman and Todd. I am afraid I do not have a spare copy but we are studying it in St Christopher's Foundation Group and are finding it very stimulating.

All good wishes for your future. I am afraid shipping companies around the world are not finding life easy and I hope you will rescue something.

Dr Andrew A. Cruikshank

Casey House Hospice, Toronto, Ontario, Canada

17 March 1988 Thank you for your letter asking me about the support we give our staff to prevent stress and "burnout".

We see very little of anything we would call "burnout" although, from time to time, we experience what we might call "battle fatigue". The hospice has now been working for 21 years and very few people have had to leave because of the continued strain of working in our field. We work very much as a fairly close-knit community with a staff development programme which includes much opportunity for appraisals and ongoing experience. From time to time we have had "support groups" but these seem to have a natural term and by far the major part of our support is given in the hand-over ward meetings that happen on a regular basis in our very stable teams.

The fact that we are a Christian foundation is important to many of the senior staff and to the whole atmosphere of the Hospice but in no way is there any pressure to conform and many people would not make such a commitment. All the same, I think this has had a major effect on the atmosphere of active involvement in caring and a constant spirit of enquiry.

To All Medical Directors

UK Hospices

April 1988 Once again I am sending a round robin and shall be most grateful if you could let me know your comments about it.

As you may have seen, Mary Baines and I are both taking part in a Conference organised by the Voluntary Euthanasia Society which is taking place at the Royal Society of Medicine with Sir Douglas Black in the Chair. We agreed to take part to present the hospice answer to terminal distress but not to be joint organisers of the Conference. However, the words "in co-operation" with the hospice movement have tended, not surprisingly, to turn in the VES's publicity spread to "in conjunction" and I would like to make it quite clear that my own position is that we cannot work together with them in the way of deliberately ending the lives of our patients at any stage.

The response I had from the last meeting of the Association of Palliative Care and Hospice Doctors leads me to believe that this position still speaks for the hospice movement but it would be a great help to me to have a few comments on the subject.

My title is "Potentials in Terminal Illness" and I will be talking about potentials in treatment, including research and education and potentials for personal growth for patient, family and staff. I will stress that whereas we do not think inappropriate treatment should be pursued and are prepared to relieve distress even though, incidentally, this may occasionally shorten life, and that we may approve of Advanced Directives signed by a patient requesting such an approach (the Living Will), we would never deliberately end a patient's life nor let it be known that we could ever take such a position. Mary will, of course, go into the details of medical management of terminal distress from the clinical stand-point.

If you agree with this position generally or have any other comments I would be pleased to know. Also, as I have requests from time to time from various parts of the country to take part in euthanasia debates, I would also be grateful to know whether or not you would be agreeable to my giving your name as an alternative suggestion as I think it important that there should be a group of speakers available.

Dr D. Murphy

St Mary's Hospital, Newport, Isle of Wight

12 May 1988 Thank you very much for your response to my round robin. So far, every single hospice person has been in agreement but only a limited number are prepared to be speakers so I am very grateful to you for that.

As you may not have seen a Living Will, I enclose a copy that was sent to me by the Working Party on the subject at Kings College, London. As you see, it is in no way asking a doctor to kill the person to whom it refers but only to desist from treatments at a stage when they are likely to be inappropriate. I think it may be important to have a proxy who can interpret general wishes in a particular instance but I myself feel that a legal provision is probably unnecessary and might, indeed, be ill advised, so here I seem to depart from the Working Party. I certainly would not respond to a Living Will which went further than this one does.

Dr H. M. O'Conor

The Hospice of St Francis, Berkhamsted, Hertfordshire

12 May 1988 Many thanks indeed for your letter and of course I totally agree with you that hospices cannot intentionally end life.

I certainly agree with you about the severely brain damaged and the long term sick but I think in their case we are talking about appropriate treatment and suitable care rather than any form of euthanasia. I agree with Professor Brian Jennett who deals so often with the brain damaged, that the phrase "passive euthanasia" should be avoided at all costs. It is used by the Society to make an active intervention to end life more "respectable" and every time I have been in discussion or debate with them over the past 20 or more years they have tried to keep pushing that line. I am very pleased to see that the BMA has taken care in definition at the beginning of their Report. I am glad indeed to have it before the meeting with the VES next week.

This, of course, also refers back to your comment on your appraisal of our Ethical and Legal Issues meeting. Once again, I think you are using "passive euthanasia" to refer to appropriate treatment when what is given to cope with pain or, more often, terminal rest-lessness may have an incidental effect of hastening the actual moment of death. I agree with Judge Devlin at this point in saying that whatever a doctor does to relieve the cause of suffering is not the cause of death in the sensible use of the term. All the same, I hope we continue to improve our skills in this area so that the very occasional decisions to maintain sedation are made by a full multi-disciplinary team with due regard for the earlier wishes of the patient and the present responses from the family. I would like to go on discussing this with you some time.

Dr Herbert S. Cohen

Ijssel, Holland

17 June 1988 I would like to add one point to what I said about hospice work at the Conference where we met recently, which arises from your interview which was broadcast on the Medicine Now programme. You said then that in England the Hospice Movement was a "doctors' Movement" and that your Movement was a "consumers' or patients' Movement". This is really not an accurate summary of the United Kingdom. This is illustrated by the fact that every hospice has grown out of demand from within its local community with enormous community support for its capital expenditure, as all the independent hospices in this country only receive 27% funding from the National Health Service. All the rest comes from public charitable giving with a limited amount from other charitable trusts. We are indeed a patients' Movement as well, although the developments in terminal care have been headed by doctor and nurse commitment.

I hope this makes my point and that you will not again refer to us as merely a doctors' Movement, which would be very unfair not only to the public but also, of course, to the nurses, social workers and others, including many volunteers, who are very much part of our work and development.

Dr Robert Kastenbaum[14]

Arizona State University, Tempe, Arizona, USA

17 June 1988 I was fascinated by your article at the end of the interesting *Omega* Vol 18. As a Practitioner, albeit nearly entirely retired, who has read only a limited amount of the American Research, I must confess to being one of those to whom you refer. However, I think you are unfair to the amount of research carried out at St Christopher's and which perpetually looks at our clinical practice and our work in the psychosocial spheres.

Two recent developments may interest you. In the first place, it looks as though Professor John Hinton's recent study which he is now writing up shows that retrospective studies of spouses' immediate memories of a terminal illness are, in the great majority, very like their views as illustrated at the time. This confirms a lot of Colin Parkes' work which was all retrospective.

Secondly, we now have a Chaplain who has done some work on staff attitudes already at another hospice and who is really looking at spiritual needs in what I think will be a very constructive way.

As I know you appreciate, the English scene is quite unlike the American hospice scene and I am only sorry that I do not now have the opportunity of visiting the States and getting myself up to date once again. However, one cannot have everything and I am extremely happy as Chairman of St Christopher's and as diligent spouse to an enchanting 87 year old.

I enclose a few reprints that may not have come your way.

Dr Herbert S. Cohen

Ijssel, Holland

5 August 1988 Thank you for your letter of the 23rd July and also for the copy of your paper. I enclose a copy of mine in return.

I am afraid I still think that there is no way that a working hospice team could suddenly change direction and deliberately bring a patient's life to an end. My speech did not mean that it was unnecessary and impossible because requests for euthanasia are virtually non-existent in hospices, although they are very rare indeed. What I did mean was that we could not suddenly change direction in this way.

I know that Dr Admiraal and others seem to be able to do this but I cannot imagine a hospice ward in which such an occasion could take place and I know that I am speaking for all the Hospice doctors who spoke from their teams in response to my request for their views.

We do not, however, consider we should prolong life at all costs, as I am sure you must have realised from what Dr Baines and I were saying. Nor do we think that a patient's

[14] Professor of Communications at Arizona State University and noted thanatologist; the two had been in contact since 1966, when as a graduate student he had been impressed by the impact her lectures were making in the USA.

"autonomy" extends to a complete freedom to ask another person to do exactly as he (the patient) chooses.

I do not see any need for angry debate between us but I am afraid I think we have to accept that we are working for very different objectives, even though we have a common desire to relieve suffering.

Professor Vittorio Ventafridda[15]

Fondazione Flioriani, Milano, Italy

7 October 1988 I understand from Robert Twycross that he has been in touch with you about the Approach that Dr Norris of the Doctors who Respect Human Life made to the European Association for Palliative Care.

I thought you would be interested to know that before taking part in a symposium organised by our Voluntary Euthanasia Society in order to present the alternative palliative care view, I wrote to the Medical Directors of all the Hospices. I have a very good response rate (between 70–80%) and they were unanimous in saying that they could not envisage the active termination of a patient's life. Like Robert Twycross, I believe that palliative care or hospice care and euthanasia are mutually exclusive.

The statement from the National Hospice Association which I checked by telephone before my meeting that "Hospice affirms life and regards dying as a normal process. Hospice neither hastens nor postpones death" remains their principle and we would ourselves agree with this.

All good wishes for your Association and for all your work.

Annette Buchan

Newtown, Wellington, New Zealand

17 October 1988 Thank you for your letter and the news of the Mary Potter Hospice. We keep in touch with people around the world through our Information Service and will shortly be sending the information about our next International Conference in July 1989.

St Christopher's has 18 single rooms in its 62 patient beds and the remainder are in four bed bays. When I visited the USA some years ago now I looked at a number of two bed rooms and felt they were most unsuitable for hospice work. Indeed, in the only hospice that had such a setting I found that frequently once a patient had died the second patient asked that there should not be another admission there as they had found it so difficult. There are, of course, problems from time to time in a four bed bay where three patients die quickly and the fourth is left feeling very upset and lonely. But if we were to build again, we would keep very much the same balance. It is far easier to keep one's privacy among four people than within just two who are inevitably eavesdroppers of each other's conversations and who also feel a responsibility for a very sick neighbour.

I think an adolescent unit probably wants to be quite separate. Any adolescents we have had have gone into single rooms and that has been reasonably satisfactory. On the whole, they need

---

[15] The pioneer of palliative care in Italy; a leading figure in the development of the World Health Organization strategy for cancer pain relief; and co-founder and Honorary President of the European Association for Palliative Care.

a rather different approach, often desperately request more active treatment however difficult it may be and generally find the atmosphere of an ordinary hospice somewhat difficult.

In spite of all that, however, one manages to make work what one has but it is nice to have a chance of looking at what to plan ahead of time.

If your architects have any specific questions, I suggest they get in touch directly with the architects to St Christopher's, who are: Messrs Stewart Hendry & Smith.

Sandol Stoddard

Holualoa, Hawaii, USA

17 October 1988 I was very glad to have your letter with the news that you probably have another book coming and I think your comment about the answer being home care plus carefully guarded beds is probably right

However, I am very sad to hear what you say about New Haven and will be interested to know what comeback you have from Florence Wald through whom I had a rather different picture a little while ago. Apparently Rosemary Hurzler was talking with her about nurse exchanges with St Christopher's. Without your comments I would have thought this very unlikely anyway and will certainly feed that back to Madeleine Duffield who is now Matron here in case Ms Hurzler gets in touch with her directly. What you say fits with one or two other comments I have heard.

It is sad that the medical professionals have simply not taken hospice on board but I suppose this is partly because of the US scene in general. We are very fortunate in spite of cuts in the Health Service and our own rather meagre NHS funding (one third of our running costs now) because we are much more recognised as proper medicine. Recently, we had the final agreement that hospice or palliative medicine should be included in Higher Medical Training.

I wonder if you would be interested in talking with Robert Fulton at the Department of Sociology, University of Vermont. He has a very wide look at the sociological scene and wrote to me recently to say how important it was that the hospice idea was about before the AIDS needs became so acute.

However, I am really very out of touch with the US scene now and my comments are not worth very much. I was very cheered at your comments on the few good places you met. I am sure there must be more about.

Marian and I are fine although my protectiveness of his age means I find it increasingly difficult to get away at all. However, I do some quite interesting talks from time to time but not evening and of course never overnight. No grumbles about that, we are blissfully happy and I am glad to hear you are too.

Dorothy Bvard

Eagle Ridge Hospital and Health Care Centre, Fort Moody, British Columbia, Canada

20 October 1988 I am so sorry to have taken such a long time to respond to your letter but it was held up in our postal strike.

I am now enclosing a note of her aims from our new Occupational Therapist and part of a chapter contributed by our Principal Physiotherapist who has been with us for many years.

St Christopher's had a trained Occupational Therapist for a few years near the beginning of its work (it opened in 1967) but after that was unable to find a trained worker and worked with a diversional therapist and many volunteers. We are only now building up our team again. In the past we have had both a Poetry Workshop and an artist visiting weekly and a considerable amount of music and other diversion. As well as our patients with terminal illness, for whom the average stay is only three weeks, we have a Wing for the frail elderly and a number of patients coming for day care and it is in these latter two groups that our long term members come from.

Our physiotherapy started as we opened and has developed until we now have over 50 hours a week made up of part-time workers who also have a considerable input into our ward meetings and teaching programme.

I am enclosing the whole of Mrs O'Gorman's chapter as it illustrates how much she knows about the treatment given by other members of our multi-disciplinary team.

Dr Sam Klagsbrun

Four Winds Hospital, Katonah, New York, USA

1 November 1988 Firstly, we really find it as difficult as ever to thank you enough for what you do for us when you come for your week. Each time I think it is especially good and I am really optimistic about ongoing results from your involvement with the one or two special problem points. Also, thank you that it is such a gift to St Christopher's in the way that you do it.

I think the Council were really stimulated in their discussion and I am glad we were able to move on from the money side into the things that it is really appropriate for us to discuss with you as well as among ourselves.

The enclosed list will, I hope, impress you as it does us. We have just heard from Mr Geoffrey Tucker's secretary that he has collected this group to meet with us. I only hope the discussion will be as fruitful as it looks potentially. As I said to you, I think it is wise for us to concentrate on our own experience but moving out from there to the voluntary sector as a whole.

Frank Hill put on a good meeting yesterday at which we looked at the importance of proper accountability and efficiency. What I think is impossible to quantify are some of the quality of life questions that have to be answered if we are going to do a proper look at our "cost effectiveness". In case you did not see Frank's paper, I enclose a copy.[16] As I tried to point out, we are not always able to compare like with like. What is done in some of our smaller hospices needs to be challenged as I think it quite often, however good the care, is organised rather carelessly as to costs and accounting.

Clifford Longley

Religious Affairs Editor, The Times, London

10 November 1988 Thank you very much for your response to my letter. I do appreciate some of your problems.

---

[16] She is probably referring here to a paper which was published the following year: F. Hill and C. Oliver, Hospice – an update on the cost of patient care, *Palliative Medicine*, **3** (1989): 1229–36.

I am afraid I have disposed of *The Times* which included the comment on Anglican Spirituality which seemed to me to question whether there was such a thing. From what you write I am sure you did not really mean this. Perhaps it is difficult to define but I think both the introduction to The English Spirit – The Little Gidding Anthology and Canon Allchin's comment on Anglicanism in *The Study of Spirituality* published by SPCK in 1986, convey what I would mean myself. Over the years in which I have belonged to different sections of the Church of England, I have felt a freedom and openness which sits very well with the development of hospice work. The emphasis both on scripture, on hymn singing and on the centrality of the Eucharist, have been very nourishing. I suppose I would take Archbishop Temple and CS Lewis as those who influenced me most in early days and I would add to them Dorothy Sayers and in particular "The Man Born to be King". Now, I have been greatly helped by Bishop John Taylor, lately of Winchester and John Austin Baker's "The Foolishness of God". These two Bishops have had considerable input to St Christopher's.

Perhaps you would be interested in our statement of Aim and Basis which as you see dates from before the Hospice opened and has been discussed on various occasions since then and hardly changed at all. As we are very much a group of the unlike, this is kept in the files and is just available if it is asked for. I suppose another example of a rather Anglican approach. I cannot remember who made the comment on conformity that "some should, all may but none must".

I also enclose something on Spiritual Pain that I presented at one of our International Conferences to a very mixed audience from nearly 30 different countries.

Dr Michael J. Cousins
President, IASP, Bedford Park, Australia

9 December 1988 Thank you very much for your letter of the 29th November and the most welcome news that the Council of the IASP [International Association for the Study of Pain] has approved my election as an Honorary Member. I greatly appreciate this honour.

I have always enjoyed reading *Pain* and am delighted to have a lifetime subscription. I am afraid, however, that I cannot travel these days and leave my now very elderly and frail husband, so I will not be able to be in Adelaide. I will be sorry to miss the proceedings and hope that the medal can reach me by another route.

Mrs S. Malblank
Paris, France

23 February 1989 Thank you for your recent telephone call about euthanasia.

In answer to your queries, the question of legalising euthanasia has been raised three times in the House of Lords of the United Kingdom Parliament. Each time it has been defeated. The dates are approximately 1936, 1955 and 1971. The last time the title was "The Incurable Patients' Bill" and it was presented by Baroness Wooton and defeated by a large majority. The other times the majority was considerably smaller. On each occasion the vote has gone across the parties but, of course a debate in the Lords is not at all the same as that in the Commons and is only a question of airing a subject. I doubt if there would be definite party support for any of them to bring forward a Bill in the House of Commons. The text of the various debates would be available from Hansard.

No law has so far been passed in any country in the world legalising the active killing of patients. The current situation in the Netherlands is that a doctor is not likely to be prosecuted but a Bill has not so far gone through their Houses of Parliament to the best of my knowledge, which extends until fairly recently.

I enclose some reprints which I hope will be of interest.

Dr Robert Buckman

Toronto-Bayview Regional Cancer Centre, Toronto, Ontario, Canada

31 March 1989 It must seem a very long time indeed since you wrote the Foreword for this second edition.[17] I have just received it but we do not have a publication date at the moment, nor a price. I think they have done it quite well. You will see that Mary took over the pain chapters and they are very neatly put in but I have left the beginning and the end much the same, taking your good advice wherever you gave it. I hope you still approve.

As you sent your foreword directly to me and I am not sure whether Oxford has your address, I am sending you this copy and if you would like some more, I will make sure they send them to you.

The Hospice goes on well. Dr Gillian Ford has left to go on to be Secretary to the Standing Committee on Post Graduate Medical Education and a doctor who did some training here before taking over a smaller hospice is taking her place. His name is Dr Anthony Smith and he has a background in surgery but 5 years solid hospice work. The teaching side goes on strongly and we now have approval from the Joint Board for Higher Medical Training for a Senior Registrar Post. Palliative medicine has therefore been officially recognised as a speciality and there will be various other posts around the country. So hopefully, we will not only have more people coming in for hospice senior posts, but also various oncologists or radiotherapists who have had time working in a training hospice.

You may be interested to know that our Foundation Group had a very good evening discussing your chapter on Spiritual Aspects and you might not have seen the enclosed reprint which comes from a talk I gave at our IVth International Conference.

Professor Franco Pannuti

Unita Sanitaria Locale Ventotto, Bologna, Italy

15 May 1989 Thank you very much for sending me your book. The earlier part is, of course, of less relevance to me than the last two chapters, with which I am very interested. I very much like your ten suggestions and I think in some ways they stand alongside the principles which I suggested in the second edition of our textbook and in one of the reprints, which I enclose. If I have sent you these already, I apologise but as I am enclosing my more philosophical ones, I thought they might be of interest to you in view of what you write in your chapter.

---

[17]   Dr Robert Buckman, the medical oncologist and well-known broadcaster, qualified in medicine at Cambridge University in 1972 before emigrating to Canada in 1985; he had written 'A foreword for people who are not experts in palliative care' which appeared in C. Saunders and M. Baines, *Living with dying: the management of terminal malignant disease*, 2nd edn (Oxford: Oxford University Press, 1989).

I think we both have a very powerful aim to help our patients to find their maximum potential in the way they live up until they die. For many of our patients this is at home for as long as possible but, of course, our hospice wards are very unlike those of a general or even an oncological hospital. There is far less pressure on acute work, although of course we are very active as we set out to relieve an often complex pattern of symptoms. It is increasingly true that we have here patients that other people have found present problems which were difficult to resolve. There is a surprisingly lively atmosphere in the wards in spite of the fact that so many of our patients come in for the last few days only.

Over the years I have found that most doctors in Europe are less likely to be really frank with their patients about their prognosis than they are in England or the United States. I am therefore very interested in your comments on truth because it seems to me you are more likely to be discussing a patient's dying with him than I understand is usual. Our experience is that whereas some patients never wish to discuss this during their whole lifetime with us, more and more are anxious to do so and are helped by facing the likely outcome of their illness and in so doing come to better communication with their families and discover strengths that none of them realised they possessed.

I do hope there will be a chance to meet with you one day and discuss our work which seems to overlap in many ways.

Dr Harold Y. Vanderpool

University of Texas Medical Branch, Galveston, Texas, USA

20 June 1989 This is a letter out of the blue for you but I finally believe I must tell you how frequently I use your paper "The Ethics of Terminal Care" from the *JAMA* in 1978 when talking about ethics with our multi-disciplinary groups who come for courses at St Christopher's and also when I am thinking round problems myself.

I well remember my trip to Galveston and meeting with you and I wonder if you have continued to work in this or related fields and whether you have written anything else on the subject. I would be very interested.

Since we met, St Christopher's has gone on developing, especially in its multi-disciplinary teaching in general and courses in particular. We continue to have a number of young staff who come here for about two years before returning to our National Health Service with this special knowledge or continue with smaller hospice teams around the country. What is the most exciting aspect is, I think, the way the general principles are interpreted in so many ways appropriate to different situations. We are about to have an International Conference to which delegates are coming from 37 different countries. It is all a long way from the very first patient who gave me the idea and although hospices are obviously of very different calibre, I feel happy about the movement as a whole.

Grace Goldin

Swarthmore, Pennsylvania, USA

2 August 1989 We were delighted to have your long letter and to know that you were going to have another lovely trip before embarking on a change of medication and so on. It sounds as though you will enjoy yourselves again and I hope the dentistry is all completed in good time.

Marian sends special love. He has just completed two excellent portraits and I have just taken a lovely still life in pastels to be framed. We are expecting family from Poland but have no word from them yet as to whether they have got either their visas or their flights.

You may be surprised at the enclosure but I had two very evangelical friends who ran the Garden Tomb just outside the Damascus Gate in Jerusalem and they connected me up with the writers of this leaflet. The preamble may strike you as extremely fundamentalist but I thought you would be interested to know that at least some of us agree with you that it is unfair reporting when we hear so much about this and so little about so many of the other conflicts. I wish the Labour group had more power and more support because they sound to me more reasonable and more likely to reach a lasting peace.

Some of the writings of Christian Friends of Israel I certainly do not go along with but at least I feel they give us a view which is rarely presented in the general press.

Professor Vittorio Ventafridda

Fondazione Floriani, Milano, Italy

10 August 1989 Thank you very much for your Newsletter. I was delighted to see the first edition coming from the European Association for Palliative Care. I enclose my Inscription Form but I have not filled in the "presented by" as I am on the list as a Foundation Member. I am not, however, quite sure about the membership fee. Should I pay the full or associated member fee as I will only be able to come to meetings that might take place in this country? My second problem is that I do not know what currency you are referring to by the letters Lit.

We have just had a very successful International Conference with a number of people attending from Europe and I wonder whether our Information Service and your group should be exchanging addresses. We have our Conferences, as you probably remember, every two years and although some of the people who came this time will not, I think, be in a position to afford much in the way of membership dues, I am sure they would be interested to know of the European Association if they do not already know of it.

Our Conference was a very stimulating occasion and we were very glad to see Dr Giorgio Di Mola from Milan.

Patrice O'Connor[18]

St Luke's Hospital Center, New York, USA

8 November 1989 Thank you so much for sending me the programme of your Service which was beautifully set out. I am delighted that Tom was able to be there. I know he was very pleased.

----

[18] Patrice O'Connor, a nurse by profession and a former nun; she had first joined the palliative care team at St Luke's Hospital Center, New York, in 1979, working closely with Carleton Sweetser and Sam Klagsbrun.

Thank you also for sending me the Nouwen article. It really is much more lively than some of the things he has written recently. I am going to share it with one or two others because I think people will find it valuable, in particular our excellent Chaplaincy.

I have just been re-reading Mother Julian [of Norwich], one published in this country by Darton, Longman and Todd but translated in the States and first published there in 1988 by the Walker Publishing company under the title "A Lesson of Love".

I am not sending it now as you have probably met it already but if you have not, let me know and I would love to send it over for Christmas.

Christopher Olsson
Swedish Council of America, Minneapolis, USA

23 November 1989 Thank you very much indeed for your letter of the 14th November and the cheque for $5,000 which I have paid into the funds of St Christopher's.[19] We are all most grateful.

I have indeed heard from my step-daughter, who telephoned me both from St Louis and as soon as she got back to San Francisco. She told me all about the dinner and obviously enjoyed herself as did my granddaughter. She is sending me a copy of the programme but I understand there were a number of photographs taken at the time and if there is one available, I would very much like to see it as would my husband.

I will look forward to seeing the Orrefors crystal bowl when Mr Lundh visits England. I will certainly consider using the presentation as a public relations opportunity.

I can only repeat again what an honour I feel it is that I should receive an Award in memory of Raoul Wallenberg.

Fr Dennis D Knight
Vatican II Institute, c/o St Patrick's Seminary, Menlo Park, California, USA

9 January 1990 Many thanks indeed for your card. I am delighted to hear you are taking a study sabbatical and hope you enjoy it. I am also delighted that you are still in hospice.

Our very stimulating and very enjoyable visits from Louvain have died out since your days. If you were ever in touch with them again and you feel that it is still something that might be helpful to the seminarians either in the six weeks during the summer or the three weeks over Christmas, I hope you will encourage the new Rector or appropriate person to think of us.

St Christopher's has expanded in home care and day hospital since your days and remains extremely busy with usually twice as many people being cared for at home as within the wards. The demand is unremitting. We have more doctors, more teaching and training, a certain amount of research and now a very strong Chaplaincy department with an excellent senior chaplain and two assistants. I hope the feeling in the wards is the same as you knew and certainly an awareness of spiritual issues is very much around.

[19] She had just been given the Raoul Wallenberg Humanitarian Award by the Swedish Council of America. Unable to attend the award-giving ceremony, in St Louis, USA, on 4 November, she had been represented by her step-daughter, Ms Daniela Faggioli.

Sister Gilberte

Communauté de Grandchamp, Neufchatel, Switzerland

22 January 1990 I was delighted to have your long letter with all your news. I am glad you will go back in the Spring to thank the Lord and the Brothers. That will be a special occasion after 27 years spent at Taizé.

I am so glad to hear your description of being cared for by your younger sisters and your remark that the whole world remains open to your prayers. I have always been conscious of your support. I am enclosing a copy of our Prayer Diary for these two months. I think it has much too much detail for you but perhaps you would like it. If you will let me know I will put you on our list.

We remain very ecumenical here, as you are. We have the head of a Catholic College talking on "Our Image of God" with our staff later this week. The last meeting was a very stimulating one on "Does Everybody Go to Heaven?" from a local evangelical Christian. He pointed out how few are the referrals to eternal fire, how there are many biblical statements which those who feel that in the end everyone will be gathered in can point to, but really came down himself to the belief that the eternal life is the gift of God and if it is refused then the soul will not continue and certainly not in eternal punishment. It was stimulating and comforting and met a need to discuss something that certainly concerns us here.

Dr X. Gomez I. Batiste Alentorn[20]

Hospital de la Santa Creu, Barcelona, Spain

13 February 1990 I am sorry to be such a nuisance but the enclosed letter is in answer to a plea for help I had from someone in your country who is thinking of committing suicide. As you will see from the enclosed envelope, his address was completed blotted out by the post office stamp. The only address he gives on the letter is Cartagena, which I presume is his town. Is there any hope of your finding his address in the telephone book or elsewhere and sending my reply on to him? I can think of no other way of trying to reach this desperate young man.

Meantime, I hope things are going well with you.

The Lord Jellicoe

House of Lords, London

13 February 1990 Professor Wall has sent me a copy of the nomination for the Nobel Peace Prize for which I know you took a great deal of trouble and care. I am really very grateful to you for your efforts on my behalf and, of course, on behalf of hospice as a whole.

It was really very moving looking at what various people have said and I would have liked very much to have shared it with so many of the patients of the past who inspired and taught me in the beginning.

We are well ahead with the booklet which we are producing from part of the Onassis prize money as an information and publicity handout and I am very pleased with it so far.

---

[20] Dr Xavier Gomez-Batiste, the architect of palliative care in Catalonia, had visited St Christopher's Hospice a few years earlier.

I think it goes together with the part of the Prize which went to support our International Conference because, as I look at it, I realise how similar we all are in principle as we practise our very different ways of giving hospice care.

Heather Greenland
Grand Falls, Newfoundland, Canada

21 February 1990 Thank you very much for your interesting letter and the photographs of your mother. I agree with you that one of them looks very much like me but the other one much less so.

It is very interesting that her maiden name was the same as my mother's and when I read that you had met some friends in South Africa I thought that there might be a link as that was where my mother was born. Her father and three of his brothers all went out to South Africa in about 1870 and my mother came back to England in the early years of this century. None of the family, so far as I know, ever went to Canada, and I don't know what part of the country my grandfather came from.

I think therefore that there probably is not a near link but inheritance does funny things and maybe there was some connection we will never discover.

Christopher Olsson
Swedish Council of America, Minneapolis, MN, USA

27 February 1990 Thank you very much for sending me the issue of Sweden & America. I was very pleased to see it having heard all about the evening from my step-daughter, Daniela.

I understood that the bowl was coming over with someone visiting London in January but I have not heard anything yet. It is very good of whoever will finally bring it to take the trouble because I am sure it must be in quite a large container. We will certainly want the local press to know when they are bringing it down here and I hope to hear about this in due course.

I thought you would be interested to know that I am spending the $5,000 award that I have already received on upgrading the room that we have for families to relax together, where there is a television for the children and where volunteers provide refreshments for them all.

Gina and Luitgarta Cadeggianni
Viola Film, Ottobrunn, West Germany

2 April 1990 Thank you very much for the film of my life which has now arrived and which I have had time to watch twice. I am very impressed by both the sensitivity of the filming that Patrick Horl organised and the way it has been edited and presented.

I do not understand about any problems you have had but I know that this is for my personal use and I am very glad to have it at last.

Dr Russell K. Portenoy

University of Wisconsin-Madison, Madison, Wisconsin, USA

4 April 1990 Thank you for sending me the good news of the bi-monthly publication of the *Journal of Pain and Symptom Management* and your thoughts about the next editions.

I am afraid the time has past when I would be thinking of contributing something myself but we have just put together a book on team working in this field from St Christopher's and I will hope to send you a copy for review in due course.

In the meantime, all good wishes to the publication.

Tina Diaz

The Australian Jewish Times, Darlinghurst, Sydney, Australia

5 April 1990 Thank you for your letter about David Tasma. I am sending a copy of my biography because it gives you more than enough about me. The chapter about David is very true and really includes all I know about him. I am sure he came back to the faith of his Fathers and tried to express this in the short poem I wrote which I also enclose. His photograph is still in my office and I never forget him each year on the anniversary of his death, January 25th. Recently, German television made a film of my life and the very diligent researcher discovered David's grave, which I had not visited since the funeral. We went there with the film crew and I laid a stone, which I believe is a Jewish tradition. I am very grateful to him. For the rest, you will find what you want in Shirley du Boulay's very sensitive biography.

Grace Goldin

Swarthmore, Pennsylvania, USA

12 April 1990 All is well with us and I do apologise for not having written for such a long time. There is really no excuse except that I had a granddaughter over from Poland for a month and have been getting two collections of other people's works together with some introductions by me for two different publishers. One has been an enlargement of the little book which I put together before which was called "Beyond all Pain" and has now turned into "Beyond the Horizon" (interesting to see yours is "Foothills"). The other is an attempt to put together something on working as a team with the disciplines all making their contributions. Marian was delighted to have his granddaughter and continues doing some really splendid portraits. The latest is one of his best.

I am sorry your feet have been such a trial and I felt for you all the way through "Foothills". The ones that made an impact on me on a first reading were number 2, the splendid number 10 and the poignant number 19. I loved that one. I liked the plea of number 20 and the firm response to your Better Angel in number 25. I felt for you over "Diabetes" and very much so about your "Friends Mislaid" number 35. When I think of your house, it is full of lovely possessions but most of all it is full of the two of you and the welcome that you give. I agree with you that number 48 is a key thought about hospice and if I may, I would love to put it in our Annual Report this year. Does that run into troubles with copyright as we do not know about publishing yet? I loved Lelar and Mr Wilson and joined with you for a deep moment about your daughter and again, later in quite a different way, about your mother. Finally, of course, I felt for the Coda.

I do hope you get these published but in the meantime they are a very deep joy to your friends.

Grace Goldin

Swarthmore, Pennsylvania, USA

20 April 1990 This is a very quick follow up from my last letter to tell you that I am talking by satellite on "Hospice as Bridge Builder" to Bal Mount's International Conference in Montreal this Fall. Among such things as emphasising that bridges go in two ways and starting off with a picture of a bridge done by one of my patients a long time ago, and so leading into bridges of listening. I am putting in a little section on bridges to history. This led me back to the History of Hospital Ward Design and pages 6 onwards which I have quoted when I have been talking about the Evolution of Hospices to the groups that visit here. I was thinking of referring to these early hospices by making a slide of the site plan of the Monastery of Turmanin. It has photocopied well from the book and I think the people who do our slides could produce a good black and white for me. I would rather use this than the Victorian painting of Fabiola, which I normally use and which is my alternative. May I have your permission to do so? I am going to talk briefly about the earlier Syria hospices as well as Fabiola and it is marvellous to have something of the fifth century to illustrate. I am then leaping to the later middle Ages and the slide you gave me years ago of a marvellous confused mix of people and a print from the nineteenth century from Jeanne Garnier's Home in France and on to St Joseph's. As I have to talk about bridges with the researchers, with the acute services, the community and to and within the family and across prejudice and into the spiritual dimension and, finally, end up with something about growth through loss including the growth of staff, all in some 40 minutes, I am going to be hard put to it. All this, of course, will have the added anxiety of whether the slides are being transmitted safely to the audience across the Atlantic.

Dr Christine Dare

St Luke's Hospice, Kenilworth, Cape Province, South Africa

25 April 1990 Your last newsletter was very cheering and I hope everything goes on well.

My reason for writing now is that I am billed to start the Montreal Conference at the end of September with a satellite presentation for which I have chosen the title "Hospice as Bridge Builder"! I will be tackling such things as acute medicine, community, families and so on and, of course, the spiritual dimension but I want to include bridges across prejudice. For this I am having a slide from an AIDS hospice and one from a Northern Ireland Hospice which simply goes across the border and works in Southern Ireland as well. I would dearly love one from you as you have done so much to bridge race difficulties. Have you got a slide of black and white patients and staff together that you could spare me? I have a slide of your building and if you have nothing I will use that but I think it would have more impact to show something in the wards if you have such a thing.

Life here never seems to stand still and I hope the new directions we are looking at in the way of both work, management and publicity are right and proper. We had the most wonderful Easter Sunday with 65 people including two patients in beds and many wheelchairs somehow tucked into the chapel, with plenty of good music.

Sister Antonia[21]

Blackrock, Dublin

8 May 1990 Many thanks indeed for your letter and please thank Sister Teresita as well. It was very good to hear from you.

I was thinking of you the other day as I selected just a few of my original notes from St Joseph's and finally threw the rest away. I still have my punch cards somewhere in the hospice and also my copies of the tape-recorded conversations but I thought it was time to get rid of the last lot of other papers. It brought back many people to me again and I have never forgotten those early days together.

I am glad Dr Kearney is doing well. I know he is very busy and I hope the improvements you mention will go on in the Hospice at Harold's Cross.

The Professor keeps well and surprisingly energetic in his 90th year and is starting a new picture today. He already has two portraits on the go.

Soon I hope to be sending you a new edition of my collection of the poetry and prose that helped me so much during all the days of preparation and planning. I am delighted that one of his pictures is going to be on the cover.

Dr Austin H. Kutscher

The American Institute of Life-Threatening Illness and Loss, New York, USA

21 May 1990 It is always interesting to know what your Foundation is doing and I was pleased to receive your April letter and Congressional Notes. I was also interested in the new name and agree with your reasons for having made the change.

I suppose we have the same problem with the word "hospice" as you have had with the word "thanatology" and certainly we have to work hard with the general public to make them realise that being enrolled in a hospice programme does not mean that death is inevitably close but may mean living with a life threatening illness for longer and, certainly, in a much better way than may be expected. We are just producing an illustrated booklet to emphasise this although the demand for our service shows how many people are happy to be referred when they are in need.

I am sorry I can never travel these days due to my husband's age and dependence but it is nice still to be in touch with another of the early pioneers.

---

[21] Sister Mary Antonia (1915–2001) had worked in St Joseph's Hospice, Hackney, at the time when Cicely Saunders was doing research and clinical work there; she lived for the last years of her life in Blackrock, near Dublin, and the two kept in close contact over the years.

Sandol Stoddard

Holualoa, Hawaii, USA

4 July 1990 Many thanks for your letter. I am delighted to read that you are producing an updated hospice book.

St Christopher's has changed quite a lot since you were here. For example, we now have some 90 patients at home which will go up to 120 at a time in January 1991 when we enlarge our visiting area again, and we have 62 in-patient beds. These, of course, are not 100% full as there are always people coming in and out and we do not fill a bed immediately after someone has died. Usually we have some 50 in-patients at any one time.

At the moment we are building a larger base for Home Care and for the Day Centre. As you were so much involved as an in-patient volunteer, I think you did not emphasise that we did, in fact, start hospice home care back in 1969, the first to do so.

Many of the rest of your questions are answered by our Annual Report, which I enclose and I think you will be able to pick up any changes. One of the main areas of expansion is teaching. Even more goes on now, both with our three doctors in training posts and in the many nurses who come here for a 1 month staff development programme. This and other developments I think you will find in the second of the Annual Reports I am sending which is the one we had for our 21st Anniversary. I am also enclosing the latest Hospice Directory which gives you the up to date information about hospice provision in this country.

We are much larger than any other hospice here apart from St Joseph's in East London. We have some 250 staff and 250 volunteers with almost the same number of volunteers running our charity shops. We have over 800 admissions a year and are more like a small hospital than the average hospice. However, I think the care goes on the same and when we have our International Conferences and hear people from different countries talking about their beginnings and where they are now, it is always recognisably the same aims and ideals that they are talking about.

Finally, my thoughts on hospice and AIDS and, indeed, any other of the disadvantaged dying. Our cancer patients are not about to go away and the demand is unremitting but we would look at any appropriate patient on an individual basis as we do with those with motor neurone disease. I think the hospice principles are very suitable for AIDS home care and for a limited number of back-up beds but think on the whole it should be new beds and new money so that we all keep our focus and really continue to learn about the work that we are doing. Symptom control, understanding of families and all ought to advance during the next 10 years and not just be the same as they are now.

Peter Kaye, of course, was a Senior Registrar here and I am very glad you are having him in on the symptom side. I wish you well with everything.

If you have any further queries, perhaps you could come back to me when you have read what I have enclosed.

Dr Josefina Magno

Southfield, Michigan, USA

5 July 1990 Thank you so much for your letter and interesting package. I had, of course, seen the article in the *Journal of Pain and Symptom Management* and we have been involved in a rather second-hand way with the WHO booklet which is so important.

However, I would like to pick up on one or two points from your article on the Hospice Concept of Care.[22]

St Christopher's planned Home Care from the beginning and went out into the homes around us before we were two years old, that is in the summer of 1969. At the present moment we have 62 in-patients beds as well as our 16 bed sitting rooms for the frail elderly and some 90 patients at home. We will be enlarging our visiting area and going up to some 120 patients at any one time as from January 1991. I have always talked to visitors about Home Care but I suppose because that has been in our bricks and mortar building, they have become fixated on that. However, I really must give credit to Barbara McNulty and Mary Baines who started the first ever Hospice Home Care Programme from St Christopher's.

Secondly, I was at your Washington Conference as well as Sandol and the others. Thirdly, you may be interested to know that Professor John Hinton did a longitudinal study of every third patient referred to Home Care, following them up right through to the end of their illness and has some fascinating data which we hope will appear soon in the general medical literature. One figure that may interest you is that the patients did, in fact, spend 80% of their time at home and only 20% as in-patients and also that those who came in for the last day or two left their families feeling, as they said to him later, that the whole care had been "home" and they felt they had, in fact, done the caring themselves throughout. Admission to St Christopher's was not thought of as being like a hospital admission but as an extension of home.

I totally agree that an oncology department should be carrying out hospice or palliative care but there are many patients and families who need the extra time and space that a Hospice Home Care Team with its own beds can offer. A study we are planning will, I hope, give some guidelines as to who should be referred from the general hospital at an earlier stage than often happens. "And then I came here and you listened" is still said to us, even from those coming from very good, but often very stressed, hospital wards.

All good wishes to the International Hospice Institute and the Academy. I am not sure if I told you before but our Joint Board for Higher Medical Training has now recognised palliative medicine as a speciality, with entry through different routes of specialised training and accreditation.

Dr Mary Eleanor Toms

Hospice Care of Rhode Island, Rhode Island, New York, USA

9 July 1990 I was very interested in your article in the May/June issue of *The American Journal of Hospice and Palliative Care* as we have been caring for patients in the terminal stages of Motor Neurone Disease, as we call it, since our first patient was admitted in 1967. You will see from the enclosed Review article that I did some years back of our first 100 patients, that we are tackling the same problems as you are, although with some slightly different medications. It seems to me that you are achieving with amytriptyline what we achieve with carefully calibrated Atropine and smaller doses of oral morphine given much earlier in the disease than is usual.

---

[22] The article referred to is J. B. Magno, The hospice concept of care: facing the 1990s, *Death Studies*, **14** (1990): 109–19.

You will see how little I wrote about some of the emotional stresses at that time and as we turn to a review of our second 100 patients, we will obviously be enlarging in that area. All the same, I thought you might be interested to read this.

If you have any other writing on the subject, we would be very interested to see it, particularly as we are having an important conference with neurologists discussing this subject early next year.

Professor Ronald Melzack

McGill University, Montreal, Canada

30 July 1990 An American friend sent my brother a copy of your article "The Tragedy of Needless Pain" and it has finally reached me. I was, of course, delighted to read it. It is a real tragedy that there is pain going on at this moment in so many parts of the world which could be relieved by the use of present knowledge, which has been well researched and demonstrated.

Just for your records, I first saw the regular giving of oral morphine at St. Luke's Hospital, originally "Home for the Dying Poor" and founded in 1893. I worked there as a volunteer from 1948–55 in the evenings. I was therefore able to introduce the regular giving of the drugs they were using already in St. Joseph's Hospice when I started to work there in 1958.

It was at our invitation and with monies already waiting for us from our Department of Health that we asked Robert Twycross in 1970 to come and carry out the comparative study between morphine and heroin. During his years with us, we also omitted cocaine and so landed up with the oral morphine mixture which we all use now.

I always want to give acknowledgement to St. Luke's where I think it was the nurses who came upon the idea of regular giving rather than the doctors. The Matron who was there in 1948 could date this back to when she first arrived in 1935 which, of course, was quite soon after the Brompton Cocktail was originally introduced. It was fascinating to arrive in St. Joseph's where drugs were given prn and to find that it was like waving a wand over the house and once we had seen the results in a limited number of patients, I never had problems again with the Irish Catholic nuns feeling we were giving the patients too much.

I very much like your two diagrams and I wonder if you would let us use them in lectures at St Christopher's If you would allow us to do this, we would photocopy it and colour it and have the slides made over here.

I am so sorry I cannot travel these days and cannot see you in Montreal or come to the International Conference. However, I will, I hope, be there via satellite and there will be excellent representation from St Christopher's with our multi-disciplinary team.

Dr Austin H. Kutscher

The American Institute of Life-Threatening Illness and Loss, New York, USA

30 July 1990 You set me a real problem in your letter asking me if I would join your Honorary Editorial Board for the beginnings of your Journal "Illness, Crises and Loss". I have always admired your work and have only been sorry that I have not been able to travel these last years and come to any of your conferences.

However, I wonder very much whether it would be wise for me to come on at this point. I am only Chairman now at St Christopher's and very much out of the clinical scene. I am therefore, rather sadly declining your invitation.

Dody Cotter

Tucson, Arizona, USA

13 August 1990 I cannot tell you how delighted I was to have the long letter about the celebration of Sister Zita Marie's Golden Jubilee. I think about her so often. Some years ago when we were crossing Westminster Bridge she asked me to pray for her every time I went over and I have never forgotten this and, as I do this frequently, it is a constant reminder but I also remember her at other times.

I loved your description of her quietness. It is the first time that I have really had a picture of how she is now and it was very precious.

I am very glad that Betty shared the extract I sent her from the life of Helen Waddell whose books have been very important for me and who also had this long time of being incommunicado.

I am not sure if you know how many times I visited with Sister Zita Marie in the States but we went twice to Gethsemane together and I also spent a few days with her in New Mexico and visited the Grand Canyon as well as two trips when we were both speaking at conferences together. But, best of all of course, I remember the nine months that she spent with us here when she was a very precious part of our most early days.

I am enclosing one or two copies of my husband's pictures and, when my collection which I have put together as a search for meaning comes out next month, I will be sending you that.

Sydney Cauveren

Glebe, New South Wales, Australia

22 August 1990 Thank you for your letter. You will find my autograph at the end of this letter and I hope this will be suitable to add to your collection.

Thank you also for your congratulations on the Order of Merit. I am afraid, however, that we only meet together about every 5 years or so and there is no group photograph that I have available as I have not yet been on such an occasion. I am sorry to disappoint you about this.

Kayumi Saito

Chiyoda-ku, Tokyo, Japan

11 September 1990 Barbara has brought me back the copy of your translation of Shirley du Boulay's biography as a present from you. I am quite fascinated to see it and very grateful to you for having given it to me and, of course, above all for all the trouble and time you must have taken in making the translation.

I am going to keep it in our bookshop here so that we can show it to Japanese visitors and encourage them to buy it when they get back to their own country.

Barbara seems to have had a very good and very busy time. It is very exciting to think of the development in hospice work that is happening in your country and it is a great credit to you and your husband and the others who have worked so hard.

Grace Goldin

Swarthmore, Pennsylvania, USA

1 October 1990 As soon as I showed your photographs to Marian he seized the best and put them in his album and asked me to tell you that he thinks you have yet again caught us both, particularly me this time.

There are a number of people asking for photographs from time to time and I would very much like to have some more copies of number 34A. I took the liberty of having some black and white copies done of the one that you liked best but there are some people who need colour and I have nothing up to date now. Is it asking too much for half a dozen?

I have re-read your wonderful description of the holiday and hope very much that you are both carrying on with the benefit of your time and Judah's time in hospital.

Marian says he has completed a series of portraits and has just done a beautiful pencilled drawing of a Catholic chaplain who is here for two months for an interregnum. I think he is going to turn to drawings for a spell and probably this is a good thing because the last portrait took him a very long time to complete, although it is certainly one of his best.

We enjoyed his granddaughters from Poland for two weeks here and only had my stepson for three days, so we did not have such a visitation as last year, when we were both of us fairly tired at the end of it all.

The Hospice seems to be busier than ever with tremendous pressure, particularly on Home Care but also on our beds. It seems to be difficult for people to realise that the hospice can actually be full and have people waiting and not be able to take somebody as an emergency, although we always try to do this for anyone who is under our Home Care Team.

I am dictating this with quite bad toothache and am about to go off to the dentist. I seem to remember that you were having a marathon going with dentistry and I hope it all finished successfully.

I did my satellite broadcast to the Montreal Conference last evening with a nice slide of the Syrian Monastery, planned to show not only the very early roots but the mix of patients who were taken in at that time. I was talking about hospice as bridgebuilder, with one bridge to history which is how that came in. I won't bother you with the whole script, which after all is dependent very much on its 68 slides. It may turn up as an article one day.

Brother Roger[23]

Taizé, Burgundy, France

9 October 1990 For many years, ever since I had a few days in Grandchamp in 1961, I have followed the development of their community and of Taizé itself with prayer and thought, especially through correspondence with Sister Gilberte, who was at Taizé as part of your hospitality. The community at Grandchamp have prayed for the developing work of

---

23 Founder of the Taizé community in France.

St Christopher's Hospice which I was planning when I visited there and which opened in 1967 and was the first of now many modern hospices throughout this country.

I have recently read "The Taizé Experience" with photographs by Vladimir Sichov. I am writing because you refer to "western homes for the dying" as being places of "abandonment and isolation". I am aware that you are referring to an all too prevalent disregard of the deprived in the west but I would like to reassure you that hospice and hospice teams out in the community and, increasingly, within general hospitals, are endeavouring to help dying people to live until they die and to do so as part of their families and part of the larger community around. St Christopher's itself is very much part of our local area and in particular has links with many churches and Christian people, some of whom are our hardworking volunteers. It is a place of life and living with a nursery for children, including those of the staff, and a wing for elderly people, with priority for our own dependants. I hope this pattern will be repeated increasingly around the world.

We do not compare with the impact that your work has had but I thought you might be comforted to know that there are many, often with a Christian commitment, who are endeavouring to care for dying people in the west and elsewhere.

Dr Gary A. Johanson
Sebastopol, California, USA

23 October 1990 Thank you very much for your letter. I am glad you appreciated both the satellite presentation and our team. I am sorry you did not have time for your question.

I am sure you use your "flexible repertoire" of responses very sensitively when dealing with the fears of the occasional physician, because there is no doubt that any kind of confrontation is counter productive. However, I suppose we have developed over the years with the philosophy that we will work hard with those who will co-operate with us and not waste too much time with those who wish to have little or nothing to do with what we have to offer. We often find that many times it is the third party, that is the co-operating physician, who will influence and persuade the others in the long run. Secondly, I suppose we can help by presenting objective data, good sound research and its writing up in general as well as specialist journals has a place here. Finally, however, I suppose we have to accept that we cannot win them all, although sometimes people will come back long after you seem to have lost touch or have any chance of altering attitudes and fears.

Dr Charles-Henri Rapin[24]
Centre des soins continues, Geneva, Switzerland

26 October 1990 It was a great pleasure and surprise to receive the telegram from the First Congress of the European Association of Palliative Care. Thank you so much for thinking of the beginnings of this movement and of us at St Christopher's.

I have heard from our participants that it was a very interesting meeting and I was also glad to hear that as well as having a large meeting there was also encouragement for smaller

---

[24] Geriatrician, pioneer of palliative care in Switzerland, and later Vice-President of the European Association for Palliative Care.

more regional meetings, especially for the type where a more limited number of participants from different countries can share their own experience both from years of work and also from the difficulties and excitements of starting palliative care in a variety of ways.

Sandol Stoddard

Holualoa, Hawaii, USA

5 November 1990 Thank you very much for the two chapters of the new book. Quite a lot is happening around the world.

I thought you might be interested in something by Dr Anne Merriman who was so much involved with Hospice Singapore in its earliest days and who, as you know, is now in Nairobi.

To bring you up to date with the United Kingdom, I enclose a copy of a paper from our Hospice Information Service.

At the moment, Help the Hospices is providing leadership of a sort for the independent hospices but we are looking carefully at a single hospice voice that may be a little stronger in negotiation with Government and in some more general fund raising and, of course, the setting of standards.

I do not know whether anyone has told you about the presentations at Montreal. I did something on Hospice as Bridgebuilder via satellite. I enclose a copy of the typescript, which of course, will not read the same without being able to see the splendid set of slides I showed. The inter-disciplinary team from St Christopher's did an excellent presentation about a family in pain in the morning and a team in pain in the afternoon. I also enclose a copy of our latest book which includes contributions by staff, some of whom were members of the team who presented in Montreal.

I suppose Lambeth is a dazzling award, although it has never struck me as being more exciting than the fact that I got the British Medical Association's Gold Medal for clinical expertise, but perhaps that is a good juxtaposition with Lambeth, which has its theological background. The one formerly given to Florence Nightingale is the Order of Merit, which is a personal award from the Monarch. There are only 24 holders at any one time and I was only the fifth woman to receive it since it was set up in 1901.

I am also enclosing a note of our latest International Conference. We hope we will top the 37 different countries who had representatives at the last conference. I am sorry you are so far away, you would enjoy meeting them all.

You are indefatigable with your writing and it was lovely to hear from you again.

Professor Vittorio Ventafridda

European Association for Palliative Care, Milan, Italy

12 November 1990 Thank you so much for your letter. The idea of seeing you to talk through some of the possibilities that lie ahead is very attractive and I hope that you will be coming to London and will get in touch with me and hopefully be able to visit St Christopher's again.

I never go away because my husband is now too frail and elderly to travel himself and neither can I leave him. However, I do have a number of commitments here and it would be helpful if you could give me some notice when you think you might be coming to London.

I enclose a copy of our latest Drug Control of Common Symptoms which Mary has just completed.

Dr Alexander Waller

Hospice, Tel Hashomer Hospital, Ramat Gan, Tel Aviv, Israel

3 January 1991 Many thanks indeed for your postcard from Montreal after the Conference. It was quite an experience being on satellite and surprising how near you seemed to me as I gather I seemed to you.

In your card you said you would send me the draft of your poster on intravenous fluids and I am looking forward to receiving this.

We had a good Christmas here. Marian is well and painting and has his 90th Name Day on 2nd February.

Renate Niebler

Koln, Germany

7 January 1991 I hope you got safely back to Germany, although I think you may be a little surprised to get a letter from me straight away.

I mentioned your interest to our Director of Nursing, Mrs Barbara Saunders, and you will be hearing from her directly offering you a place as one of our summer volunteers. She was more ready than I expected to consider your working the usual weekly stint and to use your camera in your off duty time. As she will tell you, this will mean there will be accommodation here and you will be on the spot all the time that you need to be.

I hope you will consider this because we remain very impressed by your pictures of Dachau and are always ready to try and help hospice development elsewhere, especially of course in Munich after our long connection with Father Iblacker. We would also hope to be able to use some of your photographs ourselves should they seem suitable for any of our Reports or Journals.

I hope this sounds reasonable for you. It will, of course, be some time after you expect to be in Munich which will give you a chance to be thinking around what it is you want to present.

The Rt Hon Virginia Bottomley MP

Minister for Health, London

11 January 1991 We were indeed delighted to have the news that the Government is giving nearly £17 million this coming financial year to hospice work.[25] This is very good news and we look forward to our own contacts with the South East Thames Regional Health Authority and the Districts in the South West Thames area which are served by St Christopher's.

I enclose a copy of the Report of the survey carried out by Human Perspectives for Young and Rubicam which was commissioned and partly funded by St Christopher's and which we discussed at the dinner party where I met you recently. We are finding this very

---

[25] Following a ministerial statement in late 1989, the UK government sought to move towards a full funding partnership with the country's voluntary hospices. New monies of £8 million accompanied the statement; by 1993 the government's total contribution had risen to £43 million. Well received by the hospices, the allocation came to be known as 'Bottomley monies' after the Secretary of State at the time.

useful as we plan our public relations and development and it is very opportune that we should have opened our enlarged Day Centre and Home Care base just recently.

Dr Jan Stjernsward

World Health Organisation, Geneva, Switzerland

7 February 1991 Thank you so much for sending me the Cancer Pain Relief and Palliative Care book.[26] I was very glad to receive it although I had seen Dr Mary Baines' copy briefly. I understand that there is going to be a further book on other symptom control, which of course is only touched upon in the two books published so far.

I am enclosing a book we have recently produced from here which I think adds a dimension to the literature which has not been looked at closely so far. I think that it is in working in a team and addressing a number of major problems that emerge, often more obviously once pain and symptom control has been achieved, that is the way forward.

I am delighted that palliative medicine is spreading on such a firm basis these days and much look forward to the Oxford Textbook. I think there will still be a place for hospice Home Care, Day Centre and In-Patient Teams and our experience has been very much as it was summed up by Dr Thelma Bates, the Radiotherapist and Oncologist at St Thomas' Hospital, who said that once she had her Team established "I do not use hospices less, I just use them more rationally". So long as we maintain our standards and continue with all the volunteers, research and training that is demanded of us, I think we will be a useful resource for perhaps a large number of people who will be working within more traditional medical settings.

Henry Ejike

Sacred Hearth Catholic Parish, Kogi State, Nigeria, West Africa

28 January 1991 Thank you for your letter and your interest in St Christopher's. I am enclosing a brochure about what we do and you will see that we are an ecumenical and not a Catholic hospice and we do not, therefore, have a particular concern for devotion in honour of St Christopher himself, who I understand has been demoted in the Catholic Church as being a legend rather than a historical person.

However, I think there must have been a well loved person helping people across a dangerous river to whom the legend was attached. This states that Christopher, who was very strong, heard a knock at his door one stormy night and found a child who wanted to cross the river. As he carried him across he felt an almost intolerable weight and realised that this was the Christ child himself, bearing the sorrows of the world, but that at the same time strength was coming from the child that enabled Christopher to continue the journey. He

---

[26] Dr Jan Stjernsward, as head of the World Health Organization's Cancer and Palliative Care Programme, had been working since the early 1980s on the problem of cancer pain relief, worldwide. The publication referred to here is the revised version of *Cancer pain relief* (Geneva: WHO, 1986), which appeared as *Cancer pain relief and palliative care*, Technical Report Series 804 (Geneva: WHO: 1990).

carried him safely over the river and was blessed. St Christopher has therefore become the patron saint of travellers and as we are caring for people on their last journey, we have chosen him knowing that his legend implies that people are travelling in danger to a mysterious destination but that Christ will take them there safely.

Dr Alexander Waller

Hospice, Tel Hashomer Hospital, Ramat Gan, Tel Aviv, Israel

13 February 1991 Thank you so much for your letter and the important Abstract. I am delighted to have it and am circulating it round our doctors, one of whom is interested in pursuing such a study here. This will be very helpful.

Your greetings arrived for the Professor's Name Day and he was very delighted. We had a lovely party and he managed to give a good speech on how his life was preserved when he was fighting the Bolsheviks.

We are thinking of Israel continually and certainly of you as you work under emergency conditions.

Professor Eric Wilkes

Trent Region Palliative and Continuing Care Centre, Sheffield

18 February 1991 I really must congratulate you on your masterly handling of the founding of a National Hospice Council.[27] I understand that things are going ahead, with Mike Carleton-Smith being proposed as a Vice Chairman and it seems to me that we are really on the move at long last.

I am sure the fact that it has come to hand in this way is because the time has finally come and because of the rather firm stand by the Minister and the Department, who are obviously tired of dealing with different groups all the time. I see plenty of problems ahead but at last I can view them from the sidelines as an elder statesman and from the occasional meeting with the Minister and others on a more informal basis.

We have all come a long way since we first started talking in the 1960s.

Dr H. Milberg

München, Germany

19 February 1991 Thank you for your letter which reached me this morning.

I am very interested in what you say although of course I cannot read the brochure in German.

I have a great admiration for Father Iblacker and all that he has done for hospice in Germany. However, I am not prepared to have a medal named after me. I have refused on several occasions to have a hospice called after me and I think it is very important

---

[27] This was soon to become the National Council for Hospice and Specialist Palliative Care Services.

that the movement is not just identified with one person. I would suggest, therefore, that you should call it the Hospice Medal or something similar, which no doubt you will choose.

I would certainly support the idea that Father Iblacker should be the first recipient of an award and may I tentatively suggest that perhaps a grant of money towards the work might encourage it even more.

Grace Goldin
Swarthmore, Pennsylvania, USA

18 April 1991 Thank you so much for taking the trouble to read all through my introduction of the Oxford Textbook. I agree with you about the negative spaces but that is really rather difficult in that particular setting although it is important as inaccuracies, of course, creep in and nobody else knows the full story.

I am glad you found some new things in it. The French hospices were certainly known as custodial care and it is very interesting that two or three of them are getting well involved in the new moves in France which come under the general heading of Palliative Care. We have just had a "French Day" here at the hospice with 60 enthusiastic people coming over. All the talks were given in French by English hospice workers. Our Director of Studies and Director of Social Work are both fluent French speakers and there is a Doctor at St Joseph's Hospice, a social worker from the North London Hospice and a nurse at Southampton who all speak good French. The day was very much appreciated by the French delegates.

I am delighted that you continue to use some of those early slides because they really were marvellous and although I do not do my clinical lecturing any longer, I occasionally go back to them to illustrate the sort of talks I now give which are more on the historical or philosophical side.

I am delighted about the poems because, as you say, the subject is unexplored realistically.

I hope Passover went well. You really do work hard. I imagine them from my fairly sparse knowledge but we had a good programme recently on television which gave quite a lot of the family seder of one of our more well known Rabbis over here.

We have Princess Alexandra coming next week to open what has been called the Albertine Centre, which has spacious rooms for Home Care with its clinics, family meetings as well as space for the 11 nurses and other staff who work there and a Day Centre which is being run most imaginatively and is full of life. We have about 20 people during the day time, two thirds from home and one third come across from the wards. It is a beautiful building with several rooms in an octagonal shape and unusual windows. Somehow the architect has made it fit between our ward building and the house in the middle of our whole site.

I am amazed you had not realised Marian had reached 90. He really looks very much the same as that wonderful photograph you took some three years ago. He is only rather more wobbly on his legs and needs extra care getting organised in the mornings and evenings. Today he is doing a pencil drawing of our Catholic Chaplain and he has a splendid portrait of one of his pupils who has a beard and which he is just on the point of completing.

Dr Sam Ahmedzai

Leicestershire Hospice, Leicester

9 May 1991 I was interested to see that you are doing a survey on Research in Palliative Care,[28] well remembering the time when you came to see us before we appointed Tom Walsh. Sadly, he is so busy in the States that he has never been able to send us more than an abstract of his work with antidepressants in pain, though he completed a considerable number of papers and other studies while he was with us.

I am very pleased to see that you are looking at a general view of this field, although of course there will be people who have ideas in very early stages which they are not yet quite ready to share. While it is important that we do not overlap, I think it is also helpful when people do similar work in different places.

We have a very excellent Research Committee now, including Sir Raymond Hoffenberg, Sir James Gowans and Professor Patrick Wall. I think they would all be very interested in any report you may produce as an overview of the field and I hope we will have something to hand in due course.

I hope your hospice goes well. I am sorry we are so far away and that it is not easy for me to get to the Association meetings, but I follow what is happening with continued interest.

You will, of course, be hearing of our current projects in due course but I thought I would write to you personally in the meantime.

Professor Eric Wilkes

Calver, Derbyshire

13 May 1991 You deserve all our thanks and congratulations for bringing the National Council into being. It needed you to do it and I doubt whether anyone else could have managed it, although of course you needed the backing of Anne [Duchess of Norfolk] and, in the distance, myself and others.

It will be very interesting to see how it goes although I feel the first few meetings may be quite rough and Bob Evans[29] will need a certain amount of encouragement and support. All the same, the Minister was delighted and I think an important step forward has been taken.

As I said at the HtH meeting, I was not persuaded that we needed a national organisation at an earlier stage, but I am sure we do now. This is not only because of the proliferation of hospices and the danger of there being a request for inclusion by nursing homes of dubious quality, but also because the Government is going to make us look at all the things we have been discussing if they are going to give more realistic funding.

I cannot believe that you will now merely retire to your garden and I am sure you will have some background input. No doubt I will be doing a little bit that way myself.

---

[28] The survey was published as *Palliative care research in Europe* (Leicester: LOROS Palliative Care Research Fund, 1992). Sam Ahmedzai was appointed Professor of Palliative Medicine at the University of Sheffield in 1994.

[29] The then Chairman of British Gas, who adopted the role of Chairman of the National Council for Hospice and Specialist Palliative Care Services.

Patrice O'Connor
The St Luke's/Roosevelt Hospital Center, New York, USA

23 May 1991 I was indeed sad to have your letter and it was news to me, as I had not heard from Carleton. In fact no one here has heard from him since his retirement and we were beginning to get rather worried as to how he was.

Sam Klagsbrun was here yesterday and I had some discussion with him about it and I gather that another Team has come into the same trouble as a non-revenue producing department. With our new system of contracts within our National Health Service, we may well come up against the same problem for the similar teams here. It is sad indeed that the pioneer team of them all in St Luke's should be the first to go.

I hope very much that you will be able to continue in an educational role. The Team has had such an impact on the hospital but I know how easily the things you teach could be dropped out of people's thinking.

I am so glad to hear that Carleton is on a holiday and will also be planning to come to Italy in the summer. I hope very much he may call in on us on the way. It must be difficult for him to re-organise his life after such a long service of such deep commitment.

I am sending you my enlarged Anthology with special good wishes and hopes that we will meet somewhere some time.

Catherine Musgrave
Jerusalem, Israel

29 May 1991 Thank you so much for sending me your article on acute post-operative pain. I congratulate you on your very detailed and careful look at the literature and the neat presentation of the major advances. Thank you also for the Pain Protocol which I hope will be useful to many who will not have an opportunity of seeing the WHO Cancer Pain Relief booklet, which is rather expensive though good.

Have you thought of getting some kind of thesis accepted by a University, or are you too busy in the active work and hopefully in looking at the problem of dehydration and its treatment? In case you may not have seen it, I enclose a copy of the presentation that Dr Waller made to our Advanced Symptom Control Workshop at our International Conference last week. I hope we will be looking at this problem at St Christopher's in the not too distant future.

We have thought of you in Israel a great deal recently. I do hope some solution will be found to the endless problem of threat.

The two Bulgarian doctors whom you met at a European conference have been in touch with me and duly came to our International Conference. At the moment they are visiting a smaller hospice and they will come back to us next week. They seem delightful people up against tremendous odds with an even less sympathetic milieu for work in palliative care than in Israel.

Reverend Carleton Sweetser
Teaneck, New Jersey, USA

10 June 1991 We are hoping to see something of you if you pass through London on your summer holidays this year. We have thought of you a lot and I was very sad indeed to hear of the end of the hospice team. However, a letter from Florence today tells me that Patrice, having stood firm, has been given permission to approach a Foundation for a year's grant, so perhaps it will continue and lead into a teaching programme.

It is difficult to believe that the finances are so difficult that such an important team should be closed down and we will continue to pray and hope that at least the teaching side will continue. They needed you and your position to protect them, although it is hardly helpful for me to tell you that.

In the meantime, I hope you are adjusting to retirement and as that is a kind of bereavement, I am sending the enclosed in the hope that you do not need it any more.

Marian is well and his last two portraits are particularly strong. We had a lively celebration of his 90th birthday and will shortly be welcoming his daughter over from San Francisco.

Professor Balfour Mount

Royal Victoria Hospital, Montreal, Canada

21 June 1991 I was delighted to have your long letter with the general agreement on comments about the proposed Association, or whatever it will call itself.

The news that you are going to be full time in the Palliative Care Service is indeed good and I am not surprised that those you mention are well stuck into their present post and unwilling to move. May I make one comment, and that is that I am sure it would be an enormous help to the Service if they had a really firm diary of your other activities and knew exactly when you were going to be around well ahead of time. I have the feeling, though of course I may be maligning you, that your attendance is sometimes rather mercurial and a touch unpredictable! You will have many demands on your time and I know from experience how difficult it is to have a real clinical commitment and a general role, both public and political as well as educational. Even you cannot be in two places at once!

Dr Gary Gambuti

St Luke's/Roosevelt Hospice Center, New York, USA

10 July 1991 You will probably not be surprised to hear from me with my concern at the end of the Palliative Care Team in St Luke's/Roosevelt. It is sad indeed that this first ever hospital team at the hospice/hospital interface should come to an end because of financial problems.

I understand, however, that Patrice O'Connor is trying to set up an Education Programme which would at least keep hospice care and principles to the fore. I am sure that if we are going to continue to give our terminally ill and dying patients all that they deserve in the place where so many of them are cared for, the acute general medical centres, that this important innovation should be supported. I wonder if there is any chance of the hospital at least giving Patrice a start as she looks for finances for her budget.

There are now some 40 Teams around our country and there is no doubt that they are carrying out an important educational role. None of them pre-date the St Luke's Team and many have drawn their inspiration from the news of its work. It seems to me it would be a tragedy if the hospital failed to support this initiative, especially when the situation in medicine has so many pressures that militate against optimal care at this time of a person's life.

Whatever they call this, Teams and Educational Programmes of this type are a most important growing point in the whole hospice movement.

Dr Luzito de Souza

Shanti Avedna Ashram, Bandra, Bombay, India

7 August 1991 Mary Baines tells me that you would very much like a short message for you to include in your brochure. I am not sure how much you want but I imagine it does not have to be much longer than the following:

> Those of us at St Christopher's Hospice and all those who attended our first International Conference in 1980 remember with great pleasure the visit of Dr de Souza and the imaginative plans he was putting forward for the Shanti Avedna Ashram. It is good news indeed that, not only has such good work been done in Bombay since 1986, but also that there is the development in Goa and plans for Delhi. This is a great achievement and we have all followed its progress with admiration.
>
> It is exciting now that you are holding your own International Conference and we send our very good wishes for a splendid time together and a further growth of the work for suffering people each in your own ways as East meets West.

Major General M. E. Carleton-Smith[30]

Marie Curie Cancer Care, London

27 August 1991 Many thanks indeed for sending me the circular about the National Council. I am pleased that it is coming together and it certainly looks as though the Executive Director has a relevant background and a good base from which to learn more of our own particular scene.

We would be very happy to welcome her here for one of her early visits to assess what is going on in the hospice world, particularly as, of course, we have been a centre for information for so long. This has been much drawn on by Paul Rossi and other people and, of course, we have many personal links as our Information Officers had been in post for a number of years.

I think the definition of the role of the Council has been very well set out and I hope that we will be looking at standards across the whole field, such as those our patients deserve.

We are certainly going to have to learn how to work best with the NHS reforms and I think hospices will be needing the Council in this field as in many others as it develops. I hope you will enjoy your own role.

---

[30] After his retirement from the army, Michael Carleton-Smith became Director General of the charity Marie Curie Cancer Care in 1985. He was instrumental in the early 1990s in establishing the National Council for Hospice and Specialist Palliative Care Services.

Birger Jorgensen

Oresundskollegiet, Copenhagen, Denmark

9 September 1991 Thank you for your letter all about the visit of Ingrid Monsen. I am afraid I do not remember all the details of her visit but one thing in your letter is certainly inaccurate. There is no second Guest or Visitors Book and certainly none which has only four names in it and her name as the fifth entry. We do give a separate page to our Patron, Princess Alexandra, as we did for Her Majesty The Queen, but they are in the ordinary book.

Perhaps you do not realise that we have some 3,000 visitors from overseas during the course of a year as well as a heavy teaching programme for people in our own country and our own staff. We try as much as we can to give them what they would like, although this is not always possible.

Dr Jan Deszcs

The Krakow Hospice, Krakow, Poland

23 September 1991 I wrote to you on the 31st July to say that St Christopher's Hospice would like to be twinned with The Association of Friends of the Sick in view of our long, though rather intermittent, connections. I wonder if this letter has reached you because I would very much like to have your confirmation of this and certainly to hear from you before our Annual General Meeting which takes place at the end of October.

However, I am now writing with what I am sure you will feel is very good news. I was asked by an anonymous charity to recommend an overseas hospice in need of money and I sent them your leaflet asking for support and describing the beginnings of your building of a hospice unit. I am now happy to tell you that they wish to give you a grant of £30,000 without making any conditions as to exactly what you should use it for. However, as this was in response to your leaflet, they were probably thinking that at least a major part of it would go towards your building. The money will come to St Christopher's and I now need to know how you would like it transferred to your hospice. Please could you let me know how you would like this transferred (in pounds sterling or in dollars) and your Bank details (your account number and the name of the account). If it is easier to fax me this information, our number is at the head of this letter. I would be glad to know your fax number if you have one as post to Poland still seems to be somewhat unreliable.

Robert Evans

British Gas, London

8 October 1991 Thank you once again for a splendid lunch and what I thought was a very good discussion. I was delighted to be brought so well up to date and think that matters have been resolved so far well enough to feel quite optimistic for the future of the National Council.

You mentioned the Report which goes before the European Parliament on November 7th and I can only say that I hope that they might extract the offending sentences which suggest that doctors should go ahead with deliberate and intentional killing of patients because, as you say, the rest of the statement gives a very positive view of palliative care. I think the great danger is of bringing the two together as having the same aims. In a sense I suppose they have, in that both are determined to relieve suffering, but all we have been working on in the last decades has shown that you do not have to kill the patient to kill the pain, and that you can address the further aspects of suffering in a much more positive way. For those who are finally unrelieved of their mental anguish, I think we can only stand by. Should there be a law which would make their exit possible, it would undermine the right to care for so many more.

We have a visitor from Denmark this week and I am horrified at what he says of the inept care in the Danish hospitals he knows. We have a long way to go to spread the knowledge that has been mainly developed in this country.

Patrice O'Connor
St Luke's Roosevelt Hospital Center, New York, USA

8 November 1991 I was delighted to have your letter with its good news and I hope and believe that you will have done such a good job by March 1993 that there may even be a demand for the Team to return in full but hopefully you will have made a difference to care in the meantime.

I showed the "Death Anxiety Scale" and the original article to Colin Murray Parkes yesterday. His comment was that, even though it is quoted in major studies, it is not necessarily something suitable for use with patients such as we are caring for. When he asked me whether I would be happy at presenting it to a patient at St Christopher's rather than to a fit person, possibly as young as a student looking at the future, I certainly took his point, which I am therefore passing on to you. He has been looking at various scales as he plans a study comparing care in hospice wards with care in hospital wards and is much more knowledgeable in this area than I am.

Thank you also for the article on auditing hospital records. If you have time to send me your results, I would be very interested to keep in touch over this.

I am amused that you refer to me as "Chairwoman". I really am Madam Chairman, although I am sure that would upset some feminists. I suppose I am old enough to have been really entrenched in the old phraseology!

Professor Balfour Mount
Royal Victoria Hospital, Montreal, Canada

27 February 1992 Sandol Stoddard has just written to me and I have received the updated and expanded copy of her book "The Hospice Movement".[31] Going through it at some speed as I was sitting with Marian yesterday, I was very interested to find a note about your weekly meeting called "partege". Have you written anything about this, is it still going and would you send me anything you may have on it? I would be very interested and I am sure our Chaplain, Len Lunn, would be too. He does something a bit similar in our Day Centre on a regular basis and is very imaginative in his own way.

---

[31] M. Stoddard, *The hospice movement*, rev. edn (New York: Vintage Books, 1992).

Prayers here in the mornings in chapel now take place at 8.50 am and this enables some of the nurses to come. It is well attended at the moment and is often more a "thought for the day" rather than prayers and that means we have a great variety of people taking it in a great variety of ways. Marian has been in one of the wards here for the past two months and so I have been able to go sometimes and have appreciated the chance to do so.

Marian had an acute gastro-intestinal bleed just before Christmas and lost a lot of blood. He became very ill and also confused on Cimetidine. The hospice scooped us up two days after Christmas, but he goes home this weekend, we hope for good. He had a chest infection and was very ill but is pulling up slowly. He is very weak on his legs so I cannot leave him at all. Help will be organised and once Rugby ward has been refurbished, he will be able to go back to his studio and be managed as part of their commitment during the day, which will give me a bit more freedom.

Another question I would like to ask you is whether you believe, as we have been thinking in this country, that our ethnic minorities do not on the whole want to come into hospice, whether or not it is a hospice known as a Christian Foundation, as we are. I remember when visiting the PCU [Palliative Care Unit] that it seemed that at least half of the names indicated that people came from Europe as displaced persons, or from other minority groups. Is there any difference in the attitude towards palliative care in the French and English speaking and in these other groups? Have you looked at this since you had the chapter in "Hospice – the Living Idea" from our Bar Mitzvah Conference? We would be very interested as we are getting together with Dr Sam Ahmedzai, who runs the Leicester Hospice, to look at this. He works in a very multi-ethnic society but has just the same hospice population as we do apparently.

I do hope all goes well with you both at home and at work. I like the filming that Father Iblacker did in the PCU and which he has recently sent me. I much enjoyed my visits and wonder if you have developed as much as we seem to have done, although I think, from being around the ward now for 2 months as a wife, the basics are still there.

Grace Goldin

Swarthmore, Pennsylvania, USA

26 March 1992 Here is the suggested foreword[32] which I hope is a reasonable length. I have tried to salute your incredible breadth of work, both in the early chapters and in the latter part with the modern hospice. However, you will see that I have taken the story on a bit because it is really important that we should now emphasise that hospice has widened its spiritual sights even since you last visited us. It is fascinating how you pick that up out of different strands in your second chapter about us all and how without, I believe, compromising too much, we have kept a spiritual dimension as part of our hospitality. I know Derek Doyle up in Edinburgh feels that there has been quite a secularisation of the whole hospice scene but we have had such tremendous response every time we have put on a conference on spiritual issues that we have to keep repeating it. There is no doubt that the situ-

---

[32] This appeared as C. Saunders, Foreword, in *Work of mercy. A picture history of hospitals* (ed. G. Goldin) (Ontario, Canada: The Boston Mills Press, 1994).

ations in which our patients find themselves call out questions of a very deep kind which, in this day and age, are not couched in specifically religious terms, although some people certainly turn to the more traditional prayers and services that we maintain on a voluntary basis. If you feel I have gone too far from the scene as you saw it on your journeys around, come back to me and I will do some re-writing, but I would like to make this salute to the hospice capacity for taking real note of the contributions of its very varied group of patients, family and staff.

I have very few comments on the earlier chapters except that I wonder whether you should refer to the "Iron Curtain" without perhaps qualification. I think your contrast between photographs of buildings and the details thereof and the occasional old print or revealing face is quite fascinating and I am not at all surprised that your publishers like it.

I have not had time to dig out the photographs that you took of a patient who was discharged and her husband but I am hoping to do this when Marian is in his studio on Saturday while he is painting a doctor friend. I think it is important because you hardly emphasise home care at all, which after all we began in 1969 and you have no photograph of a family member and they have been our unit of care from the beginning. That must be a real distinction between us and the older hospices. Even Dr Barrett, although he mentions the sad state of the families at home, can do little about them.

You will find I have written all over chapters 17 and 18, particularly the St Christopher's bit. I thought that was better than making a long list in a letter. I know you are hampered by words and I doubt you can put anything else in but there are a few inaccuracies which I think you wanted me to correct. Early on, as I told you on the telephone, I have pointed out that in fact the Australian hospice was after the Dublin one and both of them after Mme Jeanne Garnier in France. The Sisters of St Joseph's are sure that there was no connection and that the word "hospice" in connection with the dying in the two separate settings came from two separate inspirations. It was fascinating to have two or three people with connections to some of the few Homes that remain (there were 7 in all) at a French speaking conference we had two or three years ago. They are hoping to re-introduce true hospice principles to what have become places of custodial care. Earlier than that, we had two visitors from the Paris house, which is now called Maison Medicale de Jeanne Garnier, one the former Administrator and the other a volunteer. The former felt we had moved on from the original vision and has kept in touch, sending me good wishes every year. It was obvious that at that time the doctors had not really moved into true palliative care, but hopefully this will happen as there is quite a lively movement in France now. It is because of the alms house custodial image of hospice in mainland Europe that the word cannot helpfully be used there. In fact the Oxford Textbook, which is in preparation at the moment, will be called the *Textbook of Palliative Medicine*.

I have spoken to Mrs D on the telephone about the photograph of your 16 year old and she assures me that she and her husband will be quite happy for you to include it. She was going to ask him to call me back if he had any further thoughts when he came home but he did not call, so I was to take it that all was well.

Finally, congratulations on a magnum opus. I long to see it in proper print with all the illustrations and am only sorry I have never had a chance to see the exhibition on which it has been based.

Dr John F. Scott

University of Ottawa, Ottawa, Ontario, Canada

1 June 1992 I was reading your article "Palliative Care 2000: What's Stopping Us?" in the *Journal of Palliative Care* with great interest and am taking the opportunity to get in touch once again. There seem to be rather a lot of problems at the moment in palliative care in different countries, all including much the same things that you are facing in rather different proportions. Dr Gillian Ford's Editorial in the last issue of *Palliative Medicine*, a copy of which I enclose, highlights some of them from our point of view. We are fortunate in being rather more recognised by the medical fraternity than many countries but our heavy reliance on voluntary giving in a time of recession makes us vulnerable, as also does the new era of the open market and the negotiating of contracts, although I am happy to say that St Christopher's itself has so far had a great deal of understanding from our own Regional Health Authority. They are hopefully going to do a certain amount of ring-fencing with the small District Health Authorities with whom we relate.

Meantime I am sure the work between patient, family and staff must continue much as yours does but we have to look at the wider, more political issues if that is to be maintained.

How is life treating you? I would love to hear how your personal saga is going. Mine is happily divided between work and a lot of care now for my very frail husband, who has now reached 91 and has gone through a series of life-threatening problems. He is still painting and I bring him into the hospice to his studio every day and, with a certain amount of help am able to do some work here, though no longer on the clinical scene except very much in the background. Tom West will be retiring at the end of the year and we will be appointing his successor shortly. We have two very good candidates. It will be very much a new era for us but I have great hopes of it.

You may not have seen my Editorial on euthanasia, nor the enclosed issue of the journal Contact in which I try to tackle spiritual pain. I remember hearing you talking around that area in Montreal some years ago and I am sure you have been thinking deeply about it ever since. Have you written anything else in that field, or any other for that matter?

Professor Geoffrey Hanks[33]

St Thomas' Hospital, London

8 June 1992 You may be interested to know that last week we appointed Dr Robert Dunlop to the post of Medical Director/Chief Executive at St. Christopher's. He will be taking up the post some time in the late autumn. As you no doubt know, he was at Bart's for two years heading up the Palliative Care Team there and he has a wide experience now. We look forward to working with him. I am sure he will be in touch with you soon after he takes up the post.

---

[33] At the time recently appointed to the first chair of palliative medicine in the United Kingdom, a co-editor the following year of the first edition of the *Oxford textbook of palliative medicine*, and from 1995 to 1999 President of the European Association for Palliative Care.

I have been thinking about the Second Congress of the European Association for Palliative Care in Brussels in October. Since I wrote to you my husband has been very ill but he has recovered and I can now call on a very good care assistant, which hopefully will make it easier for me to come to Brussels at that time.

In thinking around the topic for the closing Address, my initial idea is of approaching the challenges and potential to the patient and family, particularly in the later phases of the disease, although not necessarily right at the end. Without idealising what people can make of this time, I feel this is an emphasis that could be shared by all the participants as we all try to enable our patients and families to reach their full potential. It seems to me this might pick up on some of the themes of the conference, but I would be interested in your reaction to my first thoughts.

Dr William Lamers

Malibu, California, USA

4 August 1992 Many thanks for your long letter and for the interesting Review which you enclosed. It is very sad that the worlds of technology, dying and hospice are so often separated and it does seem to me that the chronic pain group, the palliative medicine group and the hospice group in the States are not always as connected as they might be. I cannot say that we are perfect so far as the pain control group here are concerned but fortunately we have a lot of interest from Patrick Wall on the basic side and as an Editor of the Pain Journal.

We are moving into a new era with a new Medical Director coming on board at the end of the year. He is Dr Robert Dunlop from New Zealand who worked in this country for two years in the Palliative Care Team at St Bartholomew's Hospital. I think he will take us on in a stimulating and exciting way. Tom will retire to East Anglia, having worked very hard for 20 years here. I shall stay around as Chairman for the time being over the transition but perhaps more in the background than you might think.

Your home sounds beautiful and I hope the new hospice will develop well. It sounds as though you may have a transport problem but I am sure you will know how to overcome that.

Good luck as you fight the Physician Assisted Suicide ballot.

Muir Hunter

Shaftesbury, Dorset

17 September 1992 Thank you for your letter and for bringing me up to date with what is happening with the Polish Hospices Fund.[34] I am very interested in what you are doing. As you probably know, they are continuing to build a small hospice in Nova Huta and St Christopher's is in fact twinned with it and I have been able to introduce them to an anonymous European Trust who have been very generous to them. I think, having been in home care for so long now in and around Krakow itself, it is the right place for the one demonstration in-patient unit, but I am sure they will have problems with their running costs.

---

[34] Muir Hunter, together with his wife Gillian Petrie, was co-founder of the Polish Hospices Fund, a charity supporting the training and professional development of Polish doctors, nurses, and others.

Obviously, I have been very interested in the Gdansk programme as I was in touch with people there from my visit in 1978. I was very impressed with Professor Joanna Penson when she came to visit St Christopher's some months ago. I also know the health service unit in Poznan and we have had a doctor from there for training.

Having said all this, I am prepared to continue as a Patron, although I have to say my particular concern will remain with Krakow, realising at the same time that home care is the most feasible way of starting up, with all the problems of that country. My admiration for the teams who have been struggling along during the years is undiminished.

The Rt Hon Virginia Bottomley MP

Secretary of State for Health, London

18 November 1992 Before the final decision of the General Medical Council relating to the Cox case[35] was published, I was talking with Sir Raymond Hoffenberg, who is a member of our Research Committee at St Christopher's and who, in fact, was attending the GMC meeting on behalf of Dr Cox. We both felt that the most unfortunate thing about the whole episode was that he did not ask the advice of a palliative, or indeed, terminal care service at a much earlier stage and thus relieve his patient of reaching such a desperate condition. However, this case has focussed attention on such situations and Professor Hoffenberg and I both thought that the time has really come for some form of Royal Commission to look at the whole area of difficult decisions at the end of life.

Previous experience in this area has shown that unless we are extremely careful to lay down guidelines and very clear definitions of what exactly is being discussed, there will be inevitable confusion between inappropriate prolongation of life, adequate control of symptoms even at the risk of bringing forward the time of death, and the degree of autonomy a patient has in the context of the pressures not only upon their family and the staff immediately concerned, but upon society as a whole, which includes so many vulnerable and dependent people.

I have seen the draft of two of the chapters of the new book on Ethics which is being produced by the BMA and am very impressed by the careful consideration they present and the stand they are taking. I was also extremely glad some months ago to have talked around this area with Dr Fleur Fisher and Dr Natalie-Jane McDonald. This is an extremely sensitive area but as so many of the general public must have been left with the impression that the only way to relieve terminal pain was to kill the patient, as has been reported by the media in the Cox case, that I think the time has come for a carefully considered look which hopefully will give guidelines which will make it unnecessary to have a change in legislation. Whatever one thinks of abortion, I am sure it is true that the present climate in that field differs greatly from that intended by Sir David Steel when he originally brought in his Bill in 1967. One only fears that legislation relating to the end of life would have exactly the same results.

---

[35] In 1992 Dr Nigel Cox, a consultant rheumatologist in Hampshire, England, was found guilty of attempted murder, after injecting a seventy-year-old patient with potassium chloride. He was given a suspended sentence by the court and reprimanded by the General Medical Council, but allowed to continue practising medicine.

I presume, should there be a Commission, that you will be very much part of the selection committee of its members, which is why I am writing to you now, knowing of your interest in what we have been trying to do over the past 25 years to make cases such as that of Dr Cox unnecessary.

Professor Greg Wilkinson

The London Hospital Medical College, London

22 January 1993 Thank you for your letter and for inviting me to take part in the conference celebrating the retirement of Colin Murray Parkes. I would be very happy to be involved and am indeed honoured to be asked.

My only problem is that I am the carer of a very frail and elderly husband and if there should happen to be a crisis at that time it might be difficult. However, I have good helpers and certainly anticipate being able to come.

Carolyn Armitage

Hodder & Stoughton, London

26 February 1993 Thank you for your letter, which I have now had an opportunity to discuss with Shirley du Boulay. We would both be very glad to see this book in print again as we are both continually hearing of people who wish to find it and are unable to do so.[36]
Since the last edition was produced, there have been a number of new hospices and a considerable development in our field, both in this country and overseas. Our Hospice Information Service provides a quarterly Bulletin which is sent to the contact people we now have in some 60 countries, many of whom still look to St Christopher's foundation as their original inspiration. I think that suitable publicity there could produce a number of requests.

Secondly, our Librarian says that she could sell 500 copies a year either by post or from our bookshop, and our new Chief Nurse, who has spoken at two of our recent Conferences, says he could have sold 12–20 on the day, and he feels that this could happen at most of our Conferences/Seminars, particularly those we hold for clergy or theological students.

As to a particular anniversary, we have just passed our 25th Anniversary but this summer the third edition of our textbook "The Management of Terminal Malignant Disease" will be published by Edward Arnold. It is considerably wider than the first two editions and they were very keen to have another follow on and to fill the gap between the new *Oxford Textbook of Palliative Medicine*, which is coming out shortly, and other smaller paperbacks to link in with this.

Shirley does not feel there is much to update to justify a further chapter but we both agree that the lists of publications should be updated and pruned, with only those still easily available and some of the early seminal works included. I also think that the list of hospices could come out and the address of the Hospice Information Service given. They

---

[36] The revised second edition of the biography appeared as S. du Boulay, *Cicely Saunders: the founder of the modern hospice movement* (London: Hodder and Stoughton, 1994). It contained a new final chapter by Cicely Saunders in the form of an afterword, on the problems of euthanasia.

produce an annually up-dated directory of all the hospices in the United Kingdom and Ireland and I think this would be sufficient for the biography. I am not quite sure about the Further Reading and I think that could also be omitted with just the name and address of our Library for anyone who was interested in further reading.

Thirdly, of course, the new generation is well established at St Christopher's but I do not think that warrants more than perhaps a note that palliative medicine is now a specialty recognised by the Royal Colleges and has a number of overseas and regional Associations. In this country, also, the National Council for Specialist Hospice and Palliative Care Services will reach its first anniversary this autumn.

Finally, of course, I was awarded the Order of Merit by HM The Queen in 1989 and, as you will know, this is a very rare honour with only 24 of us in existence at any one time.

Marty Herrmann
New York, USA

5 March 1993 It is now quite a long time since I had your letter in December and you will have had my Christmas letter in the meantime and know that Marian and I are continuing happily. He is increasingly frail but with two excellent care assistants covering the mornings for me, we are managing.

I am sad about Jane, especially as it means that you did not come over but perhaps we may have a chance to see you this summer.

As a Vice President, you are merely saluted as a past helper, alongside many others. I do not count it as a member of the board, which is what we think of as the Council of Management. Our list of Vice Presidents includes people who are very much less in touch than you are but I will certainly take you off if you will feel happier. You made a very great difference when I was able to come over to New York and some important stimulating ideas came back from those times to us here, as well as anything that I was able to contribute in my turn.

Dr Harold Vanderpool
University of Texas Medical Branch, Galveston, Texas, USA

8 March 1993 You may remember that in the 1970s I spent a week in Galveston with the Medical Humanities Group, although this is now quite a long time ago. However, I am writing now in the hope that you may recall this as once again I have found myself using your article "The Ethics of Terminal Care" in *JAMA*. Many times I have quoted you as preferring the phrase "dying with a sense of worth" to "dying with dignity" which, as you point out, is interpreted in so many different ways. I have been using it again in a Foreword I have written to a book on counselling and pastoral care for patients with HIV/AIDS.

This is really just a thank you and an assurance that I do give you credit for this excellent phrase and to send you a recent reprint of my own, which as it was an Address, has no references. The phrase "palliative care" is used in Europe in preference to "hospice care" as so many of the older hospices turned into almshouses and because the word "terminal" is also considered unacceptable.

You may not know how widely the hospice movement has spread, sometimes under different titles, but interpreting the same basic principles in different cultures and settings. Our Information Service here is in touch with people in some 60 countries and it is fascinating to meet with people who visit here and to find that, while we are so different, yet we are talking about what is fundamentally the same thing, that is "dying with a sense of worth".

Jean Gaffin[37]

National Council for Hospice and Specialist Palliative Care Services, London

19 April 1993 Just a note to thank you so much for continuing to send me papers. I was very interested in the Draft Report and particularly in the number of discharges as compared to deaths in hospices.

Gill Ford mentioned to me yesterday that you were wondering what evidence St Christopher's was submitting to Lord Walton's Committee.[38] I wrote to him personally as soon as I saw he was going to be chairing it as I know him from MRC days and sent him the editorial I wrote for Palliative Medicine. I also asked specifically that they should look at the people who care for patients and their evidence and realise how many were in some kind of middle ground, as compared to the very polarised Voluntary Euthanasia Society and Pro-Life groups. As you may not have it to hand, I enclose a reprint of the article and also a copy of an excellent article rather more suited to a lay audience written by Sheila Cassidy for the *Tablet*. I sent a copy of that to Betty O'Gorman, who is a member of the Ethics Committee, so she may have already passed it on.

I personally hope that the law will keep out of this delicate situation and that we will continue with, if anything, the sort of case law that arose from the Tony Bland experience and much more negatively from the Dr Cox case. Our new Medical Director, Dr Robert Dunlop, who has had a great deal of experience with difficult pain problems in New Zealand, is rather more optimistic about dealing with difficult pain than I fear we may hear later from the BMA. Hopefully, we will have some work here in this area.

Again, thank you so much for keeping me so well informed.

Dr Mendez-Nunez Y. Gomez-Acebo

Asociacion Espanola Contra El Cancer, Madrid, Spain

19 April 1993 Thank you for your letter and the honour of inviting me to be the Guest speaker and open your 1st International Congress on Palliative Care in Madrid. I am very sorry but I am afraid my commitment to the care of my now very frail and elderly husband means that I do not travel. I only managed to go to Brussels for the European conference last year because I could do it within a day, but even that was a great effort and worried him considerably. I therefore reluctantly have to decline.

---

[37] The first Executive Director of the National Council for Hospice and Specialist Palliative Care Services.

[38] Published as *Report of the House of Lords Select Committee on Medical Ethics*, HL Paper 21 (London: HMSO, 1994). It recommended no change to the law on euthanasia.

I have not yet spoken to Dr Mary Baines, our Consultant Physician who has been with us for 25 years now, but I wonder whether you might not think of inviting her, as I am sure she would give you an excellent opening.

Sandol Stoddard
Holualoa, Hawaii, USA

25 May 1993 Thank you very much for sending me the cutting. I know Dr Portenoy and the team at Memorial Sloan Kettering from of old and have frequently read their papers, including one of the first when they wrote about using opiates for pain relief in non-malignant pain. It is good, however, to see it in a general publication. I will pass it on to our new Medical Director, who is particularly interested in morphine resistant pain, which often happens with nerve damage. Here one has to combine the morphine and ways of giving it with other drugs including, interestingly, the anti-depressants for non-depressive patients. The body's chemistry is fascinating. We are embarked on a study in this field at the moment using what are generally considered local anaesthetics and related drugs, more generally for patients with what is referred to as neuropathic pain.

I nearly tried to get in touch with you after your hurricane and do hope nothing too bad happened to you at that time. Now, of course, I have not been in touch since you wrote to me in January, after Peter's operation. I do hope all has gone well and that he is now fit and many of the things that happened then have fitted into the memory. The hospice is going well, as you will have seen from the literature, but I am glad to say that a lot of new things are starting up with our new Medical Director and Chief Nurse and I am very happy about the vision they both have, which really links with the vision at the beginning.

Dr Meinrad Schar
President Exit, Zurich, Switzerland

15 July 1993 Thank you for your letter and your invitation, which I am afraid I have to refuse. I cannot travel away from my very frail and elderly husband, who depends on my care.

I am interested in the name "Exit" for a hospice because, as you probably know, that was the name taken for some time by our Voluntary Euthanasia Society. A hospice in England and, so far as I know, worldwide, would not promote euthanasia but rather the alternative of good care. It would certainly confuse people in this country should a hospice take such a name and I would be very interested to have your views on the subject.

Libby Purves[39]
The Times, London

15 July 1993 I always enjoy reading your articles and as soon as I see your name I turn to them. My Personal Assistant and I were particularly delighted with your latest, "A woman's place is where she likes". A good nursing training with somebody moving up to Ward

---

[39] The journalist, novelist, and broadcaster.

Manager or Sister, which in our case is often coupled with coping with a family, is another route into being able to handle almost anything that may occur and I am also very impressed by how my hairdresser manages her salon.

I was at St Anne's[40] for two periods during the War, having gone down to nurse and then, being invalided out from that, returning to Oxford to obtain a War Degree. I have always been grateful, in my later career, for the number of things that I experienced at Oxford and very much enjoyed your article in The Ship recently.

All good wishes to the farm, which I also enjoy reading about, and please continue to give us articles like this, which improve our morale as some of us try to manage a great variety of establishments.

Dr Zbigniew Zylicz
Hospice Rozenheuvel, Rozendaalselaan, The Netherlands

4 August 1993 I was delighted to read an article in the *American Journal of Hospice and Palliative Care*.[41] It gives an excellent overview and is a change after rather too much polarised opinion and possible exaggeration.

We have just had two final year medical students from Warsaw who came because they read your translation which is obviously still important in Poland. You have done a great job.

All the very best as you open the hospice at the end of the year. I am always impressed by my contacts with the Salvation Army and admire their efficiency as well as their vision, and that gives me confidence for your future.

Dr Chris Dare
Hayfield Village, Cape, South Africa

4 October 1993 Many thanks indeed for your letter and the photographs. Marian was so delighted with the one of the two of us he insisted on putting it in his wallet. It is certainly good and thank you for taking it. I am glad to have the other photograph for my own album as a reminder of your visit.

It was very good indeed to see you and I think you should have done a great job in battling through and still getting some work done.

At the moment, we are looking with Bob Kastenbaum, a rather well known psychologist and Editor of *Omega* in the United States, at getting a book together on hospice around the world.[42] We are going to have to talk round as to which places we include in about 12 Chapters, and I wonder whether you think there should be a separate one for South Africa or whether it should be included with the very different circumstances that Ann Merriman is looking at in South Saharan Africa. Also, if you think South Africa merits something

---

[40] Her Oxford college.

[41] Z. Zylicz, Hospice in Holland: the story behind the blank spot, *American Journal of Hospice and Palliative Care*, **4** (1993): 30–4.

[42] Later published as C. Saunders and R. Kastenbaum (eds.), *Hospice care on the international scene* (New York: Springer, 1997).

special, who would speak for the place as a whole with, so far as I can gather, its rather mixed group of settings? Perhaps yourself. This is not a definite invitation because I have to keep faxing too and fro to Bob and, in any case, I am waiting for a meeting with Avril and Mary, who know the overseas scene so well.

Dr Alexander Waller

The H. Sheba Medical Centre, Tel-Hashomer, Israel

14 October 1993 Marian was delighted to see your letter and it was very kind of you to enclose a photograph to remind him, as his memory for names is more fragile than it was.

However, he is still drawing and enjoying life, even though he has a great deal less energy than before.

I hope the Hospice is going well. If you have an Annual Report in English, I would be very interested to see an overview of your activities. This is probably asking too much, but I am always interested to know what is going on.

Mr V. Prabhudas

Andhra Pradesh, India

15 November 1993 I was very touched at your letter and the description of your village and the community attempt to have a central building for prayer, education and refuge. I mentioned it at our Annual Meeting and I am sure that people will be praying for your work.

Is there any fund directly concerned with this building to which I can send a small personal donation? I do not know whether you would have a bank account or in what way I can send something directly to the village, which from your letter I understand you only visit from time to time.

Our hospice is very full at the moment with people from all parts of society with advanced illnesses, and all with a great need for welcome and care.

With all good wishes to your project.

Dr Sam Klagsbrun

Four Winds Hospital, Katonah, New York, USA

14 January 1994 Life was busy over Christmas for everybody and I took two weeks off at home with Marian and had something of a rest, so there has been some delay before I have been able to discuss your Report with Rob, and even now we have only given it a fairly cursory discussion. However, I have read it carefully myself and am responding.

You are right that we have a brand new state of circumstances and we are already addressing these as well as we can with our present team. All its new ideas fit, I think, with the Government's priorities, if they can only be made to see it, and we are well aware that that is part of what we have to do. We will go on and on about quality of service and to that end I am glad we have the Chairman of our nearest Health Authority as a member of our Council. He is very enthusiastic about the work. Sadly, the Chairman of a second Health Authority who was also on our Council died recently, so we have to start again in that area. So far as the publicity is concerned, Rob is well aware of this challenge and the present inadequacy of what stands as that department at the moment. You know how well the Information Service has done and we are wondering whether the sort of overview that you suggest might not be located there, thereby avoiding putting someone over the present fund raising department, with all the consequent fuss this would produce.

We now have on board a very bright girl for developing the respite care side of our home care work. We have taken on a local team, plus its funding, and so there is quite a lot of settling down to do in that area. At the moment, we have some 170 patients being visited at home.

So far as other marketing is concerned, the member of Council I mention above is very keen that we should produce an upgraded Prospectus and do some careful, planned visits to various Trusts to see if we can raise more reliable funding. I am sure we should not look for help in setting up an endowment fund, but I think the various projects we are looking at, including the one for the family that you mention, might strike a chord if presented in the right way and in the right place. I expect to be somewhat involved with this.

I am glad you feel that internal matters are in good order. The Management Team do not always sort out their communications as well as they might but they are full of ideas and I am very happy with Robert Dunlop and Andrew Knight and their aims and, in most cases, their ways of working.

On the Chaplaincy side, I am really more concerned with looking at the wider spiritual issues to be faced by lay staff than in tackling the seminaries, who have been so sluggish in this area. I have found the money, through a Trust who helped me originally, for Len to have a third member of his team to carry out research as enclosed in the copy of the presentation he made to the Management Team. We will soon start advertising.

We have also found at least one year's support for an enlargement in the Department of Social Work and are advertising for a Principal Social Worker at the moment. I think we will have to raise monies specifically to extend in this area because I doubt very much that we will get any statutory funding.

In nursing, I am happy to report that Andrew and his wife have just had a second son. Andrew has just made some very good appointments of new Team Leaders and I hope he will be able to be firm with his Ward Managers, but that is a fairly long term proposition. The doctors do present a problem but Rob is aware of it.

So far as I am concerned, it is always a great boost to me when you come here and, of course, I have these many years' experience of your visits now, which the new team do not have, so I suppose they do mean most to me. However, your report will be circulated and I am sure will be inspirational for everybody and, hopefully, we will respond to some of your challenges.

I am feeling much better as my arthritis has settled down quite a lot and my colitis has been treated, so I am not dragging myself around as I was and hope the New Year will give good opportunities without taking time away from Marian.

In the meantime, new things have been happening ever since you were here, in that we have been invited to produce a volume for a new series on oncology based from Guy's Hospital and links with them are being fostered. This is an example of how the original request coming via Christine, reached me and then gradually brought in Rob, who will now take it up and run with it.

Professor Balfour Mount

Royal Victoria Hospital, Montreal, Canada

11 March 1994 Your book arrived a couple of days ago and I have had time to look through it. This has made me realise that, although I am sure it has been of enormous help to you, I really do not think that an elderly lady of 76 who has to look after an even older husband of 93, who has his own ideas about food, could possibly take it on. To start with, I am constantly drinking milk to avoid the oesophagitis which has given me quite a stricture. It has been dilated twice and is at the moment, fortunately, stable. Following on from that, my very considerable collapse of lumbar vertebrae makes standing up and cooking very difficult. We therefore have very simple meals in the evenings and I do hardly any very careful cooking, such as making my own mayonnaise.

It was very good of you indeed to send the book and I am sure you are healthier because of the diet it recommends. I enjoyed seeing you and your lovely retreat by the lake when I was sent a copy of the video made for Ivan Lichter.

You will no doubt have heard that our House of Lords Select Committee on Medical Ethics came down very firmly against any legalisation of euthanasia, in a series of statements which anyone in palliative medicine would have been happy to write themselves. I am enclosing a photocopy of one page, which will give you a flavour of it, and I must add that when answering questions on the radio, Professor Lord Walton, who chaired it, said that what finally made them decide against was their visit to the Netherlands, where they saw how easily "voluntary" euthanasia had become involuntary and how impossible it was to draw a line or to ensure that the guidelines were adhered to. This is very good news for us in this country, because I do not think they will look at any legislation now for quite a while to come, although there has been quite a lot of grumbling in the other camp.

I feel very much like a combatant at the end of a long campaign who can at last relax, but something tells me this is probably being too hopeful. However, there are plenty of younger people to take up the baton now.

Dr Cynthia Goh

Hospice Care Association, Singapore

29 April 1994 Your card arrived this morning and I will await the arrival of the copy of the Annals of the Academy of Medicine in due course. As I am sure you know, our House of Lords Select Committee on Medical Ethics has come down firmly on not legalising euthanasia and in support of the development of palliative care. This is firmly stated in a really excellent report. We are delighted and were most courteously received at their Committee Hearing.

I am so glad you have responded to Professor Robert Kastenbaum. It has been really exciting as Mary, Avril and I chose 12 people from around the world who represented different ways of starting hospice and palliative care. Some are very new and some have accomplished a great deal already. Bob Kastenbaum is a most experienced Editor and I hope we will eventually finish up with a useful book.

I do hope you keep well yourself. Mary is in excellent form and is starting two sessions with Croydon Community Care next week, which is another good link between us and those around and a new thing for her at this stage of all her excellent work in hospice over many years.

Dr Franco de Conno[43]

European Association for Palliative Care, Milano, Italy

4 May 1994 I was very pleased to hear that you are already making plans for the 4th Congress of the European Association for Palliative Care and that it will take place in Barcelona. I have looked at the main headings for selection of topics and I would like to suggest under "Clinical Management" that a place is made for "Spiritual Awareness and Support." I think it is important that in an increasingly secular society, we should look very widely at this issue because there is no doubt that a great many patients and families who have no background in religious practice at all, have very searching questions about the meaning of life. I think this is not quite obvious from the heading "Emotional adjustment" or "Family support, education, involvement". As spiritual support is referred to in most of our publications, I think it would be a pity if it were completely omitted.

I am very sorry but I am afraid there is no possibility of my attending the Congress and in any case when I came to Brussels, I did touch a little bit upon this topic, which I think needs to be pursued further.

Peter Buckland

Hospice of Southern Africa, Pinelands, South Africa

12 May 1994 Thank you for your long letter and explanation of your needs. I am prepared to support your project which seems to me very important. I enclose a photograph and you may certainly use the quotation "You matter because you are you, and you matter to the end of your life. We will do all we can not only to help you to die peacefully, but to live until you die."[44]

I certainly support the development of hospice in Southern Africa, and in particular education which so often has begun in the nursing field, as hospice has developed in different cultures and countries. Any support that will help the imaginative projects which you describe will enable good care to be given to a much wider group of people than those who are directly helped by the existing hospice teams.

I hope you can take a phrase from this letter and add it to your prospectus, but if you want something longer you must come back again and I will do my best if you let me know the particular points you want made.

Mgr Zofia Kabiesz

Dusseldorf, Germany

7 June 1994 Thank you for your letter and the details of your various meetings with Marian over the years.

---

[43] A key figure in the work of the European Association for Palliative Care and head of pain therapy and palliative care in Milan's National Tumour Institute.

[44] A phrase originally used in C. Saunders, A death in the family: a professional view, *British Medical Journal*, **1**(844), (1973): 30–1.

I am afraid he does not remember anybody who he has not seen recently now and I do not really think it would be helpful for you to come and see him when you are next in England. It really worries him when people remember him and he does not remember who they are.

However, I have to say that he is happy although he is becoming much weaker.

Dr Paul Henteleff

Canadian Palliative Care Association, Ottawa, Ontario, Canada

13 June 1994 Thank you so much for sending me your brief to the Special Committee of the Senate of Canada on Euthanasia and Assisted Suicide. I congratulate you on its neatness and in exchange I am sending a copy of what our own National Council presented to our House of Lords Committee, which as you no doubt know, produced a Report which came out firmly against legislation of any kind and was very sensible in what it said about decisions to limit treatment. It also pointed out that it was on the whole unhelpful to use the phrase "passive euthanasia" for such treatment.

I would point out, in view of your quote from the *BMJ*, that "the hospice movement is too good to be true and too small to be useful"[45] that this is a very inaccurate statement. I enclose a copy of the letter from our Director of Studies here, which also appeared in the *BMJ*, pointing out that in fact as a movement (and of course our input is variable) we are in touch with well over half of those who die of cancer and have had a considerable influence on those who die of other diseases.

Obviously, our Voluntary Euthanasia Society has come back into action on seeing what was, to them, a disappointing Report, but our Government has certainly taken up its main recommendations.

Our feeling here, and I am sure it will be echoed by many in Canada, is that while there are some people whose doctors do not give them adequate care and who find themselves in a very difficult situation, yet if only people will ask for advice they will find that, with a combination of drugs and if people will accept sedation, the very small number with resistant pain and intractable distress can be rendered sleepy until death takes its own time. I know there are those who find no philosophical difference between what they term "pharmacological oblivion" and euthanasia. The point I wish to make is that the former needs expertise or good advice and no change in the law, while the latter necessitates a change in law. Any such legislation would greatly undermine the safety of vulnerable people in asking for good terminal care.

All good wishes to you as you try to battle for better palliative care services and better funding for them. I personally think that it has been a great help that we have been recognised as a specialty and I am encouraged by the number of excellent young physicians, nurses and others who are anxious to come into the field and who are already making a great contribution to it.

---

[45] This had appeared in C. Douglas, For all the saints, *British Medical Journal*, **304** (1992): 579 – an unusually vituperative attack on charitable, independent hospices.

Dr John F. Scott

Centre de Santé Elisabeth-Bruyere Health Centre, Ottawa, Ontario, Canada

21 June 1994 Thank you for your fax. It was only one or two members of the Select Committee who visited St Christopher's but one or two others visited Trinity and other hospices. I understand the thing that moved them most firmly against any legislation in this area was their visit to the Netherlands. I really do recommend you read the Report, which is available from HMSO Stationery Office, London. However, the main points are covered in the two enclosures I am faxing with this letter, which is a copy of the debate from Hansard and the Review of the Committee from the Report.

So far as organising a visit is concerned, I think it is very difficult to be sure that you will have the right patient on the right day prepared to give the right sort of comment. You may be luckier than we are but I always feel this is rather a risk, although I have never really been let down. I think it is more important to find a family member who is prepared to look back and review the change that good palliative care made to what appeared at one time to be a very difficult situation.

I may say that the Voluntary Euthanasia Society in this country are by no means staying quiet after the Report, although our Government has said they do not intend to take any steps in this direction. What the Euthanasia Society are particularly talking about are the 5% whose pain remains difficult to control but who, as we all know, can be given a peaceful end if only they will accept sedation. So often, also, they have psychological rather than physical problems, or certainly problems which compound the physical. I am sure there are a few people for whom death is preferable to life and who will never be persuaded otherwise. I am equally sure that they cannot have a law making this possible for them without undermining the right to care of a great many more vulnerable people in need of help. This help is available far more widely than in the specific palliative care unit or team. The answer is education, not legislation.

As to the real fundamental objective of the visit you are thinking of, I suppose it is the emphasis on how important life can be at its ending and how challenging and rewarding our continual learning from the patients adds to our expertise and keeps us all going.

Professor David Clark

Trent Palliative Care Centre, Sheffield

17 November 1994 Thank you very much for your very interesting letter. I am delighted that somebody is prepared to look at the foundations of the Hospice Movement.[46] I well remember Sir Geoffrey Vickers in our early days asking "does your team include an archivist?" However, we did not have the money to have somebody at that point but I have in fact kept a great deal of papers, innumerable letters and memoranda and, of course, a great deal is embedded in my own memory. The real foundations of the Hospice Movement, the patients themselves, are remembered vividly and I have pictures of many which I use frequently when talking with our Course members on the Evolution of the Hospice Movement.

---

[46] The letter had outlined plans to establish a major project on the history of hospice and palliative care.

I think you are going to have to find someone who is going to give this a considerable amount of time if you are going to give an overall view of what has happened over the last 30 years. I would obviously be happy to take part in an interview but I think as St Christopher's was the catalyst for the modern hospice movement, it would probably mean somebody visiting here for rather longer than that to go through some of the early material.

Some of this was done by Shirley du Boulay when she wrote my biography, and with access to all my materials she has pulled out a great deal of important points herself. I think it would be important for you to consider a visit with her and also have her permission to use some of the things that she spent so much time in bringing together.

I presume you have a copy of the biography, but it has recently been reprinted and I would be able to send you a copy should you wish to have one.

I think the Hospice Movement, growing as it has from a presentation of the needs of patients and of their potential for achievement, has something to say to medicine as a whole, and although we have had to fit in with the Health Service (and were, indeed, always anxious to do that from the beginning) it still has something to say about the wider personal, family and spiritual dimensions, which are so important to our patients but which are not always considered in the everyday practice of medicine.

Dr B. Lytton[47]

New Haven, Connecticut, USA

4 January 1995 Thank you very much for still remembering me for a Christmas card.

This is really just to let you know that I am still doing a certain amount of work, although not clinically, but I am an elder statesman in this field, write and talk about philosophy and ethics, battle against the very tiresome people who want to introduce legislation for voluntary euthanasia and generally try to boost hospice and palliative care. The team here is excellent and I am very pleased to see what good medicine is being practised and to see the many who have trained here and gone on to leadership positions.

Palliative medicine is now a recognised specialty in this country, since 1987, and we are more related to the mainstream than I think hospice seems to be in the USA.

My husband really became too heavy for me to care for at home and he is now in the hospice in a single room near his studio. Although he nearly died twice during the last two weeks, shortly after he was admitted, he has revived yet again and they are caring for him very well indeed.[48]

Sister Mary Antonia, who gave us those splendid lunches, is still going strong and is in one of their convalescent homes in Ireland. St Joseph's has brought itself more or less into the present day, but I do not forget where we all came from. It has been a fascinating journey.

---

[47] Bernard Lytton had worked with Cicely Saunders at St Joseph's Hospice in the early 1960s when he was a surgeon at the London Hospital; he subsequently moved to the Department of Surgery, Yale University School of Medicine. It was he who had invited her to Yale in 1963 for her first visit to the USA and indeed he had met her on arrival at the airport in New York.

[48] Marian Bohusz-Szyszko died in St Christopher's Hospice on 29 January 1995.

Professor Bernard J. Shapiro

Principal and Vice Chancellor, McGill University, Montreal, Canada

12 June 1995 It was with real shock that I heard of the news that Professor Balfour Mount has resigned as Director of the Palliative Care Programme in McGill University. He has been one of the pioneers in this field since the opening of his Palliative Care ward early in 1975. His 20 years of work have set standards which have been influential around the world and his bi-annual conferences have shown, by the numbers who attend, how much his programme has to offer. Speaking as someone who has been in this field since 1958 and earlier than that as a volunteer, I would like to say as forcefully as I can that this would be a tragedy for a very important part of total medical care.

I understand that his resignation is due above all to cut-backs in the staffing and financial support for palliative care. If there is any way in which you can re-consider these decisions, I believe it would have a great impact on both research and teaching in this field. For many years now there has been an academically recognised programme at McGill University. I hope that recognition will be matched by adequate funding.

Dr M. S. Richard

Association des Dames du Calvaire, Paris, France

3 July 1995 Thank you very much for your letter inviting me to your re-opening. That is certainly a wonderful occasion and particularly close to me as I always refer to Mme Jeanne Garnier when I talk about hospice evolution to the various groups that visit here.

My problem is that I am now very arthritic and travelling alone is difficult for me and I will certainly need to travel first class. I could travel with Dr Therese Vanier and will be in touch with her about this. I would arrange to travel on Eurostar directly from London to Paris and if you could help me with this and meet me at Paris (and as I cannot walk very great distances I may need a wheelchair at the station) I would be delighted to come and speak at your ceremony. I would like to talk briefly on the values which have been central to the development of hospice and palliative care.

I will put the date in my diary and expect to hear from you if you are agreeable to the arrangements I suggest.

Dr Cynthia Goh

Chairman, Organising Committee, Hospice Care in Asia International Conference

25 August 1995 Thank you for your fax. I have definitely decided in principle to come to your Conference. I finish my time in San Diego on February 20th and hope to stay with my step-daughter in San Francisco for a few days before coming to you. She has to wait until September to find out details of her daughter's half-term dates next year, as they always go skiing then. However, so far as you are concerned I will be flying from San Francisco to Singapore as you suggest, stopping in Hong Kong but hopefully remaining on the plane.

Going across the date line I will lose a day, so I think as I will have had quite a journey, I would like to arrive with plenty of time to acclimatise, say on the 25th or 26th February. I know I will be well looked after.

I am happy to talk to your title "When the dying demand death" for the opening ple-nary lecture but from the booklet about the Conference, it looks as though I may be tak-ing the slot given to Professor Neil MacDonald. I hope this is all right. So far as the other lecture is concerned, I am happy to take your suggestion "Can we afford not to give palliative care" because I could certainly talk around ethics, resources and appropri-ate treatment under this title. Nothing else has come to my mind, so I think I will leave it to your suggestion.

Professor Balfour Mount

Royal Victoria Hospital, Montreal, Canada

29 August 1995 Thank you very much for your letter. I hope this means that you will sort out some of the problems of the PCU and have at least most of what you feel is nec-essary for a proper service. The very best of luck as you go to China. As it happens, I had just read an article about the number of baby girls who were languishing in orphan-ages awaiting overseas adoption. I hope Bethany will be happy with you and you with her.

Thank you also for all that you sent me. I am extremely interested in it and impressed by your response to a very tiresome article. These muddles of what euthanasia really is will I suppose continue, because they are deliberately put forward by those pressing for active killing. I am glad to have it to hand, because I will be debating (yet again!) the issue for our Royal College of Nursing against Sir Ludovic Kennedy, who is the most active proponent over here. A copy of any response that you get would be gratefully received. In case you did not see it in *Palliative Medicine* some time ago, I enclose a copy of an earlier effort, which of course was superseded by our House of Lords Committee and two or three legal cases since then. However, the principles remain.

Dr Franco Pannuti

Scientific Director – ANT, Bergami, Bologna, Italy

5 September 1995 Thank you very much for your letter and the book which you sent to me. We will keep it with the overseas publications in our library.

I wonder whether you have met up with the people who are already working in this field in India. A senior nurse, Miss Gilly Burn,[49] has been visiting there for several years and has travelled around the country over many months more than once and has a number of groups who are really interested in palliative medicine, as well as developing education pro-grammes in the hope of introducing the basic principles into as many hospitals in their community as possible. I think it is important that if you are going to set out with doing anything in India you should be in touch with her. She has done a lot of work already and is continuing a long term interest with the many people she now knows. I enclose a copy of our *Hospice Bulletin* which gives an extract from a letter sent to me by a doctor who trav-elled with her for part of her last trip.

With very best wishes from us all at St Christopher's.

---

[49] Founder of the charity Cancer Relief India.

A. J. Postmes

El Vendo, Netherlands

28 November 1995 Thank you for your fax. I am sorry not to have responded more quickly but life has been very busy here recently.

As it happens, I was debating the issue of Euthanasia once again for our Royal College of Nursing yesterday. My position is that according to several studies that have now been carried out around the world, some 85% of patients do not present difficulty in pain control or control of other symptoms. However, 10%–15% demand all our resources, leaving a very small group who may present some difficulty because their pain is largely enhanced by psycho-social issues. These patients can certainly die peacefully if they and their families will accept a certain amount of sedation. I think that our practice here shows that this number is very small indeed, less than the 5% that is often suggested. For example, our Director of Home Care tells me that in the past year, out of nearly 900 patients visited by our team, they have only had one or two who needed such sedation and that was successful in giving them a peaceful death. Within the In-patient Unit, the same holds true, although the number may be very slightly larger. However, it is far more likely that terminal restlessness is the problem and not terminal pain. So I do not say that intolerable pain can never be helped. It is also interesting that the small group of patients of whom I speak are quite unlikely to be asking for euthanasia. They are usually struggling with other issues, such as a particularly difficult personal history.

I am referring here to patients with terminal malignant disease, motor neurone disease and AIDS, but we do now also see patients with other types of pain from different diagnoses. We have not had a case of intolerable pain among this group either.

We hold to our position and would agree with you about what you term "narcosis". I think the programme with Dr van Oyen showed several things quite clearly.[50] In the first place, the patient was not receiving optimal palliative care. He need not have had pain and he certainly should not have been told that he might die of suffocation. This was really a threat which our work here has shown should be considered groundless.

Secondly, he was not, according to the pharmacist, receiving any other drugs and I think he may well have been clinically depressed and could have been treated for that. Thirdly, I think what came out most clearly was the isolation of all three participants – patient, wife and doctor – and the lack of support for them all.

We continue to make a stand and may I suggest that you might write to the National Council for Hospice and Specialist Palliative Care Services and ask them for a copy of the Statement which was given to the House of Lords Select Committee on Medical Ethics, which I think covers the situation very well and puts the case against any form of legalised euthanasia.

---

[50] She is referring here to the programme *Death on Request*, which had been broadcast on BBC television on 15 March 1995 and which showed the Dutch general practitioner Dr Wilfred Van Oijen administering euthanasia to his patient, Mr Cees van Wendel de Joode.

Dr Xavier Gomez-Batiste

Rambla Hospital, Barcelona, Spain

30 November 1995 Thank you very much indeed for your letter about your project "Cancerworld". My delay in responding has been that I wanted to discuss your suggestions with Barbara Monroe first and we both seem to have been rather busy recently with outside commitments. However, we have now had time to go through your draft paper.

I am very pleased that you are anxious that St Christopher's Hospice should be one of the Regional Centres and we would certainly like to co-operate. Although I travel occasionally, I am sure you will agree that it would be much more realistic if either Barbara Monroe[51] or Robert Dunlop should represent the Hospice in further discussions.

I am interested in your list but wonder if it would not give a broader base if you included someone from Canada and/or the United States. The names that come to mind are Professor Balfour Mount from the Royal Victoria Hospital, Montreal whom I am sure you know or, possibly, Dr Ina Cummings who is now based in Nova Scotia. For the United States I suggest Dr Josefina Magno, who some years ago founded the International Hospice Institute. She already has Dr Jan Stjernsward, Dr Robert Twycross and Dr Kathleen Foley on her Advisory Council. They are looking at the international scene at present, although they are not as far on in any discussion as you are but I think it is important that we avoid unnecessary duplication. There is also, of course, Cancer Relief India (under the direction of Ms Gilly Burn). Dr Robert Twycross and Dr Jan Stjernsward are also involved with this group and it would be an important voice for the Third World.

I am not sure if you know that in this country, apart from our own international Information Service based at St Christopher's, the group British Aid for Hospices Abroad is based here in Sheffield. They can be contacted at the Trent Palliative Care Centre. Although I am not suggesting that all units should be included as Trustees in your list of names, I am sure you know that there are a number of Regional Councils around the world now who would be interested in your endeavours.

I entirely agree with you that there is no need to set up a "typical" international society and that we have plenty of national and international conferences already. Incidentally, I am speaking at the conference in Singapore early next year which is being organised by Dr Cynthia Goh, who is very well acquainted with the various initiatives in Asia.

I am delighted that your supporting organisation has a legal base and that there is a source of funds for the initial work.

Finally, I have my doubts about your title "Cancerworld". Palliative care looks beyond cancer, although we are not suggesting we should take over from other specialties but that we should encourage them to carry out their own palliative care.

I know Barbara Monroe will be discussing all this with you in Barcelona and I look forward to hearing more. I certainly wish you well with this endeavour and thank you again for taking such an initiative.

---

[51] Head of patient services, later Chief Executive of St Christopher's.

Dr Kathleen Foley

Memorial Sloan Kettering Cancer Center, New York

15 December 1995 We have a George Soros Scholar with us for a few days at the moment, Dr Nicholas Christakis from Chicago and I was extremely pleased to meet him during his time here at St Christopher's.[52]

He told me that the George Soros Foundation is not only concerned with death and dying in America but also is willing to receive applications for help from Eastern Europe. When he heard that I knew you already, he suggested that I should write to you first to see if you thought that the project I mention below is something that the Foundation might be interested in.

St Christopher's has been twinned with the Hospice in Nova Huta in Krakow for some years now. I visited there in 1978 and met some of the people who were already doing some visiting to terminally ill patients and also met people in the local oncology centre. Some years later they started a small hospice venture in Home Care and are now nearing completion of a rather ambitious building not only for in-patient care but also as a base for the education programme which they have been carrying out in a way which I think remarkable considering their many difficulties. I have managed to steer some money in their direction from a Trust in Europe and we have had a number of their team attending educational courses here.

Do you think that the Soros Foundation would be interested in further development of their education programme, for which they will have space in the Hospice?

It is nice to be in touch with you again. I hope we may meet up in Singapore next year and in the meantime look forward to hearing from you with regard to this project.

Professor Renee Fox[53]

The Wellington, Philadelphia, USA

19 January 1996 I was delighted to meet Nicholas Christakis and to know that he knew you well and was able to give me your address. Thank you so much for sending me your latest book, which I will look at with interest.

Bob Kastenbaum and I have been putting together a book on Hospice and Palliative Care Worldwide. We have a fascinating group of chapters and people starting hospice in such far flung places as Hong Kong, Columbia and the Costa del Sol. It is very interesting to see how different from each other they are, and yet how they all interpret the basic principles in a recognisable way. I am very concerned for people battling in Poland, Southern Africa and India for example, and yet it does give one a feeling of hope that while the WHO has produced guidelines and battles with governments to make analgesics available, yet

---

[52] Nicholas Christakis was a member of the first cohort of faculty scholars of the Open Society Institute's Project on Death in America, under the direction of Kathleen Foley, of Memorial Sloan Kettering Hospital.

[53] Author of *Experiment perilous: physicians and patients facing the unknown.* (Glencoe, Ill: The Free Press, 1959) – a pioneering work of medical sociology which Cicely Saunders had read in the 1960s and often quoted.

small groups of dedicated people seem to have an enormous impact. They attract the attention of the media and in most cases it seems that the message is got across without too much sentimentality. There is no doubt that large numbers of people across the world who have had a bad experience are anxious to contribute in some way for better palliative care for the people of the future. As the majority of cancer patients in the developing world present at an advanced stage, if at all, palliative care is the only reasonable and appropriate response. There is much to do but there is also a real encouragement as we look back over what has happened over the last two decades.

I refer to your "Experiment Perilous" in my own chapter for the book. It appeared in the same year as Herman Feifel's "The Meaning of Death" and my own series in our *Nursing Times* on the "Care of the Dying". Something was definitely happening in 1959!

Mrs M P

Sydney, New South Wales, Australia

13 March 1996 Thank you very much for your letter which was obviously quite difficult for you to write. I am always glad to know when *Beyond the Horizon*[54] has been helpful, because the contents were gathered over many years, often at times which I found particularly difficult. Like you, I was able to look after my husband almost to the end and it was really very important that, while he became dependent, he kept his dignity and his sharpness and humour.

Also, I am very concerned about the specialists who find it so difficult to let go treatment prolonging life and to turn to all the possibilities in palliative care, but I am encouraged that there are now 6 Professors in the field in this country and that there will be more teaching of this kind given to students and graduates.

I meet people from the Hospice field in Australia from time to time and I hope that they will continue to look at the humanistic side of medicine as well as the skills of palliative care.

Dr Kathleen Foley

Memorial Sloan Kettering Cancer Center, New York, USA

22 March 1996 It was a very great pleasure to meet up with you again, to have that stimulating discussion when we were both reviving so well from jet-lag and, most important of all, hearing you talk again. It is so important that everyone involved in palliative care in hospice keeps the best possible standards of patient care and I hope that those who attended the Singapore Conference really took the message on board.

You mentioned that you had replied to my earlier letter to you and I have been waiting to see whether it came through by surface mail, but it has not arrived yet. I would be very sad if the possibility which you talked about when we met should not reach the people that I have been trying to support in Poland. I hope you may be able to send me another copy of your letter or else put their name to the SOROS Foundation yourself, so that they may be considered.

---

54 A reference to C. Saunders, *Beyond the horizon* (London: Dartman, Longman, and Todd, 1999), a collection of poems and prose pieces and itself an expanded version of *Beyond all pain*, which had first appeared in 1983; see letter to Shirley du Boulay, 1 September 1982, p. 227.

I believe you already know of Professor Luczak, who now heads up the Council for Palliative/ Hospice Care of Poland at the Academy of Medicine, Poznan, Poland. However, I would like to strongly recommend that Dr Janina Tenner of St Lazarus' Hospice, Krakow, Poland also be suggested. The Krakow Hospice Team started out in Home Care before Poznan came on the scene and, as I said in my earlier letter, have slowly been building an inpatient unit with an education facility attached. I have managed to free some funds towards them as St Christopher's is twinned with this hospice group, but they have persevered with raising a lot of money themselves while they have continued what I believe is a very good standard of home care. If there were any funds forthcoming for the education projects, or even capital and some revenue for the education centre, it would be an enormous boost for them. They have already managed to produce a booklet on pain control and got it circulated to all General Practitioners in Poland via the Government, but the amount of Government support is very limited and I think they also need a degree of independence, as we have found valuable here.

Dr Sam Klagsbrun

Four Winds Hospital, Katonah, New York, USA

29 April 1996 First of all, belated thanks for your last visit. We were waiting to write or telephone after receiving a Report from you, which we would still much appreciate if you have time.

Reported in one of our London dailies, although not I regret, *The Times*, was notification of a ruling that doctors in New York, Vermont and Connecticut should be allowed to help the terminally ill commit suicide. You are quoted as having said that doctors "wanted the freedom to make decisions with their patients without fear of government intrusion". If by this you only mean that there should be no problem in desisting from inappropriate treatment or in giving adequate analgesia in order to control terminal pain and/or restlessness, then of course that is the position maintained by St Christopher's over the years. However, Rob and I have discussed the report, of which I enclose a copy, because we would certainly never endorse a doctor's action in specifically ending a life or giving a patient the means to do so for themselves. As I know we have discussed before, we feel strongly that there are major social dangers in any law allowing an active ending of life. So far, this remains the position in this country and we believe, along with the House of Lords Select Committee on Medical Ethics, that the line between voluntary and involuntary euthanasia is in practice impossible to draw. The situation in the Netherlands certainly endorses this, where the guidelines have changed from time to time since the first ruling that doctors would not be prosecuted should they keep to specific regulations.

I enclose a copy of a report in our *Journal of Medical Ethics* which printed the conclusions of the New York taskforce, from which I have quoted on various occasions. You will see from this that the members of that group, although not all exactly of the same position ethically, felt that a law was too dangerous in a situation where there were so many vulnerable people with less than optimum medical care.

We do, as you know, fully understand that your position is not exactly the same as ours and really only want to propose two things. Firstly, that should this go further, for example to the Supreme Court, and you still be involved, that you emphasise that the real answer to nearly all these problems is better palliative care. Secondly, that you recognise that

St Christopher's holds a different point of view from your own and holds firmly to the belief that, although there may be a tiny minority who will still want out after all the best palliative care, we do not believe that they can have legal freedom for this without undermining very many other people.

I would very much like to discuss all this with you some time and perhaps we could make a date to talk on the telephone at some stage.

Your trip over this time was very productive. The doctoring seems to be sorting itself out at last and Rob is much relieved of what was really too much on his shoulders. We have really solved the Drapers' dilemma with a report to Council this week recommending the permanent continuance of 8 beds on the ground floor with vacancies there being filled as they occur.

It was lovely to see you again, always a personal joy for me.

Dr Stan von Hooft

Deaking University at Toorak, Malvern, Victoria, Australia

11 July 1996 It is now some time since I read your article "Bioethics and caring" [*Journal of Medical Ethics*, **22**: 83–9] which I have shared with others involved with the Hospice.

I found it very interesting, as I think caring is a fundamental part of our nature as persons and should be a way of reaching the inner spiritual needs of those who are cared for. This can be done often without words.

At the present moment a senior nurse here, working for a further degree, is carrying out a research project looking specifically at spiritual need. The title of her thesis is "A Study of Sources of Meaning and Sense of Self in People who are Dying". We are also looking at ways of writing of spiritual need for a worldwide publication. The latter, and indeed both of them will, we hope, have something to say to people of different religions and of none.

Have you published more on this theme? I would be most interested to read it and in the meantime enclose a paper on the subject which I wrote a few years ago now and another from a doctor who is a former member of staff here.

Professor Jacek Łuczak[55]

Karol Marcinkowski University of Medical Sciences, Poznan, Poland

30 July 1996 Thank you very much for your fax, which arrived just before I left for Lithuania and Belarus. I did my best with the Minister for Health, whom I met in Vilnius University Hospital with the excellent Pain Relief Team there. It seems to me that they will probably get oral morphine in the end. I was very impressed with everybody I met there, particularly Professor Aldona Lukoseviciute and Dr Jane Baubliene. My visit over to Belarus was in order to meet people in the village on the estate where my husband was born back in 1901, when it was Russian occupied Poland. I met Dr Gorchakova, who is doing her best with her Children's Hospice. All of them seem to have help from the SOROS organisation and I was pleased to meet the local representative in Vilnius. I only hope that that help will continue.

---

[55] The anaesthesiologist and a central figure within the development of palliative care in Poland and across eastern Europe.

You mention in your letter that Kathleen Foley is now a director of the project on Death in America. I have known her over many years now and have a great admiration for her work. I am so glad she is going to be at your conference in Budapest in early December. I am sure you have the names of people involved with palliative care in Eastern Europe in a much fuller list than we have, but I will send our own list from the Information Service by separate mail in case there is anyone you have not met.

At the end of your letter you asked if I could contribute with a lecture in Budapest and I would be very happy to do this. Kathy Foley heard me give an opening talk at the Singapore Conference and I could repeat with something of that nature, but I would really prefer to talk with slides on *Hospice as Bridgebuilder*. You could, if you like, use the words *Palliative Care* instead of Hospice.

I am a little uncertain about travelling in December as I am now very arthritic, needing a wheelchair at the airport and for any distance, but I had such a welcome in Eastern Europe that I would make the effort to come if you felt it would be of value. I would not intend to stay for more than two or three days at the most, but of course there are many people I would like to meet.

With every good wish for all your work.

Dr Martin Klumpp
Stuttgart, Germany

30 July 1996 Thank you very much for your recent letter and for the honour of inviting me to Stuttgart next year to celebrate the 10th Anniversary of your work.

Although I am, of course, interested in your work and congratulate you on all that you have achieved during these past 10 years, I do not feel that I could make the trip to Stuttgart as you suggest. I am already committed to speaking at a conference in Cyprus in late April and early May and there is a possibility that I may be travelling to Krakow in June. I feel, therefore, that it is not realistic of me to think of adding another overseas trip at that time.

I am sorry to disappoint you and send you all my congratulations on your achievements and my good wishes for the work ahead.

Dr Kathleen Foley
Memorial Sloan Kettering Cancer Center, New York, USA

2 August 1996 I have just returned from an absolutely fascinating visit to Lithuania and Belarus. In Vilnius I met the Pain Relief Team at the University Hospital, who were rightly delighted with their help from the SOROS Foundation, which will enable them to have far better records and computing facilities. They seem to be doing a good job and were extremely welcoming to me. I met the local representative of the SOROS Foundation and also the Minister for Health, doing my best to emphasise the need for oral morphine. It certainly seems ridiculous that they have 20 patients on syringe drivers out in the community, mainly for people who could perfectly well be maintained with oral opiates. I hope to keep in touch with them. After that, I visited the small hospice in Kaunas which, although it is mainly an old-fashioned cancer nursing home, was run by wonderfully warm people and I was very impressed with the doctor who was running their Home Care service and, as far as

I could see, sorting out any community care which may be available for patients coping with severe illness and often in deep poverty.

I travelled over the border to Belarus for the day, taken by the Embassy who are keen for me to donate some of my husband's pictures as he was born in that part of the world when it was Russian occupied Poland. I had the most wonderful welcome there to the village which has now spread over what was presumably his family estate. I met Dr Gorchakova who came up from Minsk to meet us. She was extremely grateful for the help she has had from the SOROS Foundation so far but is obviously concerned with how their hospice would keep going if this funding was removed. I know the Foundation is mainly concerned with education, but of course she is not able to carry out her plans to spread the knowledge of good palliative care unless she can demonstrate what it can do to others. It seems an extremely poor country and I can only say that I was most impressed by her, although I did not see the hospice, and I hope very much that the Foundation will continue with as much support as it can. I am sure the whole of Eastern Europe is crying out for help and yet they all seem so positive in the work that they are doing and it was a great inspiration to me to meet them.

Dr Luczak faxed me a letter before I left for Lithuania to encourage me to press for oral morphine for them and also to say that you were working with him in planning a Conference in Budapest in early December. He asked if I would consider giving a lecture. In spite of my arthritis and some difficulty in travelling I would very much like to do this and hope that I might meet you there.

When we opened nearly 30 years ago now, I never imagined that we would be involved with people working in this field worldwide, but I am so glad that we started out with research as well as care, so that our education has been as objectively based as possible. It is good to be able to have papers to present about pain relief and all the potential that good symptom control can have for patients and families.

It was an enormous pleasure to meet you again in Singapore and I hope that the Budapest conference will be as exciting, although I think the participants there will be battling with considerable difficulties and many fewer resources.

S. Sikorska Ratschkie

Hampstead, London

2 August 1996 Thank you for your letter inviting me to join the Society in Tribute to Maria Sklodowska-Curie.

I would be very pleased to do this and have completed the application form as requested. Unfortunately, there is no possibility of my visiting Poland but I have visited the Oncology Institute in the past and am very interested in the spread of cancer care in Poland, particularly in the later stages of the disease.

Zelda Foster

Brooklyn, New York, USA

12 August 1996 Thank you very much indeed for sending me the article and also for returning my telephone call. As I had failed to get you, I spoke to Florence who has immediately sent me the missing pages, so please do not go to any more trouble for me. These included the piece from the doctors and I especially wanted Kathy Foley's input as she is a really powerful voice. I met her again after some years when I was at the Singapore Conference and we had a long discussion on the subject. Both of us had read "The Troubled Dream of Life" by Daniel Callahan, published by Simon and Schuster in 1993. If you want a really erudite and compassionate look at this scene, I highly recommend it if it is still in print. I hope it is as a great many people could read it with benefit.

You may have seen that Sam Klagsbrun has been involved in this area and, although he feels that doctors should very occasionally and with much thought accede to patients' requests, he has been on television and he tells me that he said that what Dr Kervorkian is doing is obscene and that it is very important that we do not have careless laws in this area. I certainly feel for the vulnerable if that should happen. On the other hand, I am afraid that American medicine goes ahead too aggressively in many end of life decisions and the great need is, as of course you agree, better education. You have been in that field since I first knew you and I am sorry that life is difficult now. I think we all of us have to try and keep battling on in our own different ways, and I am very fortunate in my situation.

Harry Von Bommel

11 Miniot Circle, Scarborough, Ontario, Canada

29 August 1996 Thank you for your letter and the copy of the manuscript of our interview. Once again, I feel that the spoken and the written word are rather different and I am not sure whether, as it stands even with my minor alterations, it is worth putting into an article unless you do quite a lot of writing around it yourself. I enclose one photograph and I feel that is quite enough. There are none of me currently with patients as, of course, I am not in clinical care now.

So far as congregating people who are devalued in some way, I think it entirely depends on how you do it and, as I am sure I must have told you, we planned home care from the beginning and started work less than two years after we opened in 1967. We now have some six times as many people being cared for at home as we have in our wards, and about 20 coming up daily for time spent in our most lively Day Centre. This proportion is most probably true for our country as a whole, although many people continue to think of Hospice as just bricks and mortar.

The advantage of bringing people together is that you can offer them a welcoming community with staff and volunteers of real interest and expertise. Another all important advantage is the opportunity to carry out research. Had we not focussed particularly on cancer pain, we would not have carried out the research which has been published widely and made such a difference to practice, encouraging many other people to do likewise.

Because of our emphasis on family care from the beginning and home care shortly afterwards, we have always involved the family as part of the caring team. We certainly have not taken over either from the ordinary community services nor, above all, from what the families have been doing themselves. However, as many of our patients are elderly, their carers may become exhausted and about half our home care patients eventually come into our wards, either for respite or for terminal care. I do not think we have professionalised dying, although that impression may have been projected upon us by others.

Professor David Barnard

Penn State University, Hershey, Pennsylvania, USA

8 November 1996 Thank you so much for your letter of the 8th October. I am sorry to have been so long in replying but, having read your review, I then went carefully through "Palliative Care Ethics – A Good Companion".[56] I know Fiona Randall well as she worked here as a doctor before taking up her present position as Medical Director of a National Health Service Hospice. I began the book agreeing with you to some degree on the danger in the distinction between intrinsic and extrinsic aims of palliative care. However, as I went on reading, I came to the conclusion that the two authors are rightly warning those who, as I know myself from various reports, are sometimes rather intrusive in their questioning of patients about their problems. I think the book is excellent and an unusual approach.

I believe the danger of encouraging people to be mere symptomatologists is recognised in this country, but I appreciate it may encourage those who wish to manage care via the shortest route and in the cheapest way possible. I am sure your Review brings up an important point. When I learnt from a patient of "total pain" I certainly did not mean that every nurse or carer should move in as a pseudo psychiatrist, but only that we should be aware of the whole situation in which a person finds themselves – physically, psychologically, socially and spiritually – and which are impossible to disentangle. Having watched Fiona Randall at work, I am sure that is her own approach.

Sir Edward Ford

Central Chancery of the Orders of Knighthood, London

2 December, 1996 Thank you so much for your recent letter with regard to a possible luncheon for members of the Order of Merit. It is extremely helpful to have notification at this time, particularly as it is likely that I will be making a visit to Japan in April next year. I can now arrange my dates around the 8th April 1997. I certainly look forward to attending the luncheon and will wait to hear further details in due time.

Christmas letter to friends and colleagues

December, 1996 Christmas Greetings to you all. Please accept a general letter with personal wishes and memories.

I have had a lot of exciting travelling during the year, hence this letter as I thought you too would find it interesting, especially if you are involved with hospice and palliative care.

It began on February 12th when I flew to Los Angeles as an "Upper Class Virgin" (with limousine supplied at each end). I stayed first with Ida (Suzie) Pearce who had been one of my flatmates in 1946, having joined the 4 of us who shared in January of that year. We've met from time to time but this was a great catching up in her delightful part of Los Angeles. She works in ophthalmology and makes the most beautiful travel videos which support

---

[56] F. Randall and R. S. Downie, *Palliative care ethics. A good companion* (Oxford: Oxford University Press, 1999; 1st edn 1996).

patients in the waiting room and elsewhere. I went with her to the Kaiser Permanente Hospice Group and had a lively morning.

She then drove me to San Diego, to another hospice occasion – the celebration dinner for Professor Doris Howell, a very early worker (as a haematologist) with mortally ill children. San Diego has a luxurious hospice which she helped to found and I spoke there as well as at her celebratory dinner. Problem questions were more lively there than at a medical meeting held earlier.

Then I flew on to San Francisco for a lovely few days holiday with my stepdaughter, Daniela, who has a beautiful house overlooking the Golden Gate Bridge, a delightful daughter and two unusual and fascinating cats.

From there it was an immensely long flight to Singapore to an International Conference. My hostess, Dr Cynthia Goh, is a real leader in the field and there were 550 enthusiastic participants. I did opening and closing speeches, learnt a lot in between and had my photograph taken with innumerable workers in our field. Although there were obvious cultural differences, there was a base of shared principles and much enthusiasm.

I was home on 4th March and soon caught up with myself – jet lag doesn't bother me too much but it was nice to be home and back in the Hospice after going round the world, with wheelchair at the airports and countless helpful people to support me.

A few weeks later the Ambassador of Belarus came to the Hospice to discuss the possibility of celebrating Marian's birth in his country with a small permanent exhibition of some of his paintings in the place where Marian was born in 1901. This was then Russian occupied Poland and he was brought up on a large estate there. Turned out with the Russian advance in 1914, he moved with his grandmother to Wilno and, although he had many photographs which he loved to look at and show others, he never went back there. The Ambassador was keen that I visit the area to see for myself. They have a good house where they have a library and a music school and where they want to dedicate a room to Marian's works. I discussed it all with the Ambassador of Poland, knowing Marian's family in Poland had doubts about the political situation in Belarus. Anyway, it seemed right to go there and in July two good friends, both doctors – Dr and Mrs Falkowski – came with me to Lithuania to stay just outside Vilnius (which was formerly the Polish town of Wilno). An Embassy representative took us to the border with Belarus where we were through with little delay and where we met Professor Maldis, the Minister for Heritage and Dr Anna Gorchakova, who runs a children's hospice in Minsk (which had been much affected by the fallout from Chernobyl). With our delightful Embassy interpreter and Dr Falkowski able to translate any Polish, we were able to communicate well. We went on through forest and farmland to Marian's village, Trokeniki. It is small, with scattered cottages round a central house. We were welcomed by a small group and greeted with bread, salt and a woven runner. Six ladies in beautiful Polish costume sang as we arrived. We all went into the house for a feast of local food. There were about 16 of us in all and various speeches were made. Professor Maldis said, "A man is what he says he is and Marian Bohusz-Szyszko said he was Pole and to us he is Pole". I did my best to respond and the ladies came and sang again. To the delight of everyone Dr Falkowski joined in the singing. The Polish Priest then spoke and invited us to his church. It was an old stone building, beautifully kept though in need of some redecorating. He celebrated (in Polish) a Requiem Mass for Marian and his parents and my parents. I am sure Marian must have been baptized there. It was very moving and I left a white stone there in the graveyard and they gave me two small granite stones, one of which I have put next to Marian's photo and one where his ashes lie in the garden at St Christopher's.

That Poles and Belarussians are living well together seemed obvious and I will give an oil painting to the Minsk Academy and drawings and prints to Professor Maldis and Trokeniki. The Ambassador is keen for me to return next summer for the presentation and possibly to be involved in a television documentary about the area. I hope very much to be able to go.

We were well entertained in Vilnius (where we had been met at the airport by other hospice workers with flowers), by a delightful Polish Professor D Falkowski I had met in London and I spent a day with the Pain Relief Team in the University Hospital and met up with the press and various VIPs. They have been working for about three years but are dreadfully short of pain killers.

All three of us were driven to Kaunas to a new hospice in an old nursing home. Again, a wonderful welcome and good work being done, especially in home care, but also a shortage of analgesia and everything else and even coping with two patients who were not only dying of cancer but who had nothing but water in their homes. Belarus was even poorer.

There is no space to tell you of an exciting conference in Athens and a Working Party near the Delphi Oracle with friends old and new. Nor of the occasion when I became a Paper Dame of St Gregory the Great! But with all the help I have from my PA, Christine Kearney, and Hanka Jedrosz, who lives in the upstairs flat in my house and my regular driver, Barry, I keep going and busy. I am at St Christopher's every day in time for morning prayers and I watch the excellent young management team and everyone else at work, as well as working hard on my own projects.

A book "Hospice on the International Scene" edited by Professor Robert Kastenbaum (in the USA) and myself will be out in February 1997. Alongside this, I manage quite a lot of writing, speaking and interviewing. I am very lucky – I hope you are too.

Sir Robert Fellowes

Buckingham Palace, London

19 May 1997 Thank you so much for sending me a copy of the photograph taken at that very memorable Order of Merit Lunch last month. I am very pleased to have it and it will, as you say, serve as a happy reminder of a very splendid occasion.

It is a great pleasure to meet The Queen and The Duke of Edinburgh amongst such a prestigious yet informal gathering. It is always a delight to meet other members of the Order with their varied interests and expertise.

My driver was particularly appreciative of the welcome that he too was given and the care that is taken of those who enable us to take part in this occasion.

Professor Tetsuo Kashiwagi

Osaka University, Osaka, Japan

19 May 1997 Many thanks indeed for sending the slides. They are excellent and I will certainly make use of them. At the moment, Avril Jackson is having them duplicated so that she can use them from the Information Service.

I really had a wonderful time in Osaka and in Tokyo and was very impressed by what you have achieved so far in Japan and the possibilities that lie ahead. One thing that struck me very much in the palliative care unit at the cancer hospital was the need for education and support. They were really hungry for the sort of things I was trying to say and the fact that half the nurses in the hospital as a whole had had to be replaced within the first 5 years, was an illustration of that need. I certainly did not feel this with you and what you are doing and I think those of you who have looked at the deeper foundations of hospice and palliative care have a real challenge to make this recognised and, as far as possible, addressed.

I have enjoyed telling everyone here all about the trip, including the meetings in your home. It was all most interesting and stimulating.

I look forward to hearing of further developments through the British Council next year and of being in touch with you all again.

Sister Antonia
Dublin

11 August 1997 Thank you so much for still writing, especially when it is now so difficult for you. I do hope your arm will go on improving.

I note your new address and hope that the change was not too difficult and that you have a congenial group in your new convent. I have changed the address with our Friends Office so that you will continue to get our news.

At this time of year I often think of Antoni Michniewicz and that time in your ward remains as vivid as ever. You were very good to us in quiet support and, although you said you did not realise what was really going on, that in itself was a comfort. It is nice to know that there is someone else who knows how special he was.

I have no news of Anna's husband or the grandchildren. He obviously did not want to get in touch, so I will not send a Christmas card again, but continue to remember them in my prayers, as I am sure their grandfather and mother are doing.

I am going to send you a copy of an article that will be coming out in the Nursing Times soon of some of the earlier writings that were published, mostly when I was still working at St Joseph's.[57] In the meantime, I enclose a copy of "Watch with me" which very much came out of my experience on the ground floor with you and all my patients.

Professor J. E. Lennard-Jones
Woodbridge, Suffolk

21 August 1997 First of all, I must apologise for not having responded more promptly to your letter and the very interesting paper on *Ethical Dilemmas of Clinical Nutritional Support.* I think you have covered the ground where it applies to palliative and terminal care. We do have dilemmas with our patients with motor neurone disease but, as you say, nutrition cannot stop the ongoing deterioration and the final decision to withdraw nutrition is not too difficult when you really know the patient and, with whatever means of communication are

---

[57] She is referring to D. Clark, Someone to watch over me; Cicely Saunders and St Christopher's Hospice, *Nursing Times*, 26 August 1997: 50–1.

available, can discuss it with them. Such patients are often more than usually sharp in mind and remarkable people to meet and well able to be involved in such decisions. When gastrostomies first started to be more easily available, we had our doubts, knowing one or two cases where the patients appeared unable to die, even though they were profoundly disabled. I was told of one particular situation in a hospice where everyone concerned agonised over this but I cannot recall a similar scenario here, certainly not recently. I think what you say is quite sufficient, unless you felt it needed a comment on communication.

I have had some conversation with Professor Millard, Professor of Geriatrics at St George's Hospital, Tooting, on the subject of gastrostomy with patients after stroke. It seems to me that the geriatricians are concerned with this much more than we are and Professor Millard certainly said to me that they could not be withdrawn unless the patient is terminally ill. It seemed to me that unless a patient developed pneumonia or some other intercurrent infection, it was difficult to make a decision. Perhaps it might be helpful for you to discuss this with a geriatrician because I really cannot speak for them.

As for the paper as a whole, I hope you will allow me to circulate it among our several doctors here in training at the moment. We have a rotation system which means we have 5 at present, all most eager to learn in a hospice with a more academic approach than those they have worked in before. I would certainly not do this unless you gave me permission, but I think they would find it valuable.

I am grateful to all the Trustees for the help that the Sir Halley Stewart Trust has given us in the past and for the latest help at looking at our archives. I was able to procure the balance for this and all the material will go up to Sheffield for a year's work with the archivist before it returns to St Christopher's refurbished Education Centre.[58]

Dr Anna Gorchakova
Belarussian Children's Hospice, Minsk, Belarus

10 March 1998 Many thanks for your letter. I am delighted to know that you are moving into creating a National Palliative Care Centre but I appreciate how many problems you must have. I heard recently on the radio that the Soros Foundation had withdrawn from Belarus. I hope that may be a mistake because it seems to me they should be really interested in your project.

I am delighted to know that my husband's pictures have been put up but also, please, would be grateful if you could check on this.

So far as the books are concerned, of course you have my permission to publish anything you may wish. If you need to check with the original publishers in this country, your publishers will obviously do that directly. If they would like me to be in touch with them, please let me know.

Sénatrice Thérèse Lavoie-Roux
The Senate of Canada, Ottawa, Canada

24 March 1998 Thank you for your letter requesting information about the guidelines used at St Christopher's Hospice. I note your particular interest in ensuring that practitioners are

---

[58] Her papers were catalogued at the University of Sheffield as part of the Hospice History Project.

protected in the *Criminal Code* when making difficult decisions about treatment for the terminal ill.

Decisions to withdraw or withhold life-sustaining treatment are often made before patients are referred for care at St Christopher's Hospice. However, there are occasions when our patients are still receiving such treatments. I presume that the issue of risk for administering pain control to alleviate suffering refers to the 'double-effect' whereby the dose required to alleviate suffering then leads to the premature death of the patient. It is important to recognise that this issue relates to other medications such as sedatives and tranquillisers. These drugs are needed to relieve the terminal agitation and distress of some dying patients.

The legal protection of health care providers in the UK is based on the 'doctrine of double effect'. This was clarified by Judge Devlin in *R v Bodkin-Adams* [1957] CLR when he said that a doctor who is aiding the sick and dying does not have to calculate '*in minutes or even hours, and perhaps not in days or weeks, the effect upon a patient's life of the medicines which he administered or else be in peril of a charge of murder. If the first purpose of the medicine, the restoration of health, can no longer be achieved there is still much for the doctor to do, and he is entitled to do all that is proper and necessary to relieve pain and suffering, even if the measures he takes may incidentally shorten life'.*

This judgement formed the basis for resolving the case of Annie Lindsell, a patient suffering from motor neurone disease. She sought a declaration from the High Court which would enable her family doctor to administer appropriate doses of diamorphine when she felt that her condition had become unbearable. She withdrew her application to the High Court when reassured that a responsible body of medical opinion supported the proposed treatment [Medical Law Monitor 1999; 4: 9–10].

The importance of a responsible body of medical opinion is based on the Bolam principle – 'a doctor is not guilty of negligence if he has acted in accordance with a practice accepted as proper by a reasonable body of medical men skilled in that particular art' [Bolam vs Friern Hospital Management Committee. 1 W.L.R. 582]. It remains illegal to administer any substance or medication with the intent to kill a patient. However, the use of appropriate doses of medication to relieve suffering is recognised as being in accordance with accepted practice, as developed within specialist palliative care settings such as St Christopher's Hospice. The problem then arises about how to determine the intent behind a treatment which shortens life-expectancy.

St Christopher's desire to assure consistent standards with respect to end-of-life decision-making is not primarily motivated by a desire to eliminate legal risks. The dignity and worth of each individual patient is central to the Hospice philosophy. This includes the right to die without suffering. The principles and practices which are used in the Hospice to preserve patient dignity also protect staff from the potential misinterpretation of the intent behind treatment decisions. This is particularly important because St Christopher's Hospice has a high media profile from its opposition to the legalisation of euthanasia.

There are several strategies which we use to assure consistent standards:

1 Training on the ethics of decision-making. The principle of patient autonomy is emphasised, along with the need to present risks and benefits to patients whenever this is possible.

2 Extensive training on the variety of options that are available for treating pain and other distressing symptoms.

3 Training in handling the distress and suffering which prompts requests such as 'Isn't there something that you can do to end my suffering?' For patients, this question almost

always disguises deeper issues such as fear of what dying might be like, depression or feelings of abandonment. None of these issues require the use of a lethal injection. For families, the question reflects their deep distress and feelings of helplessness which can be addressed by other means.

4   The use of multi-disciplinary teams to discuss the risks/benefits and to monitor patient/family understanding. The different perspectives of doctors, nurses, social workers, chaplains and others ensures a broad spread of opinion and accountability. The cases of euthanasia which have arisen in the UK have involved doctors or other health professionals who have failed to seek advice on the management of difficult problems/ suffering. Because such advice and expertise is now widely available through specialist palliative care services, it is becoming less likely that a health professional will not be prosecuted if found guilty of 'mercy-killing'. Decisions to withhold treatment or administer potentially life-shortening therapies should be clearly documented in the clinical notes.

5   We do not have a policy about what level of information is communicated to the patient, except that the individual needs of the patient must be respected. Otherwise, there is the risk that some patients will be given too much information. This is just as oppressive as giving too little. The emphasis on team work ensures that patients' information needs are kept under review.

6   The competency of patients is an important issue in palliative care. Delirium and depression are two relatively common problems which can render patients incompetent. Delirium often occurs when patients are experiencing other symptoms near to death, which is when treatments might produce the 'double-effect'. Staff are given training in recognising and assessing these problems. St Christopher's Hospice has ready access to consultant psychiatrists for additional advice and review of difficult cases.

In circumstances where patients with advanced cancer develop delirium due to reversible causes, such as infection or high levels of calcium in the blood, the decision whether to treat or not can be extremely difficult. Just because a patient is admitted to a Hospice does not mean that he is imminently dying, particularly if there is a secondary, reversible cause for the deterioration. A careful clinical review is needed, including the background to the patient's deterioration. A rapid deterioration when the patient was previously reasonably well is quite different from a patient who has been steadily declining with the features of advanced cancer. The family can provide useful information about what is happening but should not be asked to make the decision about whether to treat or not. This is a difficult burden and does not preclude the family from using considerations that are not relevant, eg the desire to get an inheritance.

The Hospice has a contract with interpreting services to ensure that patients and families from minority ethnic groups have full access to information. This service is activated whenever such patients and families are referred to the Hospice.

The regulation of withholding/withdrawing treatments and the alleviation of suffering is very difficult. Some instances may be clear, eg withdrawal of nutritional support for patients in a persistent vegetative state (PVS) requires court approval in the UK. Over-legislation will not preclude abuse (eg continued practice of non-voluntary and involuntary euthanasia in the Netherlands) and is likely to introduce complexity that actually increases suffering (eg doctors withholding treatment to alleviate suffering while a decision is confirmed or ratified).

The legislation in the UK could be construed as minimalist but it is backed by a strong Government commitment to specialist palliative care. The House of Lords Select

Committee on Medical Ethics reviewed the current legislation on euthanasia in the UK [Walton L. Report of the Select Committee on Medical Ethics. HMSO, London. 1994]. The Committee concluded that the law should not be altered but that every effort should be made by Government to ensure that the principles and practices of specialist palliative care were spread as widely as possible. The National Health Service Executive has recently required all health authorities to identify what measures are being taken to provide and develop palliative care services.

The professional bodies need to clearly demonstrate the importance of palliative care. A recent example was provided by the General Medical Council. It found two family doctors guilty of 'gross professional misconduct' for failing to visit terminally ill patients, making inadequate arrangements to monitor pain, failing to involve specialist palliative care services and prescribing morphine without visiting the patients [Riley J. *Palliative Medicine* 1997; 11:317–18]. This sends a strong message to the judiciary as well as the medical professional. In the past, leniency has been shown in cases of 'mercy-killing' because it was viewed as understandable in the circumstances of unremitting suffering. It is important that judges understand what is achievable with specialist palliative care, in order that any health professional found guilty of committing euthanasia is punished for not involving or seeking advice from speciality palliative care services.

I hope these comments and observations have been helpful. Please do not hesitate to contact me again if you need further information or clarification.

Reginald V. N. Lord

University of Southern California School of Medicine, Los Angeles, USA

14 May 1998 Thank you for your recent letter. I am delighted to respond with a certain amount of information about Norman Barrett, who I always knew by his nickname, Pasty.

From 1948–51 I was his medical social worker at St Thomas' Hospital, doubling up in the last year as his secretary. He was a most stimulating person to work for and I owe him a great deal.

I had become interested in the problems of dying patients from my social worker days and have always counted the real foundation of St Christopher's Hospice with a patient who died in February 1948, leaving me £500 "to be a window in your home", as I was even then thinking of a special place for people like him, dying alone at the age of 40.

In the summer of 1951 I was driving with Mr Barrett down to one of the hospitals where he worked and I told him I would have to get back into nursing in order to help dying patients. His response is etched on my memory – he said "Go and read medicine, it's the doctors who desert the dying and there's so much more to be learnt about pain. You will only be frustrated if you don't do it properly and they won't listen to you". More about Mr Barrett appears in the Preface to our first textbook *The Management of Terminal Malignant Illness*. I enclose a copy of that Preface.

As well as encouraging me to take the step of taking medicine at the relatively late age of 33, he helped me get into the Medical School at St Thomas's and took an interest in what I was doing thereafter. When I went to work at St Joseph's Hospice with a clinical research fellowship, I remembered what I had learnt from him about keeping records and, in the pre-computer age, had the notes of 1100 patients précised on to a punch card system, from which I was able to derive my early writings. That work enabled the detailed research on morphine and diamorphine and many other studies developed at St Christopher's later by other members of the staff here.

I would be most grateful for the address of Julia Gough, as I do not have the address in Gloucestershire but only her earlier address, I think in Dorset.

Mr Barrett was a wonderful teacher, a far better teacher I have to say than he was a surgeon. He had a witty and enquiring mind and would have made a superb Professor.

Dr Robin Fox

Editor – Journal of the Royal Society of Medicine, London

16 June 1998 At the recent "Caring for Cancer" Conference organised by the Department of Health and held on 20 April last, I attended at the invitation of the Chief Medical Officer to respond on behalf of the voluntary sector to a Concordat proposed by the Secretary of State for Health. The Conference was particularly aimed at harnessing the enthusiasm and energies of the voluntary organisations at all levels and at encouraging co-operation in strategic planning and delivery of cancer services at local level, whilst recognising the complementary service already provided by the voluntary sector. During the Conference, the Secretary of State invited the conference to commit to a Concordat which encapsulated the theme of high quality and accessible treatment provided by people working across organisations to provide the best possible care for cancer patients.

I was asked to respond on behalf of the voluntary sector and to give a brief historical perspective on how the specialty of palliative medicine has been closely involved with the Department of Health since its inception.

Sir Kenneth Calman has encouraged me to use this short paper as it includes information not readily available which would be of interest to those working in the more general field of cancer care. I am submitting it to the *Journal of the Royal Society of Medicine* in the hope that it might be considered suitable for inclusion.[59]

I believe this to be particularly apt, as in 1962 I was invited to speak about the control of terminal pain by the RSM and this was subsequently published. It was an early paper on the work that has now developed into the specialty of palliative medicine and that I should have been invited by the Society at that stage to contribute this was, I naturally believe, a very forward looking step on their part.

His Excellence the Honourable Sir James Gobbo

Governor of Victoria, Melbourne, Australia

29 July 1998 The delay in writing to thank both you and Lady Gobbo for the wonderful stay in Government House recently, was to enable me to write out the talk which I gave at that most entertaining dinner. The written and spoken words are rather different, but I hope it gives you an idea of what I tried to say about the many lessons we learn from dying people and their families.

---

[59] It was published as C. Saunders, Caring for cancer, *Journal of the Royal Society of Medicine*, **91** (1998): 439–41. The original paper in the *Proceedings of the Royal Society of Medicine* is referred to in a letter to Herman Feifel of 17 June 1963, p. 55.

The stay in Melbourne was both full and very rewarding and a wonderful introduction to our time in Australia. Sydney was also busy and interesting and now Mrs Monroe and I are back and catching up with things here at St Christopher's.

It seems to me that palliative care is developing very constructively and appropriately in Australia and I especially enjoyed meeting up with many of the people working in this field both in Melbourne and Sydney.

Above all, of course, we very much enjoyed meeting you and your wife. Thank you both for your hospitality and welcome.

Professor Janina Tenner

St Lazarus' Hospice in Krakow, Krakow, Poland

4 August 1998 I am now back from a lecture trip (which incidentally I found very difficult because of my severe arthritis) so have only just had time to watch your video of greeting. I was most touched and delighted to see it. Thank you all very much for your good wishes for my birthday. I had a wonderful time and cannot really believe how old I am now.

The team from here who came to your conference were really inspired by the work you were doing in your beautiful new hospice. We really value our links with you and, although we cannot send you practical help now, we frequently think and pray for all your work.

Please give my greetings to everyone.

Helen Tudor

London

14 September 1998 The box of Pooh's home, where he lives under the name of Saunders, was a delightful present for a Monday morning. It will live on my desk with all the other things that the poor cleaner has to move when she dusts it and I will certainly keep paper-clips in it. It was fascinating that you had met it and thought of sending it to me.

I am sorry you have had an eye test which shows you need cataract operations. I had both my eyes done last Autumn and it was really no problem as I was a day patient and it has been wonderful since then to see every detail of the twigs on the trees outside my window.

Thank you again for continuing to think of me and Marian's art. Please concentrate on your own needs now.

Christmas letter to friends and colleagues

December 1998 Christmas greetings to you all and may the next year be good for you. Please forgive another general letter but as I always enjoy those I receive from friends, I continue to do the same myself.

I am writing this as I think of beginning work again following a few weeks off after a knee replacement. I have appreciated excellent care with a few days in a local private hospital and two weeks in St Christopher's. The excellent surgical nursing in the former was impressive though my time there was marred by my difficulty in taking strong analgesics. Having spent much of my life encouraging people to take them without fear of tolerance or addiction, I find no amount of anti-nausea drugs have any effect on me. It was good to go to the Annual General Meeting in the Hospice in a wheelchair from the ward to give the

Chairman's Report with real "inside" knowledge. We have to be grateful for all the hard and sensitive work that goes on day and night in the wards (and out in Home Care) while we plan expansion to tackle unmet need and all the resources that are needed for this. I was also glad to learn that I was considered "down to earth" and not too daunting to care for! I did not, of course, try to find out anything about the other patients but could not help seeing two families come into peace in the room next to mine, nor fail to appreciate the immense demands this made on the staff and their understanding and patience.

I am putting off my second knee until the summer as I have three trips booked before then. These will be for lectures and meetings in Germany, Norway and the USA (where I hope to catch up with some longstanding friends as well as lecture). People I met in the 1960s have become very special and as they, too, have been involved in hospice development, we have watched growth and learned together in our very different settings. The Professor of Sociology who is working on the history of the Hospice Movement and who has all my extensive archives at the moment, has traced how much happened in the ten years before St Christopher's finally opened in 1967. We all learned most from listening to patients (I was making tape recordings with them as early as 1961) but Professor Clark has drawn the story of innumerable contacts from my voluminous correspondence of that time. St Christopher's was a pioneer but once again I am aware of the truth "What have you that you did not receive".

1998 included several trips: an Ethics Conference in the Netherlands which I attended together with my long term Personal Assistant, Christine Kearney, revealed how palliative care can begin to develop in spite of the acceptance of euthanasia but also how much that can be avoided by the skills in listening and care we have been learning and trying to spread. German speaking Switzerland was next and revealed how little had even begun in our field but also that there was some keen interest.

Australia was another destination and was again a special trip. Our director of Patient and Family Services accompanied me and we had three luxurious, if cold, days in the enormous Government House in Melbourne before going on to Sydney to take part in the International Work Group on Death, Dying and Bereavement. Eighty of us from around the world worked in small groups to produce papers on different topics. Once again, many old friends from the first meeting of the Working Group, which took place in 1974, joined to make it a stimulating time – if a little taxing on my knees and back.

At home I have a splendid support system and still get into the Hospice for prayers at 8.45 am each morning and spend the day in my office seeing staff, writing, some teaching and a number of meetings both within the hospice and externally.

Of course, the most exciting times for me this year were the celebrations for my 80th birthday. A full Hospice chapel for Thanksgiving, followed by a tea party in the grounds of the Hospice for staff, family and friends was a wonderful occasion. This was followed by a conference attended by over 200 at the Royal College of Physicians on "Advancing Palliative Care" which was graced by the presence of our Patron, HRH Princess Alexandra (a well kept secret – I had not expected this at all). I was also honoured by a luncheon at the Richmond home of the Princess the week previously and she had not given a hint of her attendance at the Conference.

My family keep well and busy, my Polish granddaughter has her doctorate and my stepdaughter in San Francisco calls me nearly every week. Last year, I forgot to tell you of a visit in Los Angeles with a friend with whom I shared a flat in 1946 and all the catching up we did. We did not seem to have changed very much.

Altogether I am very lucky to be so busy still but find the morning of quiet all the more important and chapel is still in its central place. We have to meet the endlessly varied spiritual needs of our patients as well as all the practical needs of the end of life and the final letting go. This is wonderfully demanding and rewarding work and we have to strive all the time to support the whole Hospice community.

Kishore S. Rao

Bangalore Hospice Trust, Bangalore, India

22 December 1998 Thank you for your recent letter. I am delighted to know that you will soon be equipping your building and that you already have a date for the opening.

I would very much have liked to join you for that but I am afraid I will be preparing for a trip to the United States at that time and so it really would not be possible for me to attend.

I am sorry to disappoint you. I send every good wish to you all for your work and for the future of your hospice.

With all good wishes for the New Year also.

Professor Jiri Vorlicek

Department of Internal Medicine/Hemato-oncology, Brno, Czech Republic

22 December 1998 Thank you so much for sending me a copy of your book on Palliative Medicine. I was very pleased to see it and to read of all the particular topics which it addresses. I hope it gets the recognition it deserves. I have passed the book over to our Library here for them to keep for any interested visitor.

I wish you every good fortune as you develop palliative care in the Czech Republic.

Dr Robert Kastenbaum

Arizona State University, USA

6 December 1999 Volume 14 of the *Hospice Journal* has just reached me and I immediately turned to your concluding article.[60] I found it, as always, fascinating and challenging. One of the principles which we have tried to promote is that people should have their own death and not one that we think 'appropriate'. Those who tackle every situation aggressively or who refuse suggestions aimed at improving care are not easy for staff to stay by. However, our work with those we help in the inner city area we support which includes many minority ethnic groups, continues to teach us. How we could research this at the moment is not clear, but I will pass a copy of your article on to Professor Irene Higginson, as it does resonate with some of the work she has been doing in this area.

I should have written to you when you gave up the Editorship of *Omega* and I hope you are enjoying some extra time for yourself, although I suspect you will have found something else to do in its place.

---

[60] R. Kastenbaum, The moment of death: is hospice making a difference? *Hospice Journal*, **14**(3/4), (1999): 253–70.

Christmas letter to friends and colleagues

December 1999 My first letters from overseas with Christmas greetings have just begun to arrive so it is time to review the year myself and also send love and greetings to all of you.

A hospice Christmas is poignant and in a few days time we will have a Thanksgiving and Memorial Service for families who were bereaved during November last year, either in the wards or whilst under the care of our Home Care Service. We expect 94 adults and 17 children so the Chapel will be very full. During the service, we light candles and read out the names of those being remembered, sing well known hymns and have special prayers and readings. More than half who come in response to an invitation from the Chaplaincy are not churchgoers but in the two appraisals we have done, we have had extremely positive responses. It seems to meet the need for a reassuring ritual around that difficult first anniversary. The children have a story and take part by blowing out the candles, which most people then take home after having tea with some of the staff following the service. I always give the welcome and find it moving each time I do it.

On the Sunday following that, I will switch on 2000 lights on our huge Christmas tree in the grounds of the Hospice, each light sponsored in remembrance of someone lost. We expect around 1000 to come to that and to sing carols as they think of those the lights represent.

This has been a busy year, with some excellent new Trustees replacing valued people who have retired. The continuity among that group over the years and in the little "foundation" discussion group which is held once a month and which dates back to 1962, retain the original vision which has gone on developing and widening. I remember that on the day that the Kings Fund met and made the decision to give us the funds for the land, the text for the day in *Daily Light* was "Thou shalt bless the Lord for the good land He hath given thee" and in the evening Psalm 37 included the verse "Dwell in the land and verily thou shalt be fed". During many vicissitudes and anxious moments the original assurance of "Get it right and it will happen" has been maintained. It has also had to be learnt that "If you don't make mistakes you don't make anything". So long as we have kept listening to the patients and their families, I believe that on the whole St Christopher's and the Hospice and Palliative Care movement for which it was the catalyst, has continued to match mind, heart and spirit.

Visits to Germany, Norway, Switzerland and the USA this year were all challenging and stimulating. I do not talk except very generally now about clinical foundations and developments but my main theme has been "Lessons in Living from the Dying", which combines various thoughts about values and priorities in life with old and new stories and insights. It has all belonged to the many people I have met and loved. "We knew we'd get it" said Louie, a patient in St Joseph's Hospice, when I rang and told her we had the grant for the land. I have the picture she embroidered with one hand beside my desk to remind me of that time.

Professor David Clark, a medical sociologist, has all my large collection of archives, including memoranda, articles and thousands of copies of letters to the innumerable people who helped in one way or another to develop the ideas. He is writing a full history in a series of articles and next year will complete a book in a sabbatical year.

When we opened we could say "Everything we have is a gift" and one day in a talk in Chapel I realised I had to say "And everyone who comes here is a gift" and that included our critics as well.

My second knee replacement in July went even better than the first and, once again I convalesced in the Hospice with superb physiotherapy and nursing. My rather crumpled spine means lecturing has to be done sitting down and I need a wheelchair for any distance. However, I have had a marvellous support system with Christine, my PA who I now share with Dr Rob Dunlop, our innovative chief Executive Medical Director; Barry who drives me everywhere, helps me shop and checks out each new venue for meetings, and Hanka, who lives in the house and who helped me so much when I was caring for Marian. My stepdaughter in San Francisco and step granddaughter in Krakow telephone me each week and my own family is well and very much in touch. I am also still in touch and meeting with my nursing set from 1940. "What have you that you did not receive" keeps coming back to me.

I hope you will all have a truly special Christmas and go well into 2000. My diary already has several overseas trips booked for next year but it is the Management Team here now who will continue to take the Hospice forward.

Correspondents' Index

General Index

Abrams, Ruth D 191
Admiraal, Dr 307
adolescent unit 308–9
AIDS 130, 258, 288, 289, 296, 299–300, 309, 321, 357
  patient care 291–2
  Regional Working Party 263
Aikenhead, Mother Mary 154, 286
Alexandra, Princess 158, 232, 243, 330, 376
Allchin, Canon 311
Allen, Sir Donald 31, 32, 35, 47, 109, 110
Alzheimer's disease 288
American Journal of Hospice Care 297, 299
American Journal of Hospice and Palliative Care 322, 347
American Journal of Medicine 187
Amulree, Lord 160
Annie W Goodrich Visiting Lectureship 100
Aristotelis Prize for Man and Society 270
Association of Friends of the Sick 335
Association of Hospice Doctors 131, 262, 270, 300
Association of Hospice Physicians 258, 303
Association of Nursing Religious 160
Association of Operating Room Nurses 153
Association of Palliative Care and Hospice Doctors 305
Association of Palliative Medicine 270

Baines, Mary 235, 253, 305, 322, 346
Baker, John Austin 311
Barrett, Howard 205, 221
Bates, Thelma 195, 329
BBC Desert Island Discs 242
BBC Songs of Praise 304
BBC Week's Good Cause 63, 215, 223
BBC Woman's Hour 112
Black, Sir Douglas 305
Bland, Tony, case 345
Bluglass, Kerry 218, 239–40, 246
Bohusz-Szyszko, Marian 132, 136, 221, 260, 290, 354
Boulay, Shirley du 235, 245, 343, 354
Bowlby, John 81, 83
British Aid for Hospices Abroad 358
British Hospital Journal and Social Services Review 10
British Medical Association 250, 327, 342

Brompton Hospital 186
  Palliative Care Unit 197
Bulletin of Narcotics 399
Burn, Gilly 356, 358

Cabot, Richard 79
Cabrini Gold Medal Award 131, 232
Cade, Sir Stanford 92, 106
Callahan, Daniel 365
Calvaire, Dames du 191, 243, 286, 303
Cambridge University, honorary degree 271
Canada
  Palliative Care Movement 293
  Senate of, Special Committee on Euthanasia and Assisted Suicide 352
Cancer Care Inc., NY 63
Cancer Relief India 358
care, total, philosophy of 165
Care of the Dying, 1972 London symposium 127
Cassidy, Sheila 298, 345
Chalmers, Judith 242
children's hospice 193, 362
Christakis, Nicholas 359
Church Commissioners 113
Church of England
  Board of Social Responsibility 128
  Commission on Euthanasia 158
Church Missionary Society 32, 40
City Parochial Foundation 32, 41, 100, 110, 115, 119
Columbia University, hon Doctor of Law 189
community, sense of 27, 128–9, 151
Copenhagen, European Congress of Anaesthetists 91, 94, 110
Copperman, Harriet 228
Council of Europe 190
Cox, Nigel, case 342, 345
Cummings, Ina 358
cystic fibrosis 186

Death Anxiety Scale 337
Dept of Health, Caring for Cancer Conference 1998 374
Dept of Health and Social Security Working Party on Terminal Care 214
Devlin, Judge 283, 306, 371